CAREER TRANSITIONS IN SPORT

CAREER TRANSITIONS IN SPORT

International Perspectives

David Lavallee, Ph.D.
UNIVERSITY OF TEESSIDE, ENGLAND

AND

Paul Wylleman, Ph.D.
VRIJE UNIVERSITEIT BRUSSEL, BELGIUM

Editors

Fitness Information Technology, Inc. • P.O. Box 4425 •
Morgantown, WV 26504-4425 • USA

Library of Congress Card Catalog Number: 00-130551

ISBN: 1-885693-21-4

Copy Editor: Sandra R. Woods
Cover Design: James Bucheimer
Cover Illustration: Michael Komarck
Developmental Editor: Geoffrey C. Fuller
Production Editor: Craig Hines
Indexer: Maria E. denBoer
Printed by: Sheridan Books
Printed in the United States of America
10   9   8   7   6   5   4   3   2   1

Fitness Information Technology, Inc.
P.O. Box 4425, University Avenue
Morgantown, WV 26504 USA
800.477.4348
304.599.3483 phone
304.599.3482 fax
Email: fit@fitinfotech.com
Website: www.fitinfotech.com

Dedication

Paul dedicates this book to Marianne, Roxanne, and Annelies.

David dedicates this book to Ruth, Gail, Carole, and Lefty.

Contents

Foreword

Early in my career as a psychologist, I found myself seated before a rather large American university football player who looked like he was about to cry. In dolorous tones, which I will never forget, he managed to say before the tears began to roll, "What I could really use now is a career-ending injury." I was stunned speechless for a few moments.

His father was a well-known football head coach at a large, Midwestern university where football truly is "king." This young man had spent years in football and had excelled (he was on an athletic scholarship) all for the sake of two seemingly contradictory, but quite compatible motives: wanting to please Dad and fear of Dad's reaction if he quit football. Earlier in high school he had derived some pleasure from the sport, but at the university level football had become a major source of pain, both physical and emotional. He wanted out, but there was no way he could just quit. His fears of the imagined repercussions (his father's anger and rejection) were overwhelming. He believed his only way out was to incur a major injury. This dark side of sport career termination was his solution to leaving sport, the only solution he could see that would not leave him bereft of his father's love.

For this football player, his sport was a source of both love and pain, a truly pathogenic combination of strong emotions that would make most of us crazy. I bring up this athlete because even though his situation is not talked about much in sport, I have a feeling his plight is not rare. He represents yet another example of how complex career transitions can be. For many athletes, their sports are sources of joy, identity, and even love, and leaving them (or even just contemplating leaving them) can become events filled with sadness, confusion, and pain. This big, strapping example of American youth crying in front of me, unfortunately, experienced both joy and his father's love along with pain and confusion in one neat package: playing football. A sport career transition was desperately needed, but the only route he could see was to damage himself seriously. His career transition was a long and convoluted passage where we explored his relationship with his father, his search for an identity, and his fears of abandonment.

The common factor with the football player and all the other international examples and case studies in this book is that we psychologists, sport psychologists, and career counselors are in the business of helping athletes (and performing artists) in transit. For some, that transit may be as easy as crossing a stream; for others, the voyage may be oceanic and stormy. Keeping with the traveling metaphor, those who assist athletes in making their journeys are like intimate and personal tour guides helping athletes explore both their internal landscapes and the new environments they find themselves in after leaving sport. I am not talking Beatrice and Dante here, but we can be likened to escorts for strangers in a strange land.

One of the maps I find useful in the process of working with athletes is the one supplied by Erik Erikson (1950, 1968). His dynamic formulations of the challenges and conflicts faced in adolescence, young adulthood, and middle adulthood can add levels of understanding and meaning to the broad intrapsychic and psychosocial contexts in which "transiting" athletes find themselves. For example, establishing an identity (a core theme running through this book) is the task of adolescence. Many adolescent athletes solve this task by developing an exclusive athletic identity. Unfortunately, this identity is one with a "use by" date, and athletes who are chronologically young adults (or even older) end up facing an adolescent conflict because the foundations for their identities have crumbled. Sometimes the conflicts and challenges of adolescence (ego-identity versus role confusion) coincide with retirement from sport. For example, it seems that women's gymnastics has become more "girls" gymnastics, and retirement from international sport at age 17 is not a rare phenomenon. This retirement occurs along with the basic adolescent question "Who am I?" Identity is often an issue for retiring athletes, but when retirement comes at 16 or 17 it lands on top of a major developmental task.

Erikson's next two stages often correspond with common retirement times. For example, in middle adulthood, questions of generativity (giving back something to the next generation) versus stagnation arise just as many athletes are finally retiring (mid 30s to 40s). The 34-year-old tennis player who is finally hanging it up may ease that transition if she also partially solves the challenge of her middle adulthood by giving something back to her sport.

Erikson, however, is just one map, and there are other masterfully presented maps in this book for working with a variety of issues and populations (e.g., athletes with disabilities), along with a fine reference source in the annotated bibliography. The reader will find maps from organizational psychology, career theory, career assessment, and even existential psychology (probably a rather foreign country for some sport psychologists). There are also some real "nuts and bolts" maps about practical and logistical issues in career transition counseling. But, as I always try to pound into my students, "the map is not the territory." The map is essential for us to move through the territory, but no matter how well-outfitted we are with all our "topographical psychologies," athletes will come along who are not on one of our maps. At that time we will have to look up, really try to "see" them, and walk with them into terra incognita, seeking some guidance from our peers and colleagues along the way.

For those of you starting out reading this book, you will find some familiar and some not so familiar maps along with the stories that accompany them. Some of those stories and maps you will use and take to practice with you; some you will leave behind, but it's going to be an interesting journey, and I'd like to say, "Have a good trip."

Now where did I put my passport?

—Mark B. Andersen
Melbourne, Australia

References
Erikson, E. H. (1950). *Childhood and society.* New York: Norton.
Erikson, E. H. (1968). *Identity: Youth and crisis.* New York: Norton.

Preface

A growing body of literature is emerging on the topic of career transitions in sport. In 1980, McPherson reported that an extensive literature search identified 20 published references on this topic. Since then, no fewer than 270 empirical and theoretical citations have been identified on sports career transitions and career transition issues (see Appendix A in this volume). Researchers and practitioners have also initiated a special interest group on career transitions (SIG-CT) in order to exchange information on investigative and applied work in the area. The SIG-CT has organized a series of symposia at international congresses in recent years (Alfermann, 1998; Stambulova, 1997; Wylleman, 1995; Wylleman & Alfermann, 1997; Wylleman & Schilling, 1997; Wylleman & Stambulova, 1999). In conjunction with the Managing Council of the European Federation of Sports Psychology (FEPSAC), the SIG-CT has also contributed to the publication of a position statement (see Appendix B) and a monograph (Aflermann et al., in press) on career transitions in sport.

The objective of this volume is to bring together international scholars to provide an overview of empirical, theoretical, and applied perspectives on sports career transitions. There are 13 chapters organized into three sections: (a) Theory and Research on Career Transitions in Sport, (b) Career Transition Interventions, and (c) Special Populations. A total of 29 authors from six countries, who work in arenas that either relate directly to, or interface strongly with, career transitions, have contributed chapters that focus on the diverse research in the area.

The book is geared toward scholars and students in sport psychology and related areas interested in career transitions and retirement from sport. It has been written to complement the growing literature on counseling athletes (e.g., Etzel, Ferrante, & Pinkney, 1996) and thus is also directed toward psychologists, career counselors, and other practitioners working (or interested in working) with athletes in transition. Finally, because career transitions are among the most significant experiences in sport (Murphy 1995), the book has been written to provide coaches, directors of sport federations and national Olympic committees, and others responsible for the well-being of athletes, with an overview of the topic. It is our hope that this book will provide a foundation for further theoretical analysis and research on sports career transitions. We also hope that this volume provides a greater understanding of the transition experience itself, an understanding that may optimize practitioners' guidance of athletes in order to achieve optimal transitions.

We wish to thank Andy Ostrow and the publishing company Fitness Information Technology, Inc., for welcoming and encouraging the production of this edited volume and for providing us "rookies" with the opportunity to assemble such a distinguished panel of authors. For all their contributions to the production of this book, we would like to thank Ruth Lavallee and Alton Leigh. In addition, acknowledgments are extended to Geoff Fuller and two external reviewers, who provided useful comments and insights regarding a draft of the book manuscript. We wish to express our genuine appreciation to FEPSAC's managing council, and in particular, Stuart Biddle and Natalia Stambulova. We also thank FEPSAC, the Australian Council for Educational Research, and Mayfield Publishing Company for permission to reproduce copyright material. Last, we would like to express our gratitude to all authors for their contribution.

—David Lavallee
Paul Wylleman

References

Alfermann, D. (Chair). (1998, August). *Career transitions in sport: Determinants and consequences.* Symposium presented at the 24th International Congress of Applied Psychology, San Francisco.

Alfermann, D., Bardaxoglou, N., Chamalidis, P., Lavallee, D., Stambulova, N., Menkehorst, H., Petitpas, A., Salmela, J., Schilling, G., van den Berg, F., & Wylleman, P. (in press). *Career transitions in competitive sports.* European Federation of Sports Psychology.

Etzel, E. F., Ferrante, A. P., & Pinkney, J. W. (Eds.). (1996). *Counseling college student athletes: Issues and interventions* (2nd ed.). Morgantown, WV: Fitness Information Technology.

McPherson, B. D. (1980). Retirement from professional sport: The process and problems of occupational and psychological adjustment. *Sociological Symposium, 30,* 126–143.

Murphy, S. M. (1995). Transitions in competitive sport: Maximizing individual potential. In S. M. Murphy (Ed.), *Sport psychology interventions* (pp. 331–346). Champaign, IL: Human Kinetics.

Stambulova, N. B. (Chair). (1997, August). *Career transitions in competitive sport.* Symposium presented at the 2nd Annual Conference of the European College of Sports Sciences, Copenhagen.

Wylleman, P. (Chair). (1995, July). *Career transition of athletes.* Symposium presented at the 9th European Congress of Sports Psychology, Brussels.

Wylleman, P., & Alfermann, D. (Chairs). (1997, July). *An international perspective on career transitions of high-level athletes.* Symposium presented at the IXth World Congress of Sport Psychology, Netanya, Israel.

Wylleman, P., & Schilling, G. (Chairs). (1997, July). *Transition from high-level competitive sport: Research and recommendations for guidance.* Symposium presented at the IXth World Congress of Sport Psychology, Netanya, Israel.

Wylleman, P., & Stambulova, N. (Chairs). (1999, July). *A European perspective on career transitions in competitive sports.* Symposium presented at the 10th European Congress of Sports Psychology, Prague.

PART
I

Theory
and Research
on Career
Transitions
in Sport

1

Theoretical Perspectives on Career Transitions in Sport

David Lavallee
University of Teesside
England

Abstract

This chapter outlines theoretical perspectives on career transitions in sport. Models that have been employed to explain this phenomenon will initially be delineated, including theories of social gerontology, thanatology, and human adaptation to transition. This will be followed by an outline of a conceptual model of sports career transition (Taylor & Ogilvie, 1998). This model focuses on how the causes of career transition, developmental experiences of the athlete, and coping resources affect the quality of adjustment to career transitions in sport.

Theoretical Perspectives on Career Transitions in Sport

The sport-scientific community has made an effort to conceptualize the career transition process ever since a debate emerged regarding the incidence of distress experienced by retiring athletes. Numerous investigations have been made into athletic career termination, with various explanatory frameworks being employed to explain the phenomenon. Theorists have, however, predominantly made parallels between career transitions in sport and social gerontological models of aging, thanatological models of death and dying, and models of human adaptation to transition.

Social Gerontological Models

Gerontology, as a scientific field of study, has been defined as the systematic analysis of the aging process (Atchley, 1991). This academic discipline consists of biological, social, and psychological subdivisions, with social gerontology concentrating on the mutual interaction between society and the aged. In its broadest sense, social gerontology attempts to explain the lives and activities of those who appear to age successfully. Numerous gerontological orientations, therefore, have been utilized to explain the general process of retirement from the labor force.

Sport theoreticians have suggested that several models of social gerontology are applicable in the study of transitions in sport (e.g., S. H. Lerch, 1981; McPherson, 1980; Rosenberg, 1981). In an attempt to understand the problems and processes confronted by retiring athletes, the career transition process has been compared to the following social gerontological perspectives: activity theory, subculture theory, disengagement theory, continuity theory, social breakdown theory, and social exchange theory.

Activity Theory

Havighurst and colleagues (Friedmann & Havighurst, 1954; Havighurst & Albrecht, 1953) were perhaps the first theorists to propose a relationship between social activity and adjustment to retirement from the work force. This pioneering conceptualization of aging, known as activity theory, suggests that individuals strive to maintain homeostatic levels of activity throughout the life span. If the adjustment process is to be successful, the once active roles that are lost upon retirement need to be substituted with new ones (Havighurst & Albrecht, 1953). Although this perspective has received empirical support in the gerontological literature (e.g., Lemon, Bengston, & Peterson, 1972), it has been suggested that activity theory, not unlike the field of gerontology itself, is based on an inadequate if not invisible theoretical foundation (Longino & Kart, 1982).

In terms of retirement from elite-level sport, some theorists have suggested that there is potential in examining the application of activity theory. McPherson (1980), for example, contends that this perspective has utility for individuals who substitute an activity for the athlete role. Rosenberg (1981) has also stated that when athletes retire voluntarily it is usually not because their skills and efforts provide the rewards they once did, but because alternatives to sport look more attractive. Activity theory, however, may not apply universally to athletic career transitions because there is usually neither a cessation of work activity nor total retirement from participation in sport. Although activity theory may explain the situation of retiring athletes who successfully adjust by retaining previous activity patterns, Baillie and Danish (1992) believe that the schedules competitive athletes adhere to during their playing careers are difficult to duplicate outside of sport.

Subculture Theory

Rose (1962) responded to a need for theory building in the area of social gerontology by theorizing that it is possible to successfully adjust to retirement from the work force with less active roles. This subculture theory, which asserts that prolonged social interactions among individuals lead to the development of a group consciousness, assumes that people can be less active and well-adjusted during retirement even if the situation is different from overall social norms. Although investigators have demonstrated an application of this perspective (e.g., Longino, McClelland, & Peterson, 1980), the widely shared view among the gerontological community is that subculture theory is most applicable when it is integrated with other social gerontological theories (Marshall, 1978).

Because athletes have fairly distinguishable (sub)cultural characteristics, Rosenberg (1981) contends that subculture theory is of value in explaining sports career termination. Although it is questionable as to whether this theory can predict successful athletic retirement, it does assist in revealing the sources of potential adjustment problems experienced by athletes in transition. This perspective, however, has received considerable criticism in the literature because the athlete in transition is moving out of, and not into, the proposed subculture (Gordon, 1995).

Continuity Theory

Continuity theory originated with Atchley (1976), who focused on the evolution of individual adaptation to normal aging. Unlike the aforementioned social gerontological models, this theory allows change to be integrated into one's prior history without necessarily causing disequilibrium. The importance of a stable pattern of previously established role behavior is assumed in this model, with an emphasis on maintaining continuity throughout the aging process. Thus, the best adjusted individuals experience minimal change and greater continuity following retirement from the labor force (Atchley, 1989).

In terms of athletic career termination, it has been proposed that continuity theory can predict the level of adjustment to retirement by examining the significance of sport in the lives of athletes (S. H. Lerch, 1981). If one's athletic role is seen as more meaningful than other roles, an athlete may experience some difficulties in redistributing them upon retirement (Rosenberg, 1981). On the other hand, if sustaining the sporting role is not a priority for the athlete in transition, the reallocation of time and energy to remaining roles will not create problems in the adjustment process. The decisive question in the application of continuity theory to athletic career termination, therefore, is whether or not retirement from sport is important enough for individuals to reorganize their hierarchy of personal goals.

The belief that retired individuals are content with less active schedules has been challenged in the sport literature. Utilizing continuity as a predictor of adjustment to retirement, S. H. Lerch (1981) empirically tested continuity theory with a sample of retired professional baseball players in the United States. In this particular study, it was hypothesized that optimal adjustment would characterize the retired athlete whose postathletic career remained connected to sports, income remained relatively stable after retirement, and level of subjective and behavioral commitment to sport was maintained. This modification of continuity theory was also supplemented with a number of variables that social gerontologists have found to be related to retirement adjustment (viz., education level, preretirement attitude, and health). S. H. Lerch found, however, that no continuity variables were significantly related to adjustment to retirement from sport.

Disengagement Theory

Cummings, Dean, Newell, and McCaffrey (1960) introduced disengagement theory as an extension of Erikson's (1950) model of life-span development. This structural-functional theory of aging, which argues that the elderly and society mutually withdraw, is based on the findings from the Kansas City Study of Adult Life (Cummings et al.). In this longitudinal investigation, it was suggested that a desired equilibrium is obtained when younger workers enter the work force and replace the disengaging older, retiring population. A system-induced mechanism allows society and the elderly to progressively retract from one another, allowing the aging population to spend their remaining years in leisure. Retirement, according to disengagement theory, is viewed as a necessary manifestation of the mutual withdrawal of society and the aging population from one another.

Because most athletes do not leave the work force permanently upon athletic career termination, retiring from elite-level sport does not appear to fit the theory of general disengagement. Whereas disengagement theory assumes that athletes and the sport structure mutually withdraw from one another, S. H. Lerch (1981) demonstrated that a large number of athletes try to hang on to their sport long after their skills have begun to deteriorate. Moreover, retiring athletes clearly cannot afford to withdraw from society (Gordon, 1995). It has been suggested, therefore, that disengagement theory offers little to the understanding of retirement from competitive sport (E. M. Blinde & Greendorfer, 1985).

Social Breakdown Theory

Social breakdown theory was adapted to gerontology by Kuypers and Bergston (1973) and details the cycle associated with the process of social reorganization after retirement. Incorporating elements of activity theory, subculture theory, and continuity theory, this conceptualization proposes that individuals become increasingly susceptible to external labeling following the loss of a retirement-related role. This social evaluation leads one to gradually reduce one's involvement in certain activities until the role is completely eliminated from one's life.

In the sport literature, it has been suggested that social breakdown theory has clear application to athletic retirement. In particular, Rosenberg (1981) has indicated that the withdrawal cycle illustrates how elite athletes are vulnerable to social judgment upon career termination, particularly unfavorable redefinition. Edwards and Meier (1984) have empirically investigated the relationship between adjustment to retirement from sport and several variables proposed to be significant in social breakdown theory, including socioeconomic status, preretirement planning, and health. In this study, the data from former professional ice hockey players in North America yielded significant support for the social breakdown paradigm. In the case of career termination, however, the retiring athlete is often aware of their deteriorating athletic skills, as well as a lack of congruence with their peers. According to the social breakdown model, this may lead the athlete to withdraw further from the sport and become susceptible to more negative evaluation. To avoid such a decline, Baillie and Danish (1992) recommend that athletes need to prepare for the redefinition of social breakdown prior to the actual retirement. This procedure, which has been referred to as social reconstruction, assists the retiring athlete in restoring and maintaining a positive self-image and, thus, reduces the impact of negative external evaluation. In career counseling with athletes, Rosenberg (1981) believes a fitting prelude to a discussion of social breakdown is exchange theory.

Exchange Theory

Exchange theory was initially developed by Homans (1961) to explain how aging individuals rearrange their activities so that their remaining energy generates maximum return. This paradigm has since been adapted to illustrate how successful aging can be achieved through the specific rearrangement of social networks and activities (e.g., Blau, 1964). Rosenberg (1981) has suggested that social exchange theory is one of the most salient gerontological theories applicable to retirement from sport. In addition, Johns, Linder, and Wolko (1990) have demonstrated in a study with former competitive gymnasts in Canada that the examination of factors that contribute to retirement from sport through a social exchange perspective has some merit. More recently, however, theorists have criticized the social exchange perspective as being inadequate when applied to athletic retirement (Gordon, 1995; Koukouris, 1991).

It has been suggested that the processes associated with exchange theory do not stand up because they deny the possibility of the development of a career after sport (Koukouris, 1991). Social exchange theory, however, may be heuristically useful in providing athletes with a perspective on what their relationship is with sport, as well as what may happen to that relationship upon career termination. As Gordon (1995) has suggested, "resources such as physical talent may be able to be exchanged for meaningful rewards from the sport system, but these resources are finite and their inevitable deterioration will affect the degree of control over the sport relationship" (p. 478).

Despite the intuitive appeal of social gerontological theories, many questions have been raised by contemporary theorists about their applicability to career transitions in sport. For example, the general assumption that athletic retirement is a system-induced mechanism that forces athletes to disengage from their sport has been criticized (e.g., Greendorfer & Blinde, 1985; Koukouris, 1991). The applicability of social theories of aging to the athlete in transition, who will continue into a postsporting career, has also been questioned in the literature (e.g., Curtis & Ennis, 1988; Werthner & Orlick, 1986). Indeed, it is difficult to compare retirement from the work force with the sports career transition that biologically and chronologically occurs at a much younger age (S. M. Murphy, 1995). Perhaps the biggest shortcoming of the analogy between athletic retirement and social gerontological models, however, is the presumption that the career transition process is an inherently negative event, requiring considerable adjustment. Although this assumption may be useful in drawing a parallel between successful retirement from sport and occupational retirement from the labor force, social gerontological theories have been unable to adequately capture the nature and dynamics of the career transition process.

Thanatological Models

Thanatology is the study of the process of death and dying. This area of research, which was introduced by Park (1912) in an outline of the biomedical causes of death, has evolved into a multidisciplinary science (Kastenbaum & Kastenbaum, 1989). Academic disciplines such as anthropology, psychology, sociology, and theology have all made significant contributions to the thanatological literature, and a total of 62 different sets of variables have been identified in the extant literature to influence the dying individual (Rando, 1986). In addition, 29 separate sets of psychological, social, and physical factors appear to influence a person's response during postdeath grief and mourning (Rando, 1984). As Feifel (1990) has suggested, thanatology is such a diverse area that the very mention of it as a field of study is a limitation. However, the sport-scientific community has suggested that several thanatological theories have implications for the career transition process, including models of social death, social awareness, and stages of death.

Social Death

Of the numerous parallels that have been drawn between career transitions in sport and models of thanatology, the majority have been examined from social points of view. For example, Kalish's (1966) concept of social death has frequently been employed as a literary device describing the psychodynamics of athletic retirement (e.g., S. Lerch, 1984; Rosenberg, 1984). This analogy, which refers to the condition of being treated as if one were dead even though still biologically alive, describes the loss of social functioning, isolation, and ostracism that may accompany athletic career termination. Whereas numerous fictitious examples of social death have been used to explain this phenomenon in sport, the nonfictional works are undoubtedly the most compelling depictions of social death (S. Lerch, 1984).

Social Awareness

Theorists have also proposed that awareness contexts have application for athletes retiring from sport (S. Lerch, 1984; Rosenberg, 1984). This perspective refers to the individuals who know about a terminal hospital patient's inevitable death. The research of Glaser and Strauss (1965) suggests that, depending upon whom knows what during this process, there are observable and predictable patterns of interaction between dying patients, family members and friends, and the medical staff. As these individuals interact over time, it is suggested that the following awareness contexts develop: closed awareness, suspected awareness, mutual pretense, and open awareness.

In closed awareness, terminal patients are not aware of the fact that they are going to die, even though other people are. Various factors may contribute to the closed awareness context, including a doctor's reluctance to tell the patient, the family's decision to not inform the dying individual, and/or the general collusion of hospital staff to avoid discussing a patient's illness with them specifically (Glaser & Strauss, 1965). Terminal hospital patients who remain in this context until they die have little chance to make future plans. When applied to sport, this context is between the retiring athlete, teammates, coaches, and management. Just as a hospital staff may prefer this context in that they do not have to discuss the inevitability of death, this could apply in situations where elite athletes are unaware of management's plan to release or trade them (Gordon, 1995; S. Lerch, 1984)

The suspected awareness context exists when the dying patient suspects the inevitable death that others know about and tries to confirm or negate that suspicion. These individuals normally try to obtain realistic information about their situation from family, friends, and the hospital staff. Factors that contribute to this awareness context, such as the patient's recognition of changing physical symptoms, may be compared to the experiences of retiring athletes. For example, suspicions of being released from a team may be aroused by the tone of coaches and/or teammates (Gordon, 1995). As in closed awareness, the possible consequences are that terminal hospital patients, as well as athletes, do not have the opportunity to express their feelings and emotions because the later awareness contexts (viz., mutual pretense and open) are never realized (S. Lerch, 1984).

In the mutual pretense context, the patient, family members and friends, and hospital staff all are aware that the patient is dying. What occurs in this context, however, is that all the people involved behave as if the inevitable death is not going to occur. In terms of athletic career transition, the individual's career termination would not be discussed among coaches and teammates. Although one of the consequences of this context is that patients may have some dignity in dying, it is possible that isolation and loneliness may occur (Glaser & Strauss, 1965).

The context of open awareness exists when all people openly acknowledge that the patient is dying. This awareness gives everyone involved a chance to discuss their feelings and, thus, gives patients a greater sense of control (Glaser & Strauss, 1965). In terms of athletic retirement, many individuals may have difficulty in accepting the knowledge of their impending career termination (Gordon, 1995). On the other hand, athletes can begin to plan their postathletic career in this context. As Rosenberg (1984) has stated, however, it is more likely to find relations between athletes and coaches to be characterized by closed and/or suspicion awareness.

Stages of Death

In describing retirement from sport, the series of stages experienced when facing death has been suggested. These psychological reactions, as outlined by Kübler-Ross (1969), grew out of a study with terminal hospital patients. The stages of dying, as applied to retirement from sport, include the following: denial and isolation, in which athletes initially refuse to acknowledge their inevitable career termination; anger, in which retiring athletes become disturbed at the overall situation; bargaining, in which individuals try to negotiate for a lengthened career in sport; depression, in which athletes experience a distress reaction to retirement; and acceptance, in which individuals eventually come to accept their career transition.

The application of the stages of death theory in sport settings has become a topic of interest in recent years. For example, a number of theorists have employed this particular model to describe the psychological pattern experienced by athletes during rehabilitation from injury (e.g., Wiese-Bjornstal & Smith, 1993). This theoretical perspective has also been supported by research with physiotherapists consulting with injured athletes who have noted that many postinjury behavioral reactions resembled the stages of the grief response (e.g., Gordon, Milios, & Grove, 1991). Although a number of theorists have used the stage theory of dying to describe the process of retirement from sport (e.g., S. Lerch, 1984; Rosenberg, 1984), only E. Blinde and Stratta (1992) have systematically documented the stages of death with a sample of retired athletes who experienced involuntary and unanticipated career terminations.

The stages of death and dying represent a descriptive rather than normative look at the stages of the terminally ill and, therefore, may not be the same as those experienced by athletes in transition. Because not every person goes through every stage in the exact sequence and at a predictable pace, it has been agreed in the literature that dying is an individualistic experience (Feigenberg, 1980; Kalish, 1966). As Kastenbaum and Weisman (1972) have demonstrated via the psychological autopsy (i.e., a methodological technique providing insight into why a patient died, how the patient died, and the psychological state of the patient before death), most individuals do not progress through the stages of death in the same manner. Nevertheless, if used in a flexible way, the stages of dying and other thanatological models can provide a useful guide in understanding the different phases that retiring athletes may go through (Baillie, 1993).

Overall, models of thanatology have been criticized as being inadequate when applied to athletic retirement. Although Baillie (1993) suggests that these models can be valuable tools in understanding the career transition process, the clinical utility of thanatological models has been criticized because they were developed with nonsport populations (Greendorfer & Blinde, 1985). A number of theorists have also questioned whether thanatological models are a generalizable disposition of what happens to the vast majority of athletes (e.g., Gordon, 1995; Taylor & Ogilvie, 1998). Indeed, there are enough anecdotal examples showing that the career transition process can be very distressful for many athletes. As with social gerontological models, however, models of thanatology provide a limited perspective by not focusing on the life-span development of athletes.

Because models of social gerontology and thanatology are unable to adequately account for the complex nature of career transition in sport, it has been suggested that alternative perspectives are needed to achieve an empirical-theoretical balance (Crook & Robertson, 1991). As such, theorists have suggested that athletic career termination may serve as an opportunity for social rebirth rather than a form of social death (Coakley, 1983), and thus, have also viewed it as a transition.

Transition Models

Whereas social gerontological models and thanatological models view retirement as a singular event, transition models characterize retirement as a process. A transition has been defined by Schlossberg (1981) as "an event or non-event which results in a change in assumptions about oneself and the world and thus requires a corresponding change in one's behavior and relationships" (p. 5). As such, a number of transition frameworks have been employed to examine the interaction of the retiring athlete and the environment, including Sussman's (1972) analytic model and Schlossberg's (1981) model of human adaptation to transition.

Although McPherson (1980) was perhaps the first to refer to the phenomenon of athletic career termination as a transition in the literature, Hill and Lowe (1974) initially suggested that Sussman's (1972) analytic model of retirement from the workforce may be useful in explaining retirement from sport as a process. In this article, Hill and Lowe asserted that the retirement process is a multidimensional conceptualization. However, because athletes are aware of the brevity of their sport careers, and thus can prepare for the transition, this particular process model does not apply to athletic retirement.

The most frequently employed theory of transition that has been outlined in the sport literature has been the model of human adaptation to transition as proposed by Schlossberg and colleagues (Charner & Schlossberg, 1986; Schlossberg, 1981, 1984). In this model, three major sets of factors interact during a transition, including the characteristics of the individual experiencing the transition, the perception of the particular transition, and the characteristics of the pretransition and posttransition environments. Although it appears that these three components interact to produce a successful or unsuccessful adaptation to transition, each factor will be described individually.

The variables that characterize the individual include such attributes as psychosocial competence, sex, age, state of health, race/ethnicity, socioeconomic status, value orientation, and previous experience with a transition of a similar nature (Schlossberg, 1981). These variables may show considerable differences across the population of athletes facing retirement from sport, and Coakley (1983) asserts that a diversity of factors influencing the athlete in transition must be acknowledged in order to understand the overall adjustment process.

Regarding the perception of a particular transition, Charner and Schlossberg (1986) have suggested that the role change, affect, source, onset, duration, and degree of stress are all important factors to consider. This aspect of the model emphasizes the phenomenological nature of transitions, in that it is not only the transition itself that is of primary importance, but also the variables that have different salience depending on the transition (Schlossberg, 1981). For retiring athletes, Sinclair and Orlick (1993) have acknowledged this position by suggesting that every career transition has the potential to be a crisis, relief, or combination of both, depending on the athlete's perception of the situation.

In consideration of the characteristics of the pre- and posttransition environments, Schlossberg (1981) has noted the importance to the evaluation of internal support systems, institutional support, and physical settings. Although several researchers have examined social support networks among injured athletes (e.g., Ford & Gordon, 1999), little research has been conducted in this area with retired athletes. A number of theorists have outlined the obligations of coaches and sport associations in preparing athletes for retirement from high-level competition (e.g., Parker, 1994; Thomas & Ermler, 1988). Once again, however, few empirical investigations have been made in this area of athletic career termination.

In an attempt to understand the career transition process of athletes, several researchers have utilized the transition models outlined by Schlossberg and her associates (e.g., Charner & Schlossberg, 1986; Schlossberg, 1981, 1984). Swain (1991), for example, has provided empirical support for Schlossberg's model in terms of the characteristics of the retiring athlete, the perception of the career transition, and the characteristics of the environments. Further evidence in support of this theoretical perspective has been documented in Parker's (1994) study with retired football players, as well as Baillie's (1992) study of former elite-amateur and professional athletes. Sinclair and Orlick (1994) have also modified the transition model of Charner and Schlossberg by reassigning specific characteristics to alternate categories. Although this perspective provides a conceptual overview of career transition in sport, it has been suggested that transition models do not provide a flexible, multidimensional approach that is needed to adequately study athletic retirement (Taylor & Ogilvie, 1994). However, Sinclair and Orlick's model of career transitions in sport appears to be helpful in assessing athletic retirement processes because it incorporates the various factors related to adjustment. Thus, sport

transition models incorporate a wider range of influence than do social gerontological and thanatological models and allow for the possibility of both positive and negative adjustment (Crook & Robertson, 1991).

Overall, the theoretical models of social gerontology, thanatology, and
transition that have been applied to athletic career termination have been instrumental in stimulating research on a number of career transition issues.
Each of these perspectives, however, possesses limitations that indicate the
need for further conceptual development in the area. As Grove, Lavallee, and
Gordon (1997) have suggested, career transition research has often made gen-
eralizations across a number of athletes and thus has not presented information about how to individualize approaches. Social gerontological and thanatological models do not indicate what factors influence the quality of
adaptation to retirement from sport. In addition, the transition models that
have been applied to sport lack operational detail of the specific components
related to the adjustment process (Taylor & Ogilvie, 1994).

For these reasons, Taylor and Ogilvie (1998) and others (e.g., Gordon,
1995; Ogilvie & Taylor, 1993; Taylor & Ogilvie, 1994) have proposed more
comprehensive conceptual models of adaptation to career transition. As indicated in Figure 1, Taylor and Ogilvie's (1998) model examines the entire course
of the career transition process and includes the following components:
(a) causal factors that initiate the career transition process, (b) developmental
factors related to transition adaptation, (c) coping resources that affect the responses to career transitions, (d) quality of adjustment to career transition, and
(e) treatment issues for distressful reactions to career transition. In the following sections, selected empirical research conducted on how the overall quality
of adjustment to career transition is influenced by causal factors, developmental experiences, and coping resources will be reviewed in order to supplement the theoretical perspectives presented. Treatment issues for distressful
reactions to career transition will be addressed in chapter 7 in this volume.

Conceptual Models
of Career Transition in Sport

A review of the career transition literature reveals that emotional, social,
financial, and occupational factors interact as an individual's response to a
career transition emerges (Ogilvie & Taylor, 1993). Clearly, each athlete in
transition deals with these factors in a very individual manner, with the reasons for the transition, developmental experiences, and coping resources
influencing the overall quality of adjustment. In terms of occupational and financial factors, it appears that a number of methods for preparing athletes for
these adjustments have been identified (cf., Koukouris, 1991; Reynolds, 1981;

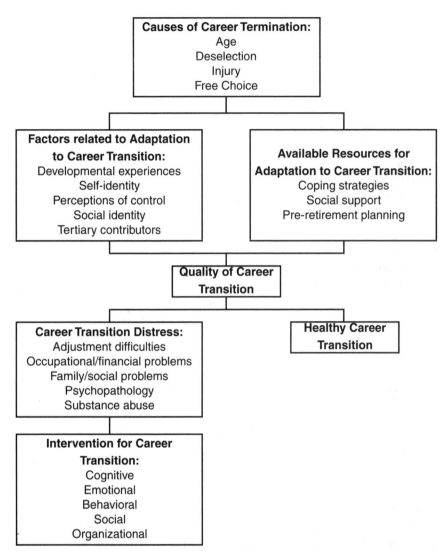

Figure 1. Conceptual model of adaptation to career transition.
Copied by permission, Taylor & Ogilvie, (1998)

Sinclair & Orlick, 1993; Werthner & Orlick, 1986). Extensive research on emotional and social adjustment has also been conducted, but these investigations have led to the considerable debate regarding the proportion of athletes who experience psychosocial adjustment difficulties upon athletic career termination (Curtis & Ennis, 1988; Greendorfer & Blinde, 1985). It is, however, the very discrepancies of this debate that reveal the need for further investigation into the overall phenomenon of career transitions in sport.

The debate regarding the prevalence of difficulties experienced during career transitions in sport appears to run parallel to the general literature on retirement from the labor force. Due to an absence of methodological rigor in the sport-related literature, it has been impossible to make a conclusive judgment about the prevalence of adjustment difficulties for athletes in transition. A number of the earliest studies suggested that retiring from sport is an inevitable source of emotional distress (e.g., Haerle, 1975; Mihovilovic, 1968; Weinberg & Arond, 1952). This research, however, tended to focus on male professional athletes in specific sports (i.e., baseball, boxing, and soccer) and emphasized the dysfunctional issues that athletes are occasionally confronted with after retirement (e.g., alcoholism).

As empirical data began to accumulate in the area, several sport theorists challenged the widespread assumption that athletic career termination is inherently stressful. For example, Coakley (1983) advanced a developmental perspective in describing how retirement from interscholastic, amateur, and professional sport is not always a traumatic event. Along the same lines, Gorbett (1985) suggested that it is naive to assume that former athletes are universally overwhelmed by retirement-induced stress. Although these pioneering points of departure in the literature led the sport-scientific community to speculate that the majority of athletes do not experience considerable distress upon career termination, a number of contemporary researchers have empirically demonstrated that the career transition process can be an inevitable source of adjustment.

Svoboda and Vanek (1982) have reported that 83% of their sample of former Czechoslovakian Olympic athletes experienced difficulties following retirement from sport. In addition, Werthner and Orlick (1986) conducted in-depth interviews with a sample of Canada's most successful amateur athletes and found that 78.6% felt some degree of difficulty in making the transition out of sport. In a survey of former Canadian junior male hockey players, Curtis and Ennis (1988) reported that 63% experienced some feelings of loss after disengaging from organized sport. Some of the most detailed support in this area of research, however, comes from a survey conducted by McInally, Cavin-Stice, and Knoth (1992) with retired professional male football players in the United States. In this study, 88% of the former athletes indicated that they found the overall career transition process to be extremely problematic. More specifically, moderate to severe problems were reported in regards to financial/occupational adjustment (31%), emotional adjustment (26%), and social adjustment (23%). Considering this evidence of adjustment difficulties experienced by former athletes upon retirement, 67% of the McInally et al. sample reported that they would still want professional football careers for their sons, and 85.6% of the Curtis and Ennis sample would prefer their sons to be as heavily involved in competitive hockey as they had been.

At the same time, other researchers have advanced the notion that chronicling athletic retirement as a painful event is an inadequate depiction of the experience. Blinde, Greendorfer, Kleiber, and colleagues conducted a series of surveys in the United States with female collegiate athletes who competed in various individual and team sports between 1976 and 1982, and male collegiate basketball and football players who competed between 1970 and 1980 (E. M. Blinde & Greendorfer, 1985; Greendorfer & Blinde, 1985; D. Kleiber, Greendorfer, Blinde & Sandall, 1987; D. A. Kleiber & Brock, 1992). In these separate but comparable studies, it was determined that approximately 90% of the athletes surveyed looked forward to life after competitive sport. This result, combined with comparable findings at the high school, collegiate, and professional levels reveals that the degree of career transition difficulty varies considerably among athletes representing different levels of achievement.

Despite the extensive amount of empirical and theoretical literature on career transition issues, there still exists considerable debate among contemporary scholars about how athletes adapt to career transition. As has been suggested outside of sport, however, every person experiencing a transition requires some degree of adjustment (Antonovsky & Sagy, 1990; Schlossberg, 1981). For athletes in transition, these adjustments can be financial, occupational, emotional, and/or social in nature, and as outlined in Taylor and Ogilvie's (1998) conceptual model of career transitions in sport, a raft of interrelated variables mediates the overall quality of adjustment.

Although each of these factors can have a significant impact on the response to retirement, it has been suggested that career transition research should focus on three areas (Gordon, 1995; Taylor & Ogilvie, 1998). The first area involves the causes of retirement and should include research on voluntary and involuntary reasons for career termination. The second needs to examine the developmental factors related to the adaptation process, focusing specifically on identity-related issues. The third, and final, area should consider the various coping strategies that mediate the response to athletic career transition.

Causes of Career Transition

Career transitions in sport have been found to be a function of a variety of involuntary and voluntary reasons. Although it has been suggested that the causes are influenced by the structure of sport, researchers have demonstrated that the most common of these causal factors are career-ending injuries, chronological age, deselection, and personal choice (S. M. Murphy, 1995; Ogilvie & Taylor, 1993; Werthner & Orlick, 1986).

Involuntary Reasons

Injury. Unexpected and sudden career transitions out of competitive sport often arise from injuries. Empirical research supports the notion that athletic retirement is difficult when caused by injury because it is something for which individuals are seldom prepared (e.g., Werthner & Orlick, 1986). In addition, D. A. Kleiber and Brock's (1992) study of athletes who suffered career-ending injuries demonstrates that an injury need not be severe to force athletes out of continued participation in competitive sport. As Ogilvie and Taylor (1993) have suggested, "elite athletes perform at such a high level that even small reductions in their physical capabilities may be sufficient to make them no longer competitive at the elite level" (p. 766). Consequently, injuries have the potential to be the most distressful reason for athletic career transition.

Age. Research by Mihovilovic (1968) with former Yugoslavian athletes has shown that retirement from sport is largely a function of the advancement of chronological age. In this descriptive survey of former professional soccer players, which was one of the first empirical attempts to analyze athletic career termination, the decline in performance accompanying the aging process was identified as one of the major causes for ending careers in the world of sport. Ogilvie and Taylor (1993) maintain that retirement due to age is one of the most significant reasons because psychological motivation, social status, and physical capabilities can all complicate an athlete's ability to continue competing at an elite level.

Deselection. Related to the physiological consequences of chronological age is the structural factor of failing to progress to the next highest level of elite competition. This deselection process is largely a function of a "survival of the fittest" philosophy (i.e., athletic Darwinism) that occurs at most levels of competitive sport (Pearson & Petitpas, 1990; Stevenson, 1989). McInally et al.'s (1992) finding that 27% of their sample were deselected from their teams demonstrates that this involuntary reason is a significant contributor to career transitions in sport.

Voluntary Reasons

The final predominant factor that describes the transition process of athletes is that of voluntary choice. Research by Wylleman, De Knop, Menkehorst, Theeboom, and Annerel (1993) with ex-Olympic Belgian athletes has demonstrated that many individuals freely elect to disengage from elite-level sport for a combination of personal, social, and psychological reasons. Some athletes may decide to retire because of financial complications, ethnic/gender-related issues, and/or an overall lack of life satisfaction, whereas others may simply want to spend more time with their families and friends (Allison & Meyer,

1988; Baillie, 1993). Although the voluntary decision to retire from sport is perhaps the most appealing reason, it should not be assumed that ending an athletic career voluntarily eases the career transition process (Taylor & Ogilvie, 1998).

As outlined by Alfermann in chapter 3 of this volume, the nature of each transitional athlete's adjustment depends on a complex interaction of factors. Consistent with findings outside of sport, Koukouris (1991, 1994) found that no single factor is primarily responsible for ceasing participation in sport among a sample of former Greek athletes. In addition, research by Stambulova (1994) with retired elite-level Russian athletes has shown that career transition occurs for a combination of reasons. Nevertheless, there still exists a lack of research on the specific reasons for career transition, as well as the impact voluntary and involuntary reasons have on the overall adjustment process (Lavallee, Grove, & Gordon, 1997).

Developmental Factors

The quality of adjustment to career transitions in sport also appears to be determined by a range of developmental factors. Several of these components have been shown to be psychosocial in nature, with developmental experiences that occur during the athlete's career contributing to the adaptation to the transition (McPherson, 1980; Pearson & Petitpas, 1990; Taylor & Ogilvie, 1994). The social identification and athletic identification with sport, however, appear to be two of the most fundamental of these issues related to the career transition process.

Social identity. The way athletes adapt during the career transition period appears to be dependent upon the diversity of their social identification with sport. Brewer (1993) has shown that individuals whose socialization process occurs in an athletic environment may assume a narrow social identity and be characterized as role restricted. Participation in high-level competition can also play an important role in the development of life skills, and many athletes may become severely inhibited in their ability to assume nonathletic roles (S. M. Murphy, 1995). Researchers outside of sport have discussed the importance of recognizing that close identification with one's job may lead to adjustment difficulties upon retirement from the labor force (e.g., Bosse, Aldwin, Levenson, & Workman-Daniels, 1991). This view has also been indirectly supported by studies in the sociology of sport literature on achievement motivation in which social identity acts to reinforce an athlete's decision to continue his or her commitment in sport (e.g., Donnelly & Young, 1988; Messner, 1992). In addition, a number of career transition researchers have suggested that athletes with narrow social identities require greater adjustment during retirement from sport than do those with broad-based identities (e.g., Grove et al., 1997; Werthner & Orlick, 1986). Hence, as suggested by Brewer, Van Raalte, and Petitpas in chapter 2 in this volume, a need exists for some athletes to gradually resocialize out of a strong "athletic identity" and into nonsport participatory roles.

Athletic identity. The influence of athletic participation on life-span development has become an important issue in the sport psychology literature. Although developmental research on career transitions in sport is somewhat scarce, an individual's athletic identity, which has been defined as the degree to which an individual defines herself or himself in terms of the athlete role (Brewer, Van Raalte, & Linder, 1993), has been hypothesized to have both positive and negative consequences for participants in sport.

By way of interviews with former Greek and French athletes, Chamalidis (1995) has demonstrated that those who ascribe great importance to their involvement in sport are more at risk to experience retirement-related difficulties than are those who place less value on the athletic component of their self-identity. In addition, several other researchers have shown how individuals who strongly commit themselves to the athlete role may be less likely to explore other career, education, and lifestyle options (Baillie & Danish, 1992; Werthner & Orlick, 1986). Along these lines, G. M. Murphy, Petitpas, and Brewer (1996) have demonstrated that both athletic identity and identity foreclosure are inversely related to career maturity among a sample of intercollegiate athletes. Identity foreclosure, which is the process by which individuals make commitments to roles without engaging in exploratory behavior (A. Petitpas, 1978), has the potential to hinder the development of coping strategies that are essential during career transitions (Crook & Robertson, 1991; Gordon, 1995; Pearson & Petitpas, 1990). One psycho-educational model that has been developed to assist athletes in developing these coping skills is life development intervention (S. Danish & D'Augelli, 1983). This primary preventive framework asserts that positive action taken before retirement will minimize or prevent difficulties and focuses specifically on the enhancement of coping strategies to deal with the transition process (S. J. Danish, Petitpas, & Hale, 1993, 1995). However, as outlined in the following section, limited empirical research has been conducted on how athletes cope with career transitions.

Coping Resources

Whereas many athletes make successful and satisfying career transitions, others may face severe difficulties for a variety of reasons. In the individual's attempt to manage the career transition process, theorists have suggested that those high in coping resources will tend to experience less stress than will athletes with few coping skills (S. M. Murphy, 1995; Pearson & Petitpas, 1990;

Taylor & Ogilvie, 1994). It appears likely, therefore, that the overall quality of adjustment to athletic career transition is influenced by the amount of coping resources available to athletes upon retirement from competitive sport.

In the general literature outside of sport, contemporary scholars have defined coping as "constantly changing cognitive and behavioral efforts to manage specific external and/or internal demands that are appraised as taxing or exceeding the resources of the person" (Lazarus & Folkman, 1984, p. 141). Empirical and theoretical investigations on coping processes initially examined how people cope with stress in their lives from a trait-oriented perspective. This approach adopted a belief that variations in stressful occurrences are of little importance, and thus ignored the specific context in which coping takes place (Folkman, Lazarus, Dunkel-Schetter, DeLongis, & Green, 1986).

More recently, personality and social psychology researchers have challenged this viewpoint by focusing on the actual coping processes that people utilize when stressful episodes occur. In this process-oriented perspective, an emphasis has been placed on global coping strategies used under particular circumstances, rather than how one reacts generally to a stressor. For example, Folkman, Lazarus, and colleagues have suggested that there are two broad coping strategies, namely problem-focused coping and emotion-focused coping (Folkman et al., 1986; Lazarus & Folkman, 1984). Endler and Parker (1990) have also proposed avoidance-oriented strategies as a third general class of coping resources. On the other hand, Carver, Scheier, and Weintraub (1989) and Costa and McCrae (1989) believe that an examination of specific strategies might be more informative than an examination of global coping strategies. However, all of these researchers are in agreement that coping is a complex, dynamic process.

In the career transition literature, a number of theorists have discussed how coping resources influence the overall quality of adjustment to retirement from sport (e.g., Crook & Robertson, 1991; Gordon, 1995). Several studies have also reported that many athletes turn to alcohol as a way of coping with their career transition (Koukouris, 1991; Mihovilovic, 1968). Sinclair and Orlick (1993), however, found that keeping busy, training/exercising, and a new focus were the most beneficial coping strategies utilized during the career transition phase among a sample of former elite Canadian athletes. These results confirm the earlier findings of Werthner and Orlick (1986) and Baillie (1992), who found that having a new focus after retirement predicted better adjustment. These collective results, combined with the available data on social support and preretirement planning, have shown the importance of transition-related coping resources in the athletic retirement process.

Social support. As previously discussed with regard to Schlossberg's (1981) model of transitions, the adaptation to athletic career transition depends largely on the availability of social support. Social support has been defined as "an exchange of resources between at least two individuals perceived by the provider or the recipient to be intended to enhance the well-being of the recipient" (Shumaker & Brownell, 1984, p. 13). The importance of social support networks among both active and injured athletes has been outlined in the literature (e.g., Ford & Gordon, 1999; Rosenfeld, Richman, & Hardy, 1989). In regard to career transitions in sport, however, very little empirical research has been conducted on the issue of social support.

Reynolds' (1981) study of former professional football players in the United States was one of the first to outline the general importance of social support during athletic retirement. In recent years, several other career transition researchers and theorists have documented the importance of the social support among friends, family, and teammates (e.g., Stambulova, 1994; Swain, 1991). Alfermann (1995) has also reported that coaches were the main social support agent among a sample of former track and field athletes from former West Germany. However, Kane's 1991 study of former male professional American athletes in the midst of a career transition demonstrated that the social support networks of athletes also suffer following retirement from sport (cited in Kane, 1995). Therefore, as S. M. Murphy (1995) asserts, social support could be the key to an optimal athletic career transition.

Preretirement planning. It has been asserted that preretirement planning is an effective coping skill for career transitions among elite athletes (Gorbett, 1985; Ogilvie & Taylor, 1993). Research outside of sport has demonstrated that such planning is significantly related to more effective adjustment following retirement from the labor force and that activities such as occupational counseling, continuing education, and social networking can all have a positive impact on the adaptation process (e.g., Fretz, Kluge, Ossana, Jones, & Merikangas, 1989). Studies on participation motivation in sport have also suggested that individuals who plan alternative areas in which to direct their attention are more likely to experience healthy career transitions (e.g., Haerle, 1975; Svoboda & Vanek, 1982). Despite the fact that retirement from sport is one of the only certainties in an athletic career, a recurring theme in the career transition literature is the resistance on the part of athletes to plan for and develop a career prior to their retirement (Sinclair & Orlick, 1993; Wylleman et al., 1993). For an outline of career development theory, the reader is directed to chapter 11 by Patton and Ryan in this volume

An empirical study by Haerle (1975) with retired professional baseball players in the United States has demonstrated that 75% of the athletes surveyed did not consider their postathletic occupations until they retired from sport. Utilizing the Professional Athletes Career Transition Inventory (PACTI;

Blann & Zaichkowsky, 1989), Blann and Zaichkowsky also reported that only 37% of professional ice hockey players and 25% of professional baseball players had a postsport career plan before retirement. Although this career indecision among retired athletes has also been illustrated in other research projects (e.g., McInally et al., 1992; Swain, 1991; Wylleman et al., 1993), it has become clear that the sport structure that requires excessive time and energy commitments leaves athletes with little time for planning during their careers (E. M. Blinde & Greendorfer, 1985). It appears, therefore, that further research is needed on how the career development of athletes is influenced by the sporting environment in which they participate.

In Australia, the Australian Athletes Career Transition Inventory (AACTI; Hawkins & Blann, 1993) and the Australian Coaches Career Transition Inventory (ACCTI; Hawkins, Blann, Zaichkowsky, & Kane, 1994) were developed to assess the career transition needs and postathletic career awareness of both athletes and coaches. In one study, 57% of coaches considered preretirement planning to be an essential part of the career transition process for athletes, but believed that the athletes themselves must take responsibility for the utilization of available programs (Hawkins et al., 1994). On the other hand, 98.2% of athletes surveyed indicated that they were primarily responsible for the utilization of programs offered, and that this could have a significant impact on their playing careers (Hawkins & Blann, 1993).

These findings are supported by the results of a survey conducted by A. Petitpas, Danish, McKelvain, and Murphy (1990) with athletes in the United States who attended workshops organized by the Career Assistance Program for Athletes (CAPA). In this study it was reported that some athletes believed that investing effort in the career development process would detract from their sport performance. Sinclair and Orlick (1993) have also reported how athletes consider that "coaches and institutional networks should treat retiring/retired athletes with respect rather than as disposable commodities" (p. 146). Although some coaches may have fears that the promotion of preretirement planning programs will distract athletes from their focus on high-level achievement, several others may envision that such preparation can ultimately contribute to the success of athletic teams (Crook & Robertson, 1991). As S. M. Murphy (1995) has suggested, many athletes believe that planning for another career actually decreases their anxiety regarding the transition process because it allows them to concentrate more fully on their sport. Therefore, as Gordon (1995) suggests, "the influence of coaches, who are often prone to operate as ideologists and focus on winning rather than as educators promoting discussions about career transition issues, may be the most significant determinant of the effectiveness of available preretirement programs" (p. 486).

In recent years, there has been a growing interest in preretirement programs for elite athletes. This increase in attention coincides with the development of primary preventive programs for retirement from the labor force, and follows Thomas and Ermler's (1988) suggestion that sporting institutions should provide support to retiring athletes during the career transition process. As outlined by Anderson and Morris in chapter 4 in this volume, several career assistance programs have been designed in countries around the world to help resolve the conflict that many athletes face in having to choose between pursuing their sporting and postathletic career goals. For example, the Olympic Athlete Career Centre in Canada was designed in 1985 to help Olympic-caliber athletes in the preparation for retirement (Olympic Athlete Career Centre, 1991). In addition, the Lifeskills for Elite Athletes Program was launched in Australia in 1989 and has since merged with the Athlete Career and Education Program to provide a nationally consistent career and education service for Australia's elite athletes (Australian Institute of Sport, 1996). The Olympic Job Opportunities Program has also been initiated in the United States, Australia, and South Africa to assist Olympic athletes who are committed to developing a professional career as well as achieving their sport-related goals (Olympic Job Opportunities Program, 1996).

Conclusion

The literature on career transitions in sport has predominantly focused on the adjustment difficulties experienced by athletes in transition. Numerous studies have revealed that a significant proportion of elite athletes experience difficulties upon career termination. Although these writings have proposed that distressful career transition experiences are manifested in a variety of dysfunctional ways, several contrasting studies have revealed minimal or no evidence of difficulties associated with the career transition process. In an effort to gain a better understanding of the athletic career transition phenomenon, sport theorists in the application of various explanatory models have addressed this discrepancy. For example, social gerontological theories of aging have been applied to sport in order to equate the process of athletic career termination with retiring from the workforce. Thanatological models, in a similar fashion, have utilized theories of death and dying to explain distressful reactions to athletic retirement. Both of these perspectives have been criticized, however, because they tend to view career termination as a singular event and more or less ignore the possibility of identity development outside of sport. Transition models have also been proposed as an alternative framework for research in the area, but these models have been criticized for failing to offer a holistic view of the career termination process. As Taylor and

Ogilvie (1994) have stated, "the theoretical models which have been applied to retirement from sport do not indicate what factors lead to the traumatic responses or what enables individuals to progress through the respective stages to reach closure" (p. 4).

With these criticisms in mind, conceptual models that explain the factors specifically related to adaptation to career transition have been developed (e.g., Gordon, 1995; Taylor & Ogilvie, 1998). These models outline how the overall quality of adjustment to career transition is influenced by the causal factors that initiate the transition process, developmental factors related to transition adaptation, and coping resources that affect the responses to career transitions. As Taylor and Ogilvie (1998) have suggested, the strength of these conceptual models is that once specific transition difficulties are demonstrated, appropriate therapeutic interventions can be recommended.

References

Alfermann, D. (1995). Career transitions of elite athletes: Drop-out and retirement. In R. Vanfraechem-Raway & Y. Vanden Auweele (Eds.), *Proceedings of the 9th European Congress of Sport Psychology* (pp. 828–833). Brussels: European Federation of Sports Psychology.

Allison, M. T., & Meyer, C. (1988). Career problems and retirement among elite athletes: The female tennis professional. *Sociology of Sport Journal, 5,* 212–222.

Antonovsky, A., & Sagy, S. (1990). Confronting developmental tasks in the retirement transition. *The Gerontologist, 30,* 362–368

Atchley, R. C. (1976). *The sociology of retirement.* Cambridge, MA: Schenkman.

Atchley, R. C. (1989). A continuity theory of normal aging. *The Gerontologist, 29,* 183–190.

Atchley, R. C. (1991). *Social forces and aging: An introduction to social gerontology* (6th ed.). Belmont, CA: Wadsworth.

Australian Institute of Sport (1996). *Athlete career and education program: A balanced approach to sporting excellence.* Canberra: Author.

Baillie, P. H. F. (1992, October/November). *Career transition in elite and professional athletes: A study of individuals in their preparation for and adjustment to retirement from competitive sports.* Colloquium presented at the annual conference of the Association for the Advancement of Applied Sport Psychology, Colorado Springs, USA.

Baillie, P. H. F. (1993). Understanding retirement from sports: Therapeutic ideas for helping athletes in transition. *The Counseling Psychologist, 21,* 399–410.

Baillie, P. H. F., & Danish, S. J. (1992). Understanding the career transition of athletes. *The Sport Psychologist, 6,* 77–98.

Blann, F. W., & Zaichkowsky, L. (1989). *National Hockey League and Major League Baseball players' post-sport career transition surveys.* Final report prepared for the National Hockey League Players' Association, USA.

Blau, P. (1964). *Exchange and power in social life.* New York: John Wiley.

Blinde, E., & Stratta, T. (1992). The "sport career death" of college athletes: Involuntary and unanticipated sports exits. *Journal of Sport Behavior, 15,* 3–20.

Blinde, E. M., & Greendorfer, S. L. (1985). A reconceptualization of the process of leaving the role of competitive athlete. *International Review for the Sociology of Sport, 20,* 87–94.

Bosse, R., Aldwin, C. M., Levenson, M. R., & Workman-Daniels, K. (1991). How stressful is retirement? Findings from the Normative Aging Study. *Journal of Gerontology, 46,* 9–14.

Brewer, B. W. (1993). Self-identity and specific vulnerability to depressed mood. *Journal of Personality, 61,* 343–363.

Brewer, B. W., Van Raalte, J. L., & Linder, D. E. (1993). Athletic identity: Hercules' muscles or Achilles' heel? *International Journal of Sport Psychology, 24,* 237–254.

Carver, C. S., Scheier, M. F., & Weintraub, J. K. (1989). Assessing coping strategies: A theoretically based approach. *Journal of Personality and Social Psychology, 56,* 267–283.

Chamalidis, P. (1995). Career transitions of male champions. In R. Vanfraechem-Raway & Y. Vanden Auweele (Eds.), *Proceedings of the 9th European Congress of Sport Psychology* (pp. 841–848). Brussels: European Federation of Sports Psychology.

Charner, I., & Schlossberg, N. K. (1986, June). Variations by theme: The life transitions of clerical workers. *The Vocational Guidance Quarterly,* 212–224.

Coakley, J. J. (1983). Leaving competitive sport: Retirement or rebirth? *Quest, 35,* 1–11.

Costa, P. T., & McCrae, R. R. (1989). Personality, stress, and coping: Some lessons from a decade of research. In K. S. Markides & C. L. Cooper (Eds.), *Aging, stress, and health* (pp. 269–285). New York: Wiley.

Crook, J. M., & Robertson, S. E. (1991). Transitions out of elite sport. *International Journal of Sport Psychology, 22,* 115–127.

Cummings, E., Dean, L. R., Newell, D. S., & McCaffrey, I. (1960). Disengagement: A tentative theory of aging. *Sociometry, 23,* 23–35.

Curtis, J., & Ennis, R. (1988). Negative consequences of leaving competitive sport? Comparison findings for former elite-level hockey players. *Sociology of Sport Journal, 5,* 87–106.

Danish, S., & D'Augelli, A. R. (1983). *Helping skills: II. Life development intervention.* New York: Human Sciences.

Danish, S. J., Petitpas, A. J., & Hale, B. D. (1993). Life development intervention for athletes: Life skills through sports. *The Counseling Psychologist, 21,* 352–385.

Danish, S. J., Petitpas, A. J., & Hale, B. D. (1995). Psychological interventions: A life developmental model. In S. Murphy (Ed.), *Sport psychology interventions* (pp. 19–38). Champaign, IL: Human Kinetics.

Donnelly, P., & Young, K. (1988). The construction and confirmation of identity in sport subcultures. *Sociology of Sport Journal, 5,* 223–240.

Edwards, J., & Meier, K. (1984, July). *Social breakdown/reconstruction and athletic retirement: An investigation of retirement and retirement adjustment in National Hockey League players.* Paper presented at the annual meeting of the Olympic Scientific Congress, Eugene, OR, USA.

Endler, N. S., & Parker, J. D. A. (1990). Multidimensional assessment of coping: A critical evaluation. *Journal of Personality and Social Psychology, 58,* 844–854.

Erikson. E. (1950). *Childhood and society.* New York: Norton.

Folkman, S., Lazarus, R. S., Dunkel-Schetter, C., DeLongis, A., & Gruen, R. J. (1986). Dynamics of a stressful encounter: Cognitive appraisal, coping, and encounter outcomes. *Journal of Personality and Social Psychology, 50,* 992–1003.

Ford, I. W., & Gordon, S. (1999). Coping with sport injury: Resource loss and the role of social support. *Journal of Personal and Interpersonal Loss, 4,*

Fretz, B. R., Kluge, N. A., Ossana, S. M., Jones, S. M., & Merikangas, M. W. (1989). Intervention targets for reducing preretirement anxiety and depression. *Journal of Counseling Psychology, 36,* 301–307.

Friedmann, E. A., & Havighurst, R. J. (Eds.). (1954). *The meaning of work and retirement.* Chicago: University of Chicago Press.

Glaser, B. G., & Strauss, A. L. (1965). *Awareness of dying.* Chicago: Aldine.

Gorbett, F. J. (1985). Psycho-social adjustment of athletes to retirement. In L. K. Bunker, R. J. Rotella, & A. Reilly (Eds.), *Psychological considerations in maximizing sport performance* (pp. 288–294). Ithaca, NY: Mouvement.

Gordon, S. (1995). Career transitions in competitive sport. In T. Morris & J. Summers (Eds.), *Sport psychology: Theory, applications and issues* (pp. 474–501). Brisbane: Jacaranda Wiley.

Gordon, S., Milios, D., & Grove, J. R. (1991). Psychological aspects of the recovery process from sport injury: The perspective of sport physiotherapists. *Australian Journal of Science and Medicine in Sport, 23,* 53–60.

Greendorfer, S. L, & Blinde, E. M. (1985). "Retirement" from intercollegiate sport: Theoretical and empirical considerations. *Sociology of Sport Journal, 2,* 101–110.

Grove, J. R., Lavallee, D., & Gordon, S. (1997). Coping with retirement from sport: The influence of athletic identity. *Journal of Applied Sport Psychology, 9,* 191–203.

Haerle, R. K. (1975). Career patterns and career contingencies of professional baseball players: An occupational analysis. In D.W. Ball & J.W. Loy (Eds.), *Sport and social order* (pp. 461–519). Reading, MA: Addison-Wesley.

Havighurst, R. J., & Albrecht, R. (1953). *Older people.* New York: Longmans, Green.

Hawkins, K., & Blann, F. W. (1993). *Athlete/coach career development and transition.* Canberra: Australian Sports Commission.

Hawkins, K., Blann, F. W., Zaichkowsky, L., & Kane, M. A. (1994). *Athlete/coach career development and transition: Coaches' report.* Canberra: Australian Sports Commission.

Hill, P., & Lowe, B. (1974). The inevitable metathesis of the retiring athlete. *International Review of Sport Sociology, 4,* 5–29.

Homans, G. (1961). *Social behavior: Its elementary forms.* New York: Harcourt Brace.

Johns, D. P., Linder, K. J., & Wolko, K. (1990). Understanding attrition in female competitive gymnastics: Applying social exchange theory. *Sociology of Sport Journal, 7,* 154–171.

Kalish, R. (1966). A continuity of subjectivity perceived death. *The Gerontologist, 6,* 73–76.

Kane, M. A. (1995). The transition out of sport: A paradigm from the United States. In R. Vanfraechem-Raway & Y. Vanden Auweele (Eds.), *Proceedings of the 9th European Congress of Sport Psychology* (pp. 849–856). Brussels: European Federation of Sports Psychology.

Kastenbaum, R., & Kastenbaum, B. (Eds.). (1989). *Encyclopedia of death.* Phoenix, AZ: Oryx Press.

Kastenbaum, R., & Weisman, A. (1972). The psychological autopsy as a research procedure in gerontology. In D. Kent, R. Kastenbaum, & S. Sherwood (Eds.), *Research, planning, and action for the elderly.* New York: Behavioral Publications.

Kleiber, D., Greendorfer, S., Blinde, E., & Sandall, D. (1987). Quality of exit from university sports and subsequent life satisfaction. *Journal of Sport Sociology, 4,* 28–36.

Kleiber, D. A., & Brock, S. C. (1992). The effect of career-ending injuries on the subsequent well-being of elite college athletes. *Sociology of Sport Journal, 9,* 70–75.

Koukouris, K. (1991). Quantitative aspects of the disengagement process of advanced and elite Greek male athletes from organized competitive sport. *Journal of Sport Behavior, 14,* 227–246.

Koukouris, K. (1994). Constructed case studies: Athletes' perspectives on disengaging from organized competitive sport. *Sociology of Sport Journal, 11,* 114–139.

Kübler-Ross, E. (1969). *On death and dying.* New York: Macmillan.

Kuypers, J. A., & Bengston, V. L. (1973). Social breakdown and competence: A model of normal aging. *Human Development, 16,* 181–220.

Lavallee, D., Grove, J. R., & Gordon, S. (1997). The causes of career termination from sport and their relationship to post-retirement adjustment among elite-amateur athletes in Australia. *The Australian Psychologist, 32,* 131–135.

Lazarus, R. S., & Folkman, S. (1984). *Stress, appraisal, and coping.* New York: Springer.

Lemon, B. W., Bengston, V. L., & Peterson, J. A. (1972). An exploration of the activity theory of aging: Activity types and life satisfaction among in-movers to a retirement community. *Journal of Gerontology, 27,* 511–523.

Lerch, S. (1984). Athlete retirement as social death: An overview. In N. Theberge & P. Donnelly (Eds.), *Sport and the sociological imagination* (pp. 259–272). Fort Worth: Texas Christian University Press.

Lerch, S. H. (1981). The adjustment to retirement of professional baseball players. In S. L. Green-dorfer & A. Yiannakis (Eds.), *Sociology of sport: Diverse perspectives* (pp. 138–148). West Point, NY: Leisure Press.

Longino, C. F., & Kart, C. S. (1982). Explicating activity theory: A formal replication. *Journal of Gerontology, 37,* 713–722.

Longino, C. F., McClelland, K. A., & Peterson, W. A. (1980). The aged subculture hypothesis: Social integration, gerontophilia, and self-conception. *Journal of Gerontology, 35,* 758–767.

Marshall, V. W. (1978). No exit: A symbolic interactionist perspective on aging. *International Journal of Aging and Human Development, 9,* 345–358.

McInally, L., Cavin-Stice, J., & Knoth, R. L. (1992, August). *Adjustment following retirement from professional football.* Paper presented at the annual meeting of the American Psychological Association, Washington D.C.

McPherson, B. D. (1980). Retirement from professional sport: The process and problems of occupational and psychological adjustment. *Sociological Symposium, 30,* 126–143.

Messner, M. A. (1992). *Power at play: Sports and the problem of masculinity.* Boston: Beacon Press.

Mihovilovic, M. (1968). The status of former sportsmen. *International Review of Sport Sociology, 3,* 73–93.

Morris, T. (1995). Sport psychology in Australia: A profession established. *Australian Psychologist, 30,* 128–134.

Murphy, G. M., Petitpas, A. J., & Brewer, B. W. (1996). Identity foreclosure, athletic identity, and career maturity in intercollegiate athletes. *The Sport Psychologist, 10,* 239–246.

Murphy, S. M. (1995). Transition in competitive sport: Maximizing individual potential. In S. M. Murphy (Ed.), *Sport psychology interventions* (pp. 331–346). Champaign, IL: Human Kinetics.

Ogilvie, B. C., & Taylor, J. (1993). Career termination issues among elite athletes. In R. N. Singer, M. Murphey, & L. K. Tennant (Eds.), *Handbook of research on sport psychology* (pp. 761–775). New York: Macmillan.

Olympic Athlete Career Centre (1991). *Guide to the administration of the Olympic Athlete Career Centre.* Toronto: Author.

Olympic Job Opportunities Program (1996, March). *Opportunities,* p. 3.

Orlick, T., & Werthner, P. (1987). *Athletes in transition.* Toronto: Olympic Athlete Career Center.

Park, R. (1912). Thanatology. *Journal of the American Medical Association, 58,* 1243–1246.

Parker, K. B. (1994). "Has-beens" and "wanna-bes": Transition experiences of former major college football players. *The Sport Psychologist, 8,* 287–304.

Pearson, R. E., & Petitpas, A. J. (1990). Transitions of athletes: Developmental and preventive perspectives. *Journal of Counseling and Development, 69,* 7–10.

Petitpas, A. (1978). Identity foreclosure: A unique challenge. *Personnel and Guidance Journal, 56,* 558–561.

Petitpas, A., Champagne, D., Chartrand, J., Danish, S., & Murphy, S. (1997). *Athlete's guide to career planning: Keys to success from the playing field to professional life.* Champaign, IL: Human Kinetics.

Petitpas, A., Danish, S., McKelvain, R., & Murphy, S. M. (1990). A career assistance program for elite athletes. *Journal of Counseling and Development, 70,* 383–386.

Petitpas, A. J., Brewer, B. W., & Van Raalte, J. L. (1996). Transitions of the student-athlete: Theoretical, empirical, and practical perspectives. In E. F. Etzel, A. P. Ferrante, & Pinkney, J. W. (Eds.), *Counseling college student-athletes: Issues and interventions* (2nd ed., pp. 137–156). Morgantown, WV: Fitness Information Technology.

Rando, T. A. (1984). *Grief, dying, and death: Clinical interventions for caregivers.* Champaign, IL: Research Press.

Rando, T. A. (1986). *Loss and anticipatory grief.* Lexington, MA: Lexington Books.

Reynolds, M. J. (1981). The effects of sports retirement on the job satisfaction of the former football player. In S. L. Greendorfer & A. Yiannakis (Eds.), *Sociology of sport: Diverse perspectives* (pp. 127–137). West Point, NY: Leisure Press.

Rose, A. M. (1962). The subculture of aging: A topic for sociological research. *The Gerontologist, 2,* 123–127.

Rosenberg, E. (1981). Gerontological theory and athletic retirement. In S. L. Greendorfer & A. Yiannakis (Eds.), *Sociology of sport: Diverse perspective* (pp. 119–126). West Point, NY: Leisure Press.

Rosenberg, E. (1984). Athletic retirement as social death: Concepts and perspectives. In N. Theberge & P. Donnelly (Eds.), *Sport and the sociological imagination* (pp. 245–258). Fort Worth: Texas Christian University Press.

Rosenfeld, L. B., Richman, J. M., & Hardy, C. J. (1989). Examining social support networks among athletes: Description and relationship to stress. *The Sport Psychologist, 3,* 23–33.

Schlossberg, N. K. (1981). A model for analyzing human adaptation to transition. *The Counseling Psychologist, 9,* 2–18.

Schlossberg, N. K. (1984). *Counseling adults in transition: Linking practice with theory.* New York: Springer.

Shumaker, S. A, & Brownell, A. (1984). Toward a theory of social support: Closing conceptual gaps. *Journal of Social Issues, 40 (4),* 11–36.

Sinclair, D. A., & Orlick, T. (1993). Positive transitions from high-performance sport. *The Sport Psychologist, 7,* 138–150.

Sinclair, D. A., & Orlick, T. (1994). The effects of transition on high performance sport. In D. Hackfort (Ed.), *Psycho-social issues and interventions in elite sports* (pp. 29–55). Frankfurt: Lang.

Stambulova, N. B. (1994). Developmental sports career investigations in Russia: A post-perestroika analysis. *The Sport Psychologist, 8,* 221–237.

Stevenson, C. L. (1989). Perceptions of justice in the selection of national teams. *Sociology of Sport Journal, 6,* 371–379.

Sussman, M. B. (1972). An analytical model for the sociological study of retirement. In F. M. Carp (Ed.), *Retirement* (pp. 29–74). New York: Human Sciences.

Svoboda, B., & Vanek, M. (1982). Retirement from high level competition. In T. Orlick, J. T. Partington, & J. H. Salmela (Eds.), *Proceedings of the 5th World Congress of Sport Psychology* (pp. 166–175). Ottawa: Coaching Association of Canada.

Swain, D. A. (1991). Withdrawal from sport and Schlossberg's model of transitions. *Sociology of Sport Journal, 8,* 152–160.

Taylor, J., & Ogilvie, B. C. (1994). A conceptual model of adaptation to retirement among athletes. *Journal of Applied Sport Psychology, 6,* 1–20.

Taylor, J., & Ogilvie, B. C. (1998). Career transition among elite athletes: Is there life after sports? In J. M. Williams (Ed.), *Applied sport psychology: Personal growth to peak performance* (3rd ed., pp. 429–444). Mountain View, CA: Mayfield.

Thomas, C. E., & Ermler, K. L. (1988). Institutional obligations in the athletic retirement process. *Quest, 40,* 137–150.

United States Olympic Committee (1993). *Positioning yourself for success: An employment counseling handbook for athletes.* Colorado Springs: Author.

Weinberg, S. K., & Arond, H. (1952). The occupational culture of the boxer. *The American Journal of Sociology, 57,* 460–469.

Werthner, P., & Orlick, T. (1986). Retirement experiences of successful Olympic athletes. *International Journal of Sport Psychology, 17,* 337–363.

Wiese-Bjornstal, D. M., & Smith, A. M. (1993). Counseling strategies for enhanced recovery of injured athletes within a team approach. In D. Pargman (Ed.), *Psychological bases of sport injuries* (pp. 149–182). Morgantown, WV: Fitness Information Technology.

Wylleman, P., De Knop, P., Menkehorst, H., Theeboom, M., & Annerel, J. (1993). Career termination and social integration among elite athletes. In S. Serpa, J. Alves, V. Ferreira, & A. Paula-Brito (Eds.), *Proceedings of the VIII World Congress of Sport Psychology* (pp. 902–906). Lisbon: International Society of Sport Psychology.

2

Self-Identity Issues in Sport Career Transitions

Britton W. Brewer,
Judy L. Van Raalte,
and Albert J. Petitpas
Springfield College

Abstract

This chapter reviews research on self-identity in sport context (i.e., athletic identity) as it pertains to sport career transitions. Individual differences in athletic identity are examined along with the role of athletic identity in adjustment to sport career transitions and the effects of sport career transitions on athletic identity. Recommendations for research and practice are provided.

Self-Identity Issues in Sport Career Transitions

During the course of their involvement in sport, athletes may experience a number of transitions. Among the more common transitions encountered by athletes are injury, deselection (e.g., being "cut"), and sport career termination, all of which may require considerable personal adjustment. In Schlossberg's (1981) model of adaptation to transitions, which has been widely extrapolated to sport career transitions (e.g., Crook & Robertson, 1991; Gorbett, 1985; Pearson & Petitpas, 1990; Swain, 1991), adjustment to transitions is thought to be influenced by cognitive appraisals of the transitions, personal factors, and environmental characteristics. One personal factor that has consistently been deemed relevant to the sport career transition process is self-identity (Crook & Robertson; Gordon, 1995; Pearson & Petitpas; Taylor &

994). Self-identity not only may *influence* adjustment to sport sitions, but also may be *influenced by* the transitions themselves. Before describing research on self-identity specific to sport and sport career transitions, however, it is instructive to discuss self-identity in general.

Self-Identity

"Self" is defined in *Webster's New Collegiate Dictionary* (1981) as "the union of elements (as body, emotions, thoughts, and sensations) that constitute the individuality and identity of a person" (p. 1040). The self has long been a topic of inquiry in psychology. More than a century ago, James (1892) wrote eloquently on the processes underlying the self. Cooley (1902) described the "looking glass self" in which self-perceptions are determined by reflected appraisals from a social mirror of significant others. Empirical study of the self has exploded in recent years, as evidenced by the proliferation of descriptors with the "self-" prefix (e.g., self-actualization, self-image, self-control, self-efficacy, self-help) in the literature. A search of *Psychological Abstracts* illustrates this point. In 1969, eight descriptors with the "self" prefix were referenced; in 1979, 19 descriptors were referenced; and in 1989, 33 descriptors were referenced (Hoare, 1991).

Given the growing array of descriptors with the "self" prefix, it is useful to highlight the distinctions among key self-related terms. Self-identity and self-concept both address the question, who am I? However, whereas self-concept is the collection of self-descriptive roles and attributes that constitute the self (Fox, 1997), self-identity is more elaborate and distinct (Brettschneider & Heim, 1997), referring to "a clearly delineated self-definition . . . comprised of those goals, values, and beliefs which the person finds personally expressive, and to which he or she is unequivocally committed" (Waterman, cited in Brettschneider & Heim, 1997, p. 207). In contrast, self-esteem is "the evaluative and affective component of the self-concept" (Weiss, 1987, p. 88). In other words, self-esteem is how people feel about themselves. Thus, self-identity pertains to self-definition rather than self-evaluation.

Self-Identity in Sport

Although the self has traditionally been considered a unidimensional construct (e.g., Coopersmith, 1967; Piers, 1969), recent theory and research have treated the self as a multidimensional entity, with self-perceptions varying as a function of the content domain under consideration (e.g., Fox & Corbin, 1989; Gergen, 1971; Harter, 1990; Markus & Wurf, 1987; Marsh & Shavelson, 1985). For example, people may think or feel differently about themselves depending on whether they are considering their "social" selves or their "academic" selves. Moreover, the value or importance placed on a given self-concept domain is thought to determine the relationship between performance in that domain and self-esteem, affect, motivation, and, ultimately, behavior (Harter, 1990; James, 1892; Rosenberg, 1979).

Given the salience of self-evaluation in the physical and athletic domains across the life span (Harter, 1990), it is not surprising that the trend toward increased theoretical and empirical attention to the self in general psychology has been evident in sport and exercise psychology as well (cf. Fox, 1997, 1998). Self-identity in the sport domain (or "athletic identity," as it will be referred to in this chapter) can be defined as the degree to which an individual identifies with the athlete role (Brewer, Van Raalte, & Linder, 1993). Athletic identity is conceptualized as comprising the athletic portion of a multidimensional self-concept.

Correlates of Athletic Identity

Although self-identity in sport is a relatively recent topic of scientific study, significant relationships between athletic identity and several personal factors that may harm or contribute to adjustment to sport career transitions (McPherson, 1984; Schlossberg, 1981) have been documented. In particular, differences in athletic identity as a function of gender, age, race/ethnicity, and personality have been obtained.

Gender

Across a number of studies, men have consistently been found to have higher athletic identity scores than those of women (Brewer, Van Raalte, & Linder, 1991, Study 2; Brewer et al., 1993, Studies 1 and 2; Curry & Parr, 1988; Curry & Weiss, 1989, Austrian sample; Good, Brewer, Petitpas, Van Raalte, & Mahar, 1993; Matheson, Brewer, Van Raalte, & Andersen, 1994; Mehlhorn, 1996; Schroeder & Lantz, 1996; Wiechman & Williams, 1997). Closer inspection of the data, however, reveals that the majority of studies in which significant gender differences in athletic identity have been obtained have consisted of samples of individuals varying in level of sport involvement. Indeed, within-study gender comparisons by level of sport involvement have indicated that the magnitude of gender differences in athletic identity has been greater among individuals at low levels of sport involvement (e.g., nonathletes, recreational athletes) than among individuals at higher levels of sport involvement (Brewer et al., 1993, Study 1; Good et al., 1993). Consistent with these findings, seven investigations with competitive athlete samples have failed to show gender differences in athletic identity (Curry & Weiss, 1989, United States sample; Deiters, 1996; Hale, Stambulova, & James, 1996; Hale & Waalkes,

1994; G. M. Murphy, Petitpas, & Brewer, 1996; Neyer, 1996; Van Raalte & Cook, 1991). Curry (1993) even found competitive female athletes to have higher athletic identity than that of competitive male athletes.

Although male and female competitive athletes are likely to be comparably self-invested in sport participation, it is possible that the processes underlying athletic identity may differ somewhat for men and women. Brewer et al. (1991, Study 2) examined the relationship between athletic identity and gender roles in a sample of college students enrolled in an introductory psychology course. For men, athletic identity was significantly correlated with neither masculinity ($r = .07$) nor femininity ($r = .09$). For women, athletic identity was significantly correlated with masculinity ($r = .34$), but not with femininity ($r = .00$). These findings suggest that athletic identity is a salient gender-role issue for women, but not for men. In another study indicating a potential difference in how men and women experience athletic identity, Van Raalte and Cook (1991) administered a measure of athletic identity to male and female intercollegiate athletes individually or in a small group setting either before or after practice. It was found that although prepractice and postpractice athletic identity did not differ for men, prepractice athletic identity was significantly lower than postpractice athletic identity for women. Van Raalte and Cook concluded that the athlete role may not be as salient for women outside the sport context.

Age

Little research has examined the relationship between age and athletic identity. Nevertheless, negative associations between age and athletic identity have been obtained in two cross-sectional studies, one with college students (Brewer et al., 1993, Study 1) and one with patients at a sports medicine clinic (Brewer, 1993, Study 3). Although the correlations between age and athletic identity were weak (i.e., in the $r = -.2$ range) in both studies, they are suggestive of a pattern of decreasing identification with the athlete role as the individual matures and becomes exposed to a variety of activities and influences. Consistent with these results, Greendorfer and Blinde (1985) reported a decline in the perceived importance of sport from high school to postcollege among former intercollegiate athletes in a retrospective investigation. Similarly, the longitudinal findings of Krauss, Dittman, and Camas (1998) indicate that emotional attachment to, investment in, and importance of sport decreased for former high school athletes in the 5 or 6 years following graduation. Clearly, there is much work to be done in examining athletic identity across the life span. Further research on age and athletic identity should consider the role of environmental factors in athletic identity development. Factors such as encouragement from others to pursue sports (Cutler & Meyer, 1995), absence of emphasis on books in the childhood home (Dollinger, 1994), and emphasis on sports and social life in the childhood home (Dollinger, 1994) have been associated with higher levels of athletic identity in college students.

Race/Ethnicity

As with age, there has been little systematic investigation of the relationship between race/ethnicity and athletic identity. In a cross-cultural study, Matheson et al. (1995) found no difference between British and Malaysian elite badminton players. Hale et al. (1996), however, found that athletes from Russia scored higher on exclusivity of athletic identity than did athletes from the United Kingdom and the United States. Hale et al. also reported that national-level athletes from the United States and international- and national-level athletes from Russia scored higher on the social aspects of athletic identity than did local-level athletes from Russia and international-, national-, and local-level athletes from the United Kingdom.

Within United States culture, three studies have found higher athletic identity among Caucasian student-athletes than among African-American student-athletes (Anderson, 1996; Brown, 1993; Wiechman & Williams, 1997). Mexican-American high school student-athletes were found to have greater athletic identity than their Caucasian and African-American peers in one study (Wiechman & Williams, 1997). Anderson suggested that the athletic identity of African-American student-athletes and Caucasian student-athletes may differ because other identities (e.g., racial identity) are more salient for African-American student-athletes than for Caucasian student-athletes. Brown argued that college sport may serve a functional purpose (i.e., a means to an end, such as a college education) to a greater extent for African-American student-athletes than for Caucasian student-athletes. These hypotheses warrant further empirical attention.

The Anderson (1996) study and an investigation by Tubilleja (1998) provide additional evidence that athletic identity may serve different purposes for different racial and ethnic groups. In addition to the difference in athletic identity between African-American student-athletes and Caucasian student-athletes noted previously, Anderson found that athletic identity was positively correlated with identity foreclosure, a construct involving commitment to roles without engaging in exploratory behavior (Marcia, 1966; A. J. Petitpas, 1978), for Caucasian student-athletes but not for African-American student-athletes. Similarly, although he found no differences in athletic identity between African-American and Caucasian student-athletes, Tubilleja documented a significant positive correlation between athletic identity and an index of psychosocial development ("establishing and clarifying purpose") for Caucasian student-athletes but not for African-American student-athletes. The findings of Anderson and Tubilleja suggest that athletic identity is independent of other aspects of identity development for African-American student-athletes but not for Caucasian student-athletes. Further research is needed, however, to verify this speculation and establish its meaning within a broader theoretical framework.

Personality

In the few studies that have examined the relationships between athletic identity, a relatively stable characteristic, and other personality traits, several significant associations have been documented. Positive correlations have been found between athletic identity and extraversion (Dollinger, 1994), social identity (Buntrock & Brewer, 1994; Dollinger), and ego involvement (Baysden, Brewer, Petitpas, & Van Raalte, 1997). Dollinger found that athletic identity was negatively correlated with openness to experience. The one consistency in these otherwise isolated findings is that athletic identity seems to be associated with an external, socially focused orientation.

Self-Identity and Adjustment to Sport Career Transitions

Although maintenance of a strong, exclusive athletic identity may have a positive effect on sport performance (Danish, 1983; Werthner & Orlick, 1986), there may also be risks associated with such a pattern of self-identification. Outside the sport literature, several contemporary models of reactive depression and stress and coping are consistent with the idea that a strong, exclusive identification with a given role is a risk factor for difficulties (e.g., emotional disturbance) in adjusting to transitions involving that role (Dance & Kuiper, 1987; Klinger, 1977; Lazarus & Folkman, 1984; Oatley & Bolton, 1985; Pyszczynski & Greenberg, 1987). Linville's (1985, 1987) empirical work on self-complexity and affective extremity, which suggests that people who organize information about themselves in a unidimensional, nondiversified way are vulnerable to dysphoria in response to stressful events, lends credibility to her warning, "Don't put all of your eggs in one cognitive basket."

In the sport realm, theorists have also ascribed a critical role to patterns of self-identification in influencing adjustment to sport career transitions, such as sport injury (e.g., Brewer, 1994; Deutsch, 1985; Eldridge, 1983; Heyman, 1986; Little, 1969; Ogilvie, 1989; Pearson & Petitpas, 1990; A. Petitpas & Danish, 1995; Wiese-Bjornstal, Smith, Shaffer, & Morrey, 1998) and sport career termination (e.g., Baillie & Danish, 1992; Blinde & Greendorfer, 1985; Crook & Robertson, 1991; Gordon, 1995; Lavallee, Grove, Gordon, & Ford,

1998; McPherson, 1980; Ogilvie & Howe, 1986; Orlick, 1980; Pearson & Petitpas, 1990; Schafer, 1969; Taylor & Ogilvie, 1994; Werthner & Orlick, 1986). Further, a growing body of empirical literature suggests that individuals who invest strongly in sport to the exclusion of other pursuits are vulnerable to difficulties in adjusting to transitions involving the athlete role. Research has focused on the relationship between athletic identity and adjustment to sport injury, adjustment to sport career termination, and career development.

Sport Injury

Direct support for the hypothesis that maintaining a strong, exclusive athletic identity is associated with increased risk for problems adjusting to sport injury was obtained by Brewer (1993). In a series of four studies, Brewer found that athletic identity was positively correlated with depressive reactions to actual and hypothetical sport injuries. Results of investigations conducted by Little (1969) and Kleiber and Brock (1992) augment the findings of Brewer. In a clinical investigation, Little found that physical injury was more likely as a precipitating event in the neuroses of individuals who excessively and exclusively valued athletic prowess than in the neuroses of individuals who did not overvalue athletic prowess. Kleiber and Brock assessed the self-esteem and life satisfaction 5 to 10 years postinjury of college student-athletes who incurred a career-ending injury. It was found that only those student-athletes with a high investment in playing professional sport (who were presumably high in athletic identity) tended to report lower self-esteem and life satisfaction. Although there are limitations with each of the investigations, the research of Brewer, Little, and Kleiber and Brock provide preliminary evidence that athletic identity plays an important role in how athletes adjust to sport injury.

Sport Career Termination

Several studies have examined the relationship between athletic identity and adjustment to sport career termination. In an investigation of former competitive gymnasts, Hinitz (1988) found that gymnasts who strongly identified with the role of "gymnast" and who considered involvement in their sport a central source of self-definition experienced difficult adjustments to sport career termination. In a retrospective study of retired elite athletes, Grove, Lavallee, and Gordon (1997) found that athletic identity at the time of retirement was positively correlated with the degree of emotional and social adjustment required and the amount of time required to adjust emotionally and socially during the transition out of elite sport involvement. Similarly, Schmid and Schilling (1997) found that both strength and exclusivity of athletic identity were associated with greater anticipated difficulty adjusting to a hypothetical forced disengagement from sport participation among physical education students. These results strongly suggest that maintenance of a strong and exclusive athletic identity may be maladaptive in the process of leaving a sport career.

Indirect support for the hypothesized relation between athletic identity and adjustment to sport career termination has been obtained in studies in which adoption of identities outside of the sport domain were associated with more favorable adaptations to sport career termination. In a study of former Canadian Olympic athletes, Werthner and Orlick (1986) found that individuals with an alternative pursuit in which to commit and invest energy made smoother transitions out of the athlete role than did individuals without such an alternative pursuit. Similar findings were obtained in investigations by Baillie (1992), Schmidt and Schilling (1997), and Sinclair and Orlick (1993). Bolstering these results, Lavallee, Gordon, and Grove (1997) found that reductions in athletic identity following retirement were associated with greater overall success in coping with sport career termination and less negative affect among former elite athletes. In contrast to the data showing adjustment benefits for investing in new identities and shedding athletic identity in the sport career termination process, Chamalidis (1997) reported that some former French elite male athletes encountered difficulties adjusting to retirement even when adopting new social roles and patterns of identification. Identification with new roles, therefore, may not guarantee problem-free sport career termination, especially when the roles are closely connected with one another at a conceptual level (Linville, 1985, 1987).

In addition to the research linking athletic identity to the quality of adjustment to sport career termination, there is evidence that athletic identity is related to the process by which athletes adjust to retirement from sport. Specifically, Grove et al. (1997) found that athletic identity at the time of retirement was associated with certain coping strategies used by elite athletes during the retirement process. Relative to former elite sport participants low in athletic identity, former elite sport participants high in athletic identity tended to report using more venting of emotions, mental disengagement, behavioral disengagement, denial, seeking of instrumental social support, suppression of competing activities, and seeking of emotional social support during retirement. Thus, there appear to be clear differences as a function of athletic identity in the coping strategies that athletes enlist in the sport career termination process. One other study that does not pertain directly to sport career termination warrants mention. Dollinger (1994) documented a significant positive correlation between athletic identity and self-reported alcohol use, a coping strategy that could prove maladaptive if adopted during the transition out of competitive sport.

Career Exploration

Failure to explore other vocational identities and prepare adequately for careers outside sport may contribute to the difficulties encountered by individuals strongly invested in the athlete role whose sport careers are ending. For example, Owens (1994) found that college student-athletes who identified strongly with the roles of both "athlete" *and* "student" had significantly higher levels of career exploration than did college athletes who identified strongly only with the role of "athlete," suggesting that individuals with a strong and exclusive athletic identity may fail to explore career options prior to sport career termination. G. M. Murphy et al. (1996) documented an inverse relationship between athletic identity and career maturity, indicating a tendency for student-athletes high in athletic identity to have inhibited career decision-making skills. Consistent with the findings of Owens and G. M. Murphy et al., Grove et al. (1997) found that athletic identity at the time of retirement was positively correlated with anxiety about career exploration and negatively correlated with preretirement career planning for elite athletes. Thus, greater athletic identity has been consistently associated with a maladaptive orientation toward the career decision-making process.

Findings regarding the relationship between identification with the athlete role and the tendency to commit to an occupation or ideology without first engaging in exploratory behavior (i.e., identity foreclosure) add support for the claim that individuals high in athletic identity are less likely than individuals low in athletic identity to consider thoughtfully a wide array of career possibilities prior to sport career termination. In particular, athletic identity has been positively correlated with identity foreclosure in three studies of college students and student-athletes (Anderson, 1996; Good et al., 1993; Wurster, 1996) and one study of high school student-athletes (Varisco, Gaa, Swank, & Rudisill, 1998). Longitudinal research is needed to examine more thoroughly the connections between patterns of self-identification and vocational behavior in sport populations.

Effects of Sport Career Transitions on Self-Identity

Consistent with views of the self as relatively enduring and resistant to change (e.g., Markus, 1977), self-identity in sport has been treated as a dispositional, traitlike construct in the previous two sections of the chapter. Because current theory also considers the self as a dynamic, mutable entity that is subject to social and environmental influences (Cantor, Markus, Niedenthal, & Nurius, 1986; Markus & Kunda, 1986), there is merit to examining athletic identity from a situational perspective. Such an approach is especially warranted in the context of sport career transitions given that transitions, particularly those involving loss, can fundamentally alter the way in which people define themselves (Harvey, 1996).

Several recent investigations provide evidence of situational influences on athletic identity. As noted above, Van Raalte and Cook (1991) found that athletic identity was lower before practice than after practice for women college student-athletes. Antshel (1995) documented changes in athletic identity over the course of the competitive season for college swimmers. In two independent samples, Brewer, Selby, Linder, and Petitpas (1999) showed that college student-athletes who were dissatisfied with their performances during the competitive season decreased their identification with the athlete role to a greater extent than did those who were satisfied with their performances during the competitive season.

The malleability of athletic identity has also been demonstrated in the domain of sport career transitions. In a study by Allison and Meyer (1988), elite athletes consistently reported that they experienced identity loss as a consequence of sport career termination. Grandisson and Vezina (1997) found that the athletic identity of retired elite athletes was significantly lower than that of active elite athletes. Grandisson and Vezina's finding suggests that competitors tend to reduce their identification with the athlete role following sport career termination, a process shown to be adaptive by Lavallee, Gordon, and Grove (1997). Finally, Fish, Grove, and Eklund (1997) found that individuals who were not selected for an elite sport squad decreased their athletic identity, whereas individuals who were selected maintained their preselection levels of athletic identity. Together, the results of investigations by Allison and Meyer, Grandisson and Vezina, Lavallee et al. (1997), and Fish et al. provide support for the claim that sport career transitions can affect patterns of self-identification.

Recommendations for Research and Practice

Based on the literature reviewed in this chapter, it is clear that self-identity is relevant to sport career transitions. Further inquiry is needed to gain a more complete understanding of how athletic identity influences adjustment to sport career transitions, how sport career transitions affect athletic identity, and how individual difference variables (e.g., gender, age, race/ethnicity, personality) moderate the relationship between athletic identity and sport career transition processes. In conducting future research, it will be important to attend to methodological considerations, such as including appropriate control groups, implementing longitudinal research designs, and using both general and sport-specific measures (A. J. Petitpas, Brewer, & Van Raalte, 1996).

Given the consistent inverse relationship obtained between athletic identity and adjustment to sport career transitions, one potentially fruitful avenue of intervention is to assist athletes in transition to reduce their exclusive identification with the athlete role and to invest in other sources of identification. Because athletes can perceive themselves as happier and more competent in the sport role than in other roles (Griffin, Chassin, & Young, 1981), athletes may be reluctant to engage in such "expansion of self-identity" (S. M. Murphy, 1995, p. 342). It may be necessary to promote the acquisition of self-efficacy in other domains before athletes are willing to invest in alternative identities. Consequently, it is vital to consider athletic identity as part of a multidimensional self-concept in future research and practice, assessing and directing interventions toward not only athletic identity but other self-concept domains as well. Research by Fischer (1994) and Stambulova (1998) provide examples of this sort of approach. Fischer demonstrated that a time management intervention increased academic identity and decreased athletic identity relative to a control condition in a sample of student athletes. Stambulova documented an inverse relationship between athletic identity and invalid identity among athletes with disabilities. Through further research and the development, implementation, and evaluation of interventions focusing on self-identity, sport career transition specialists may be able to help athletes adjust more effectively to sport career transitions and experience growth that transfers to other domains outside the sport arena (A. J. Petitpas et al., 1996).

References

Allison, M. T., & Meyer, C. (1988). Career problems and retirement among elite athletes: The female tennis professional. *Sociology of Sport Journal, 5,* 212–222.

Anderson, E. (1996). *Identity foreclosed thinking, athletic identity, and the Black collegiate athlete.* Unpublished master's thesis, Springfield College, MA.

Antshel, K. M. (1995). *The effect of time of season on the athletic identity in collegiate swimmers.* Unpublished master's thesis, University of North Carolina, Chapel Hill.

Baillie, P. H. F. (1992). *Career transition in elite and professional athletes: A study of individuals in their preparation for and adjustment to retirement from competitive sports.* Unpublished doctoral dissertation, Virginia Commonwealth University, Richmond.

Baillie, P. H. F., & Danish, S. J. (1992). Understanding the career transition of athletes. *The Sport Psychologist, 6,* 77–98.

Baysden, M. F., Brewer, B. W., Petitpas, A. J., & Van Raalte, J. L. (1997). Motivational correlates of athletic identity [Abstract]. *Journal of Applied Sport Psychology, 9* (Suppl.), S67–S68.

Blinde, E. M., & Greendorfer, S. L. (1985). A reconceptualization of the process of leaving the role of competitive athlete. *International Review for the Sociology of Sport, 20,* 87–93.

Brettschneider, W. D., & Heim, R. (1997). Identity, sport, and youth development. In K. R. Fox (Ed.), *The physical self: From motivation to well-being* (pp. 205–227). Champaign, IL: Human Kinetics.

Brewer, B. W. (1993). Self-identity and specific vulnerability to depressed mood. *Journal of Personality, 61,* 343–364.

Brewer, B. W. (1994). Review and critique of models of psychological adjustment to athletic injury. *Journal of Applied Sport Psychology, 6,* 87–100.

Brewer, B. W., Selby, C. L., Linder, D. E., & Petitpas, A. J. (1999). Distancing oneself from a poor season: Divestment of athletic identity. *Journal of Personal and Interpersonal Loss, 4,* 149–162.

Brewer, B. W., Van Raalte, J. L., & Linder, D. E. (1991, June). *Construct validity of the Athletic Identity Measurement Scale*. Paper presented at the annual meeting of the North American Society for the Psychology of Sport and Physical Activity, Monterey, CA.

Brewer, B. W., Van Raalte, J. L., & Linder, D. E. (1993). Athletic identity: Hercules' muscles or Achilles' heel? *International Journal of Sport Psychology, 24,* 237–254.

Brown, C. (1993). *The relationship between role commitment and career developmental tasks among college student athletes*. Unpublished doctoral dissertation, University of Missouri, Kansas City.

Buntrock, C. L., & Brewer, B. W. (1994, August). *Social and personal aspects of athletic identity*. Paper presented at the annual meeting of the American Psychological Association, Los Angeles, CA.

Cantor, N., Markus, H., Niedenthal, P., & Nurius, P. (1986). On motivation and the self-concept. In R. M. Sorrentino & E. T. Higgins (Eds.), *Handbook of motivation and cognition* (pp. 96–121). New York: Guilford Press.

Chamalidis, P. (1997). Identity conflicts during and after retirement from top-level sports. In R. Lidor & M. Bar-Eli (Eds.), *Proceedings of the IX World Congress of Sport Psychology* (pp. 191–193). Netanya, Israel: International Society of Sport Psychology.

Cooley, C. H. (1902). *Human nature and the social order*. New York: Scribner's.

Coopersmith, S. (1967). *The antecedents of self-esteem*. San Francisco: Freeman.

Crook, J. M., & Robertson, S. E. (1991). Transitions out of elite sport. *International Journal of Sport Psychology, 22,* 115–127.

Curry, T. J. (1993). The effects of receiving a college letter on the sport identity. *Sociology of Sport Journal, 10,* 73–87.

Curry, T. J., & Parr, R. (1988). Comparing commitment to sport and religion at a Christian college. *Sociology of Sport Journal, 5,* 369–377.

Curry, T. J., & Weiss, O. (1989). Sport identity and motivation for sport participation: A comparison between American college athletes and Austrian student sport club members. *Sociology of Sport Journal, 6,* 257–268.

Cutler, R. P., & Meyer, R. G. (1995, August). *Athlete identity salience and adjustment in Division I collegiate athletes*. Paper presented at the annual meeting of the American Psychological Association, New York.

Dance, K. A., & Kuiper, N. A. (1987). Self-schemata, social roles, and a self-worth contingency model of depression. *Motivation and Emotion, 11,* 251–268.

Danish, S. J. (1983). Musing about personal competence: The contributions of sport, health, and fitness. *American Journal of Community Psychology, 11,* 221–240.

Deiters, J. A. (1996). *Social psychological correlates of sport commitment and anticipated retirement difficulty among college athletes*. Unpublished master's thesis, University of Northern Colorado, Greeley.

Deutsch, R. E. (1985). The psychological implications of sports related injuries. *International Journal of Sport Psychology, 16,* 232–237.

Dollinger, S. J. (1994). [Correlations between athletic identity and selected autophotographic, personality, demographic, and life experience variables]. Unpublished raw data.

Eldridge, W. D. (1983). The importance of psychotherapy for athletic related orthopedic injuries among adults. *International Journal of Sport Psychology, 14,* 203–211.

Fischer, K. E. (1994). *The effects of learned time management skills on the academic and sport identities of NCAA Division III women student-volleyball athletes*. Unpublished doctoral dissertation, Ohio State University, Columbus.

Fish, M. B., Grove, J. R., & Eklund, R. C. (1997). *Short-term changes in athletic identity as a function of deselection*. Manuscript submitted for publication.

Fox, K. R. (1997). Introduction: Let's get physical. In K. R. Fox (Ed.), *The physical self: From motivation to well-being* (pp. vii-xiii). Champaign, IL: Human Kinetics.

Fox, K. R. (1998). Advances in the measurement of the physical self. In J. L. Duda (Ed.), *Advances in sport and exercise psychology measurement* (pp. 295–310). Morgantown, WV: Fitness Information Technology.

Fox, K. R., & Corbin, C. B. (1989). The Physical Self-Perception Profile: Development and preliminary validation. *Journal of Sport & Exercise Psychology, 11,* 408–430.

Gergen, K. J. (1971). *The concept of self.* New York: Holt, Rinehart & Winston.

Good, A. J., Brewer, B. W., Petitpas, A. J., Van Raalte, J. L., & Mahar, M. T. (1993). Athletic identity, identity foreclosure, and college sport participation. *Academic Athletic Journal, 8,* 1–12.

Gorbett, F. J. (1985). Psycho-social adjustment of athletes to retirement. In L. Bunker, R. J. Rotella, & A. S. Reilly (Eds.), *Psychological considerations in maximizing sport performance* (pp. 288–294). Ithaca, NY: Mouvement.

Gordon, S. (1995). Career transitions in competitive sport. In T. Morris & J. Summers (Eds.), *Sport psychology: Theory, applications and issues* (pp. 474–501). Brisbane: Jacaranda Wiley.

Grandisson, A., & Vezina, J. (1997). Psychological consequences of retirement on high level amateur athletes [Abstract]. *Journal of Applied Sport Psychology, 9* (Suppl.), S98.

Greendorfer, S. L., & Blinde, E. M. (1985). "Retirement" from intercollegiate sport: Theoretical and empirical considerations. *Sociology of Sport Journal, 2,* 101–110.

Griffin, N., Chassin, L., & Young, R. D. (1981). Measurement of global self-concept versus multiple role-specific self-concepts in adolescents. *Adolescence, 16,* 49–56.

Grove, J. R., Lavallee, D., & Gordon, S. (1997). Coping with retirement from sport: The influence of athletic identity. *Journal of Applied Sport Psychology, 9,* 191–203.

Hale, B. D., Stambulova, N., & James, B. (1996). *Determining the dimensionality of the Athletic Identity Measurement Scale: A "Herculean" cross-cultural undertaking.* Manuscript submitted for publication.

Hale, B. D., & Waalkes, D. (1994). Athletic identity, gender, self esteem, academic importance, and drug use: A further validation of the AIMS [Abstract]. *Journal of Sport & Exercise Psychology, 16* (Suppl.), S62.

Harter, S. (1990). Causes, correlates and the functional role of global self-worth: A life-span perspective. In R. J. Sternberg & J. Kolligian (Eds.), *Competence considered* (pp. 67–97). New Haven, CT: Yale University Press.

Harvey, J. H. (1996). *Embracing their memory: Loss and the social psychology of storytelling.* Needham Heights, MA: Allyn & Bacon.

Heyman, S. R. (1986). Psychological problem patterns found with athletes. *The Clinical Psychologist, 39,* 68–71.

Hinitz, D. R. (1988). *Role theory and the retirement of collegiate gymnasts.* Unpublished doctoral dissertation, University of Nevada, Reno.

Hoare, C. H. (1991). Psychosocial identity development and cultural others. *Journal of Counseling and Development, 70,* 45–53.

James, W. (1892). *Psychology: The briefer course.* New York: Holt, Rinehart & Winston.

Kleiber, D. A., & Brock, S. C. (1992). The effect of career-ending injuries on the subsequent well-being of elite college athletes. *Sociology of Sport Journal, 9,* 70–75.

Klinger, E. (1977). *Meaning and void.* Minneapolis: University of Minnesota Press.

Krauss, I. K., Dittman, S. M., & Camas, T. C. (1998, August). *Changing athletic participation patterns following successful high school competition.* Paper presented at the annual meeting of the American Psychological Association, San Francisco.

Lavallee, D., Gordon, S., & Grove, J. R. (1997). Retirement from sport and the loss of athletic identity. *Journal of Personal and Interpersonal Loss, 2,* 129–147.

Lavallee, D., Grove, J. R., Gordon, S., & Ford, I. W. (1998). The experience of loss in sport. In J. H. Harvey (Ed.), *Perspectives on loss: A sourcebook* (pp. 241–252). Philadelphia: Brunner/Mazel.

Lazarus, R. S., & Folkman, S. (1984). *Stress, appraisal, and coping.* New York: Springer.

Linville, P. W. (1985). Self-complexity and affective extremity: Don't put all of your eggs in one cognitive basket. *Social Cognition, 3,* 94–120.

Linville, P. W. (1987). Self-complexity as a cognitive buffer against stress-related illness and depression. *Journal of Personality and Social Psychology, 52,* 663–676.

Little, J. C. (1969). The athlete's neurosis—a deprivation crisis. *Acta Psychiatrica Scandinavica, 45,* 187–197.

Marcia, J. E. (1966). Development and validation of ego-identity status. *Journal of Personality and Social Psychology, 3,* 551–558.

Markus, H. (1977). Self-schemata and processing information about the self. *Journal of Personality and Social Psychology, 35,* 63–78.

Markus, H., & Kunda, Z. (1986). Stability and malleability of the self-concept. *Journal of Personality and Social Psychology, 51,* 858–866.

Markus, H., & Wurf, E. (1987). The dynamic self-concept: A social psychological perspective. *Annual Review of Psychology, 38,* 299–337.

Marsh, H. W., & Shavelson, R. (1985). Self-concept: Its multifaceted hierarchical structure. *Educational Psychologist, 20,* 107–123.

Matheson, H., Brewer, B. W., Van Raalte, J. L., Andersen, B. (1995). Athletic identity of national level badminton players: A cross-cultural analysis. In T. Reilly, M. Hughes, & A. Lees (Eds.), *Science and racket sports* (pp. 228–231). London: E & FN Spon.

McPherson, B. D. (1980). Retirement from professional sport: The process and problems of occupational and psychological adjustment. *Sociological Symposium, 30,* 126–143.

McPherson, B. D. (1984). Sport participation across the life cycle: A review of the literature and suggestions for future research. *Sociology of Sport Journal, 1,* 213–230.

Mehlhorn, C. A. (1996). *The relationship between intercollegiate student-athletes' sport identity and their drinking behavior.* Unpublished master's thesis, Springfield College, MA.

Murphy, G. M., Petitpas, A. J., & Brewer, B. W. (1996). Identity foreclosure, athletic identity, and career maturity in intercollegiate athletes. *The Sport Psychologist, 10,* 239–246.

Murphy, S. M. (1995). Transitions in competitive sport: Maximizing individual potential. In S. M. Murphy (Ed.), *Sport psychology interventions* (pp. 331–346). Champaign, IL: Human Kinetics

Neyer, M. (1996). Identity development and career maturity patterns of elite resident athletes at the United States Olympic Training Center. *Dissertation Abstracts International, 56, No. 11,* 4328-A.

Oatley, K., & Bolton, W. (1985). A social-cognitive theory of depression in reaction to life events. *Psychological Review, 92,* 372–388.

Ogilvie, B. C. (1989, April). *Traumatic effects of sports career termination.* Paper presented at the Western Psychological Association/Rocky Mountain Psychological Association Joint Annual Convention, Reno, NV.

Ogilvie, B. C., & Howe, M. (1986). The trauma of termination from athletics. In J. M. Williams (Ed.), *Applied sport psychology* (pp. 365–382). Palo Alto, CA: Mayfield.

Orlick, T. (1980). *In pursuit of excellence.* Champaign, IL: Human Kinetics.

Owens, S. S. (1994, October). *The relationship between student-athlete identity and career exploration.* Paper presented at the annual conference of the Association for the Advancement of Applied Sport Psychology, Lake Tahoe, NV.

Pearson, R. E., & Petitpas, A. (1990). Transitions of athletes: Developmental and preventive perspectives. *Journal of Counseling and Development, 69,* 7–10.

Petitpas, A., & Danish, S. J. (1995). Psychological care for injured athletes. In S. M. Murphy (Ed.), *Sport psychology interventions* (pp. 255–281). Champaign, IL: Human Kinetics.

Petitpas, A. J. (1978). Identity foreclosure: A unique challenge. *Personnel and Guidance Journal, 56,* 558–561.

Petitpas, A. J., Brewer, B. W., & Van Raalte, J. L. (1996). Transitions of the student-athlete: Theoretical, empirical, and practical perspectives. In E. F. Etzel, A. P. Ferrante, & J. W. Pinkney (Eds.),

Counseling college student-athletes: Issues and interventions (2nd ed., pp. 137–156). Morgantown, WV: Fitness Information Technology.

Piers, E. (1969). *Manual for the Piers-Harris Children's Self-Concept Scale.* Nashville, TN: Counselor Recordings and Tests.

Pyszczynski, T., & Greenberg, J. (1987). Self-regulatory preservation and the depressive self-focusing style: A self-awareness theory of reactive depression. *Psychological Bulletin, 102,* 122–138.

Rosenberg, M. (1979). *Conceiving the self.* New York: Basic Books.

Schafer, W. E. (1969). Some social sources and consequences of interscholastic athletics: The case of participation and delinquency. In G. S. Kenyon (Ed.), *Aspects of contemporary sport sociology* (pp. 29–44). Chicago: The Athletic Institute.

Schlossberg, N. K. (1981). A model for analyzing human adaptation to transition. *The Counseling Psychologist, 9,* 2–18.

Schmid, J., & Schilling, G. (1997). Identity conflicts during and after retirement from top-level sports. In R. Lidor & M. Bar-Eli (Eds.), *Proceedings of the IX World Congress of Sport Psychology* (pp. 608–610). Netanya, Israel: International Society of Sport Psychology.

Schroeder, P. J., & Lantz, C. D. (1996). Examination of athletic identity and gender-role orientation in university varsity student-athletes and non-athlete students [Abstract]. *Journal of Applied Sport Psychology, 8* (Suppl.), S169.

Sinclair, D. A., & Orlick, T. (1993). Positive transitions from high-performance sport. *The Sport Psychologist, 7,* 138–150.

Stambulova, N. (1998, August). Sports career transitions of Russian athletes: Summary of studies (1991–1997). In D. Alfermann (Chair), *Career transitions in sport: Determinants and consequences.* Paper presented at the 24th International Congress of Applied Psychology, San Francisco, CA.

Swain, D. A. (1991). Withdrawal from sport and Schlossberg's model of transitions. *Sociology of Sport Journal, 8,* 152–160.

Taylor, J., & Ogilvie, B. C. (1994). A conceptual model of adaptation to retirement among athletes. *Journal of Applied Sport Psychology, 6,* 1–20.

Tubilleja, K. (1998). *Psychosocial development and athletic identity among student-athletes in NCAA Division I revenue producing sports.* Unpublished master's thesis, Springfield College, MA.

Van Raalte, N. S., & Cook, R. G. (1991, June). *Gender specific situational influences on athletic identity.* Paper presented at the annual meeting of the North American Society for the Psychology of Sport and Physical Activity, Monterey, CA.

Varisco, A. J., Gaa, J. P., Swank, P. R., & Rudisill, M. (1998, August). *Athletic identity and identity foreclosure as predictors of academic motivation.* Paper presented at the annual meeting of the American Psychological Association, San Francisco, CA.

Webster's new collegiate dictionary. (1981). Springfield, MA: Merriam.

Weiss, M. R. (1987). Self-esteem and achievement in children's sport and physical activity. In D. Gould & M. R. Weiss (Eds.), *Advances in pediatric sport sciences* (Vol. 2, pp. 87–119). Champaign, IL: Human Kinetics.

Werthner, P., & Orlick, T. (1986). Retirement experiences of successful Olympic athletes. *International Journal of Sport Psychology, 17,* 337–363.

Wiechman, S. A., & Williams, J. M. (1997). Relation of athletic identity to injury and mood disturbance. *Journal of Sport Behavior, 20,* 199–210.

Wiese-Bjornstal, D. M., Smith, A. M., Shaffer, S. M., & Morrey, M. A. (1998). An integrated model of response to sport injury: Psychological and sociological dimensions. *Journal of Applied Sport Psychology, 10,* 46–69.

Wurster, K. (1996). *Identity foreclosure, athletic identity, goal directedness, and psychological differentiation in collegiate athletes.* Unpublished master's thesis, Springfield College, MA.

3

Causes and Consequences of Sport Career Termination

Dorothee Alfermann
University of Leipzig
Germany

Abstract

When considering transitions during a sport career there is no doubt that career termination and the transition to a postcareer has received the most attention in sport psychology research and practice. In this chapter the process of career termination is investigated: how it comes to the decision, which causes lead to career termination, and what is known about the adjustment to the life after elite sports. Special emphasis is given to the distinction between voluntary and involuntary drawback from sports, as it has consequences on the adjustment process. Results from the literature, as well as data of research conducted by the author, are presented.

Causes and Consequences of Sport Career Termination

Athletes' career development is a fascinating field of psychological research, intervention, and counseling. To work with athletes means not only supporting them in growth and development, but also preparing them for career termination. All athletes are supposed to leave the field of elite sports one day and to find a new way of living. Career termination is thus an event that will happen sooner or later in every athlete's life. From the standpoint of sport psychology, intriguing questions are when and why athletes withdraw and how they adjust to their postcareer life.

Most of the explanatory models of career transitions are concerned with the stage of career termination and the beginning of a postcareer. From the standpoint of a transition model, career termination can be seen as a critical life event that has to be coped with. The result should be either successful adjustment or a crisis calling for professional advice. A somewhat similar approach is presented by S. S. Greendorfer (1992) emphasizing socialization perspectives. She argues that "factors influencing involvement could also be related to those influencing withdrawal" (p. 212). This would mean that transitions at any phase in an individual's sport career are influenced by the same factors.

Studies done so far about the process of career transitions have mainly concentrated on the *reasons for* and the *adjustment to* career termination, which very often results in a higher engagement in other domains, mainly job (including sport-specific jobs) and social relationships, including family. The reasons for career termination are manifold (Boothby, Tungatt & Townsend, 1981; Bussmann & Alfermann, 1994; Koukouris, 1991; Ogilvie & Taylor, 1993b), and they seem to play a crucial role in adjustment to postcareer life. This is especially true for the subjective feeling of freedom of choice (Coakley, 1983; Taylor & Ogilvie, 1994; Webb, Nasco, Riley & Headrick, 1998). Data so far show quite clearly that an involuntary drawback may have complicating or even devastating consequences for the adjustment process shortly after career termination (e.g., Blinde & Stratta, 1992; Wheeler, Malone, Van-Vlack, Nelson & Steadward, 1996). This can be especially true if retirement is regarded as an "offtime" life event due to externally determined causes (Pearson & Petitpas, 1990). A subjective feeling of control thus seems to facilitate the transition to postcareer life. Later on, data will be presented from the literature and from our own research showing how deeply this subjective feeling of control vs. helplessness can influence the transition responses of the athlete. In addition it also contributes to differences in the quality of the reasons for career termination.

When speaking of causes and consequences of career termination, it is important to note the distinction between offtime and ontime life events that is discussed by Pearson and Petitpas (1990) with regard to career transitions. Offtime life events are those that occur "at a developmentally atypical point" in life and are supposed to cause more stress than ontime events (Pearson & Petitpas, p. 8). This seems to be a plausible distinction that would correspond to the difference between dropout (i.e., a premature career termination before the athlete has reached full potential) and retirement (i.e., an ontime event after a long-term career). Though there should be a high overlap, nevertheless, what is ontime or offtime depends on the athlete's subjective definition and experience. From the athlete's viewpoint, any career termination might come offtime. When the literature is scanned, the term *retirement* is usually reserved for career termination of adults (presumably ontime). The term *dropout* is preferred for attrition or withdrawal of young athletes from sports or a sport group. Whereas the latter is discussed by Wylleman, De Knop, and Ewing in chapter 9 in this volume, this chapter will concentrate on career termination in elite sports be it voluntarily or not. Therefore, the more neutral term of *career termination*, be it ontime or offtime, voluntary or not, is preferred in this chapter.

Besides this, the interindividual differences at the amateur and the professional level need to be examined. Though it is to be expected that the professional athlete might face more difficulties with transition out of sport, it is not easy to test this hypothesis due to the scarcity of the literature about professionals. In addition, gender as a variable that might contribute to differences in the transition process, but has been rather neglected so far, will be examined. In fact it is evident that more studies about career termination (in youth and adulthood) are directed to and concerned with male athletes. As female subjects are underrepresented in the sport psychology and sport sociology research literature in general (Birrell, 1984; Wann & Hamlet, 1995), so is the case in career transition research. Samples with males only (e.g., Curtis & Ennis, 1988; Koukouris, 1991, 1994; Lerch, 1981; Perna, Zaichkowsky, & Bockner, 1996; Reynolds, 1981; Robinson & Carron, 1982; Sands, 1978) outnumber the studies with females only (e.g., Allison & Meyer, 1988; Brown, 1985; Brown, Frankel, & Fennell, 1989; Bussmann & Alfermann, 1994). Those studies that do make comparisons between male and female athletes actually find some differences in reasons for career termination and in postcareer development (Alfermann, 1995; Hastings, Kurth & Meyer, 1989), as well as similarities (S. L. Greendorfer & Blinde, 1985).

Causes of Career Termination

In their overview of career termination research, Ogilvie and Taylor (1993a, 1993b; Taylor & Ogilvie, 1994) emphasize four main causes of career termination, and these are age, deselection, injury, and free choice. The first three of these causes mean that the athletes were unable to continue competition due to performance decrements. Thus, they seemed to have had no choice in withdrawal or not, but were forced to do so. They had to leave due to circumstances that were out of their control. In addition, Ogilvie and Taylor mention free choice as a fourth category of causes. Webb et al. (1998) even reduce the number and dichotomize the causes of career termination "into two categories— retirements that are freely chosen and those that are forced by circumstances" out of the athletes' control, like decreasing performance or injuries (p. 341). The subjective feeling of control over events has been a crucial part of social psychological theories of health and illness. In fact subjective controllability not only fosters mental health and a successful development (Seligman, 1991), but it is also strongly correlates to heightened feelings of self-efficacy, which play a key role in behavior change and adjustment (Bandura, 1997). So it can be postulated that free choice retirement will influence adjustment to it. Nevertheless the dichotomy of causes as suggested by Webb et al. needs further clarification. First, within the category of no choice, there are differences. The decision to retire due to performance loss may be qualitatively different from retirement due to an injury. An athlete in the former situation might have reached the top during his or her career, whereas an athlete in the latter situation may not have. Data suggest that injury-related retirement causes more adjustment problems than do other retirement reasons (Webb et al. 1998). Second, the two categories seem to be not exhaustive. As will be shown later, researchers have shown that there are more reasons for retirement. Lastly, what should count the most is the subjective feeling of freedom of choice of an athlete, and this is often not assessed. When studying the causes of retirement, the distinction between choice and no choice may be not sufficient, though, but could prove useful as a starting point when studying interindividual differences in the transition process of athletes.

Professional and Nonprofessional Athletes

Studies with professional athletes are rare, and those that exist unfortunately do not always ask for causes of career termination or do not report them. Those studies that give information show that male professionals seem to retire due to causes that can be classified as external, namely injuries (Reynolds, 1981; Rosenberg, 1981) or lack of contract (Reynolds, 1981). Though it might seem plausible that professional athletes only quit their job when forced to do so, qualitative studies done with small samples show that only a minority retire from sport involuntarily. Allison and Meyer (1988) point to 35% out of a sample of 20 female tennis players, and Swain (1991), in a sample of 10 former professionals, found voluntary retirees only. Both studies cite a variety of reasons for leaving the sport career including negative experiences on tour (Allison & Meyer), as well as positive alternatives the athletes want to realize, mainly family relationships and job opportunities (Swain). In addition, it is pointed out that retirement typically is a process, and not a single event. Athletes are constantly reminded throughout their career that it is short term and not lifelong. Thus, not a single event but a multitude of events may be responsible for career termination (Swain).

This process-oriented analysis of reasons for career termination applies even more to nonprofessional sports. In correspondence with transition theory, the process of retirement (instead of a single event) is typically emphasized (Sinclair & Orlick, 1994). The main reason for retirement in amateur, intercollegiate and junior elite sports is the necessity to pursue a postcareer. Thus, obtaining educational or vocational training and finding a job for earning a living are the top reasons for these athletes to terminate their sport career (cf. Bussmann & Alfermann, 1994; S. L. Greendorfer & Blinde, 1985; Hastings et al., 1989; Sack, 1980). As this is in fact an important contributor to life satisfaction after sports, several authors suggest a dual-role model during the sports career (i.e., sport and education) in order for the athlete to be better prepared for life after sport (Crook & Robertson, 1991; Emrich, Altmeyer, & Papathanassiou, 1994; Ogilvie, 1987).

Whereas family and job obligations are typical reasons for a free-choice retirement, there are forced-choice retirements that are mainly attributable to external or internal constraints. Among these, injuries and increasing age are mentioned most often (cf. Bussmann & Alfermann, 1994; Ogilvie & Taylor, 1993b), followed by a lack of financial support (Koukouris 1991, 1994; Werthner & Orlick, 1986). Typical psychological factors that may also contribute to career termination are a lack of social support, both of coach and of family members (e.g., Brown, 1985; Singer, 1992), the feeling that time is ripe for a change, and a loss of motivation (cf. Burton, 1992; Bussmann & Alfermann; Hastings et al., 1989; Sands, 1978; Sinclair & Orlick, 1994). But again it should be highlighted that career termination rarely is a single cause decision. Instead it is the result of a variety of factors inside and outside the sport domain, which have to combine in order to lead to the termination of a sports career (Alfermann, 1995; Brown, 1985; Lindner, Johns, & Butcher, 1991). In addition this is only the final point of a long-term process whereby the risks and disadvantages of high performance sport gain more and more significance while at the same time the need for educational and vocational training becomes apparent (Singer, 1992). In the end, leaving sport is often accompanied by increased efforts to get an education and to enter the job market.

Do Male and Female Athletes Quit the Sport Arena for Different Reasons?

Though gender-role socialization has been becoming increasingly similar with regard to boys' and girls' sport participation, there still exist differences in gender-role expectations toward males and females in society. The core of these expectations can be summarized in the way that males are expected to be strong and powerful and earn the family income whereas females are expected to be nurturing and sensitive and care for the family's emotional support and household duties (cf. Eagly, 1987). As elite sport may contradict these expectations in the case of women (Harris, 1987), it would be plausible to assume that women are more apt to leave the scene prematurely, at an earlier age and for different reasons than males do. The evidence in this area is scarce at best. What seems to happen is that women who enter the elite sport level are well prepared and experience no role strain (for a critical discussion of the literature see Birrell, 1988). These athletes might be a selective sample of women with a higher amount of instrumental, masculine traits than noncareer women of comparable age possess. As masculine traits are more functional for a successful career than feminine traits are, the demands of the athletic role foster competence motivation, competitive attitudes, and masculine traits. Only those women who have such masculine traits succeed and survive in sport (Gill, 1994; Harris, 1987; Jackson & Marsh, 1986). Therefore, the psychological differences between female and male athletes are expected to be small when it comes to reasons for career termination. Differences that are found can be explained by different gender-role expectations and differences in biological age. Typically female athletes not only enter the scene at a younger age than that of the males, but they also leave it at a younger age (cf. Alfermann, 1995; Hastings et al., 1989), more often mention family obligations as reason for retirement (Hastings et al.; Sack, 1980), less often expect financial or job incentives from their sport career (Alfermann; S. L. Greendorfer & Blinde, 1985; Holz & Friedrich, 1988), and less often have a job in the labor market or find a job in the sport system as a coach, manager, etc. after retirement than their male counterparts do (Alfermann; Hastings et al.). Thus, the typical differences in gender-role expectations toward the adult woman and man are reflected in elite athletes when it comes to postcareer decisions.

Adjustment to Retirement

In correspondence with the shift in theoretical models of retirement, a shift in emphasis on and data about retirement as a "normal" kind of transition phase can be observed. Whereas in earlier studies the main impetus of research and practice was the hypothesis of adjustment difficulties and how to cure them (Ogilvie & Howe, 1986), the last two decades have seen a growing number of studies trying to show retirement as a life event that can lead to growth and development. Two kinds of research studies may be differentiated. First are descriptive studies looking for the athletes' further life development, mainly in terms of occupational success and life satisfaction (Alfermann, 1995; Curtis & Ennis, 1988; S. L. Greendorfer & Blinde; 1985; Hastings et al., 1989; Koukouris, 1991; Lerch, 1981; Perna et al., 1996; Reynolds, 1981; Sands, 1978;

Snyder & Baber, 1979). These studies typically show that former athletes are not less successful in life than nonathletes or than representative samples are (Curtis & Ennis; Snyder & Baber) and that females can be found less often than males and are less successful in the labor market than males are (Alfermann; Hastings et al.). When measures of satisfaction are considered, satisfaction is generally reported as quite high (S. L. Greendorfer & Blinde; Lerch; Reynolds), and only a minority of the athletes are described as reporting transition problems (Alfermann; S. L. Greendorfer & Blinde; Koukouris; Sands).

A second kind of research is dedicated to the psychological processes associated with retirement. It is more concerned with the quality of the transition process as seen by the athletes, with coping efforts and with possible adjustment difficulties (Allison & Meyer, 1988; Bussmann, 1995; Grove, Lavallee & Gordon, 1997; Parker, 1994; Sinclair & Orlick, 1994; Swain, 1991; Webb et al., 1998; Werthner & Orlick, 1986). These studies allow a more in-depth analysis of athletes' transitional processes. Interestingly, these studies show a less brilliant picture of this process than do the descriptive studies. Instead, authors emphasize that retirement may be a critical life event (e.g., Ogilvie, 1987; Sinclair & Orlick). Like any critical life event, retirement has to be coped with, and this may take time. Though most athletes adjust quite well to their situation, nevertheless, most of them have to cope intensely with the new situation that has been regarded as moderately stressful (Sinclair & Orlick) and as a "complex interaction of stressors" (Ogilvie & Taylor, 1993b, p. 769). In a symposium on career transitions, it became obvious in several contributions that there seems to be a minority of athletes (up to 15%) facing serious difficulties after career termination (Wylleman, 1995). In one survey study with former athletes in Germany, nearly 13% of the sample was found to report feelings of depression, helplessness and other symptoms of psychological disturbances (Alfermann, 1995), but on the other hand, there were also athletes reporting relief and enthusiasm for their new life outside the sport arena. Why do athletes differ so tremendously in their adaptation to career termination?

The adjustment process appears to be determined by several psychological, social, and structural factors, the most important of which may be summarized as follows (Ogilvie & Taylor, 1993b). Athletes tend to adjust better to a post-career life if they

- retire voluntarily—that means by their own choice (Webb et al., 1998; Wheeler et al., 1996)—instead of being forced to retire (e.g., due to injuries or loss of contract).
- are prepared for a life after sport and have made plans for the future (Crook & Robertson, 1991; Ogilvie, 1987; Pearson & Petitpas, 1990; Werthner & Orlick, 1986).

- have a multiply defined identity, that is, an identity that is not exclusively defined by their success in sport, but also by social relationships, experiences, and successes outside the sport domain (Baillie & Danish, 1992; Brewer, Van Raalte, & Petitpas, this volume; Brown, 1985; Grove et al., 1997; Sands, 1978; Webb et al., 1998).

- feel comfortable with the social support/encouragement and the social relationships they are involved in (Brown, 1985; Brown et al., 1989; Bussmann & Alfermann, 1994; Robinson & Carron, 1982; Sinclair & Orlick, 1994).

One consequence of these results has been a growing number of sport psychologists and other practitioners pleading for professional advice and mental preparation of athletes for their postcareer (e.g., Baillie, 1993; Danish, Petitpas, & Hale, 1993; Ogilvie, 1987; Taylor & Ogilvie, 1994; Thomas & Ermler, 1988).

Voluntary or Involuntary Retirement: What Difference Does It Make?

As several authors emphasize the distinction between voluntary and involuntary retirement and its consequences, a field study about this topic by Alfermann and Gross (1998) is described in more detail. The aim of this study was to investigate differences in the adjustment process of elite athletes after retirement. It was expected that voluntarily retired athletes would report more positive memories and emotions with regard to career termination and a more active and optimistic coping style than would athletes who retired involuntarily. In 1996, questionnaires were sent by mail to 132 former athletes of national or international top level (43 women and 89 men) in Germany. Thirty-four women and 56 men, belonging to 20 disciplines in amateur sports, returned the questionnaires. The return rate was 68%, and the sex ratio is quite representative for elite sports. The educational level of our sample was high and higher than can be found in the normal population (which is a typical phenomenon in amateur sports in Germany). The mean age of our sample was 26 years (27 for men and 24.6 for women). The men had begun their career at a mean age of 11 and had terminated their career at the age of 24 (women: from 10 to 21 yrs.). Thus, the mean duration of the careers of our participants was 13 and 11 years, respectively. Of the 90 athletes, 51 retired by free choice, and 35 quit sports involuntarily. The remaining 4 athletes could not be classified appropriately. Both groups of athletes did not differ in career duration and successes. Our dependent measures consisted of a standardized inventory assessing 19 coping strategies (Janke, Erdmann, & Kallus, 1985) and several rating scales, as well as open-ended questions about the feelings and coping behaviors after career termination.

First, the athletes were asked to describe the reasons for retirement. As expected, athletes who retired involuntarily more often mentioned performance loss and health problems including injuries, and less often job and school obligations than did the voluntarily retiring athletes (Figure 1). When asked to describe their most characteristic emotional state after career termination, characteristic differences emerged. The answers were content analyzed and could be sorted into seven different categories. Four of them revealed significant differences (Figure 2). Athletes who retired by free choice ("volunteers") reported more often positive and less often negative reactions than did the forced-choice retirees ("nonvolunt"). No differences could be found for "sadness," "uncertainty," and "satisfaction." Comparable results were found when the answers to a 10-item scale measuring positive vs. negative feelings after career termination (e.g., eagerness, feeling free, optimism vs. sadness, lack of self-confidence, anxiety) were summarized. The volunteers reported more positive and less negative feelings (Figure 3).

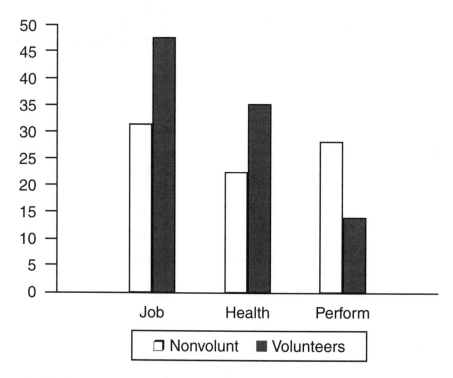

Figure 1. Reasons for career termination among voluntarily ("volunteers") and involuntarily ("nonvolunt") retired athletes (in percent of the two groups).

Note. Values represent mean percentages of dropouts and retired athletes respectively. Participants were asked to indicate on 19 forced-choice items how they coped with their career termination.

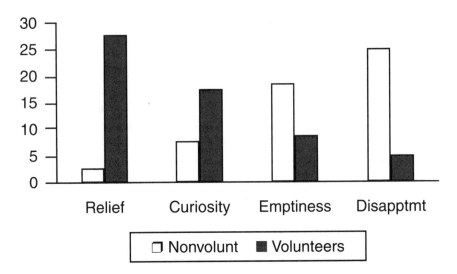

Figure 2. Mean differences in emotional reactions to career termination among voluntarily ("volunteers") and involuntarily ("nonvolunt") retired athletes (in percent of the two groups).

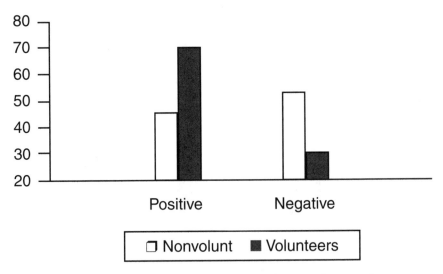

Figure 3. Overall differences in positive and negative emotional reactions to career termination among voluntarily ("volunteers") and involuntarily ("nonvolunt") retired athletes (in percent of the two groups).

Did both groups of athletes also differ in their coping strategies? The most noticeable difference existed in the quantity of strategies; forced retirees reported having used significantly more strategies than volunteers used. Individuals who are in a negative psychological condition are more in need of coping than are those who feel at ease, but there were also differences in the quality of coping. Forced retirees more often reported defense mechanisms and passive strategies (e.g., reevaluation, distraction, playing down), and they were more inclined to seek social support (Figure 4). Voluntarily retired athletes preferred active strategies showing that they were willing to begin a new life with new activities (e.g., job involvement and leisure activities).

In summarizing the results of the study by Alfermann and Gross (1998), the following conclusions can be drawn:

• Athletes who terminated their career voluntarily and who had made a conscious decision more often reported positive emotions and a more active coping process and lifestyle after career termination than did non-volunteers.

• Athletes who had terminated their career involuntarily reported more negative feelings, a higher number of coping strategies and more passive strategies as well as a higher need for social support than did voluntarily retired athletes.

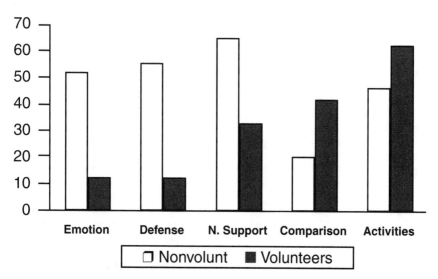

Figure 4. Differences in coping strategies among voluntarily ("volunteers") and involuntarily ("nonvolunt") retired athletes (in percent of the two groups)

Conclusion

The results of this and other studies suggest that the adjustment process of athletes to a life after career termination partly depends on the perceived amount of freedom of choice with regard to retirement. Attribution of control thus seems to improve coping with the transition to a postcareer, a result that is corroborated by other data (cf. Taylor & Ogilvie, 1994; Wheeler et al., 1996).

What about gender differences in coping strategies and adjustment to postcareer? Apart from differences in occupational success, no gender differences could be found in the existing literature or in studies done in our laboratory. Nevertheless, it should be reemphasized that this question needs further clarification, due to sample restrictions.

In summarizing the existing literature, it can be concluded that career termination is a critical life event for athletes that initiates a process of adaptation. Though the reasons for retirement often are manifold, it seems safe to conclude that voluntary retirement leads to a smoother adjustment to the new situation. Most athletes cope successfully with retirement, but a minority show emotional and behavioral problems that sometimes require professional counseling and advice.

References

Alfermann, D. (1995). Career transitions of elite athletes: Drop-out and retirement. In R. Vanfraechem-Raway & Y. Vanden Auweele (Eds.), *Proceedings of the 9th European Congress on Sport Psychology* (pp. 828–833). Brussels: European Federation of Sports Psychology.

Alfermann, D., & Gross, A. (1997). Coping with career termination: It all depends on freedom of choice. In R. Lidor & M. Bar-Eli (Eds.), *Proceedings of the IX World Congress on Sport Psychology* (pp. 65–67). Netanya, Israel: International Society of Sport Psychology.

Alfermann, D., & Gross, A. (1998). Erleben und bewaeltigen des karriereendes im hochleistungssport [How elite athletes perceive and cope with career termination]. *Leistungssport, 28 (2)*, 45–48.

Allison, M. T., & Meyer, C. (1988). Career problems and retirement among elite athletes: The female tennis professional. *Sociology of Sport Journal, 5*, 212–222.

Baillie, P. H. F. (1993). Understanding retirement from sports: Therapeutic ideas for helping athletes in transition. *The Counseling Psychologist, 21*, 399–410.

Baillie, P. H. F., & Danish, S. J. (1992). Understanding the career transition of athletes. *The Sport Psychologist, 6*, 77–98.

Bandura, A. (1997). *Self-efficacy: The exercise of control*. New York: Freeman.

Birrell, S. (1984). Studying gender in sport: A feminist perspective. In N. Theberge & P. Donnelly (Eds.), *Sport and the sociological imagination* (pp. 125–135). Fort Worth: Texas Christian University Press.

Birrell, S. (1988). Discourses on the gender/sport relationship: From women in sport to gender relations. *Exercise and Sport Science Reviews, 16*, 459–502.

Blinde, E. M., & Stratta, T. M. (1992). The "sport career death" of college athletes. *Journal of Sport Behavior, 15*, 3–20.

Boothby, J., Tungatt, M. F., & Townsend, A. R. (1981). Ceasing participation in sports activity: Reported reasons and their implications. *Journal of Leisure Research, 13*, 1–14.

Brown, B. A. (1985). Factors influencing the process of withdrawal by female adolescents from the role of competitive age group swimmer. *Sociology of Sport Journal, 2*, 111–129.

Brown, B. A., Frankel, B. G., & Fennell, M. P. (1989). Hugs or shrugs: Parental and peer influence on continuity of involvement in sport by female adolescents. *Sex Roles, 20,* 397–412.

Burton, D. (1992). Why young wrestlers "hang up" their singlet: An exploratory investigation comparing two models of sport attrition. *Journal of Sport Behavior, 15,* 209–226.

Bussmann, G. (1995). *Dropout in der frauenleichtathletik* [Drop-out in women's track-and-field athletics]. Koeln: Sport und Buch Strauss.

Bussmann, G. & Alfermann, D. (1994). Drop-out and the female athlete: A study with track-and-field athletes. In D. Hackfort (Ed.), *Psycho-social issues and interventions in elite sport* (pp. 89–128). Frankfurt: Lang.

Coakley, J. J. (1983). Leaving competitive sport: Retirement or rebirth? *Quest, 35,* 1–11.

Crook, J. M., & Robertson, S. E. (1991). Transitions out of elite sport. *International Journal of Sport Psychology, 22,* 115–127.

Curtis, J., & Ennis, R. (1988). Negative consequences of leaving competitive sport? Comparative findings for former elite-level hockey players. *Sociology of Sport Journal, 5,* 87–106.

Danish, S. J., Petitpas, A. J., & Hale, B. D. (1993). Life development intervention for athletes: Life skills through sports. *The Counseling Psychologist, 21,* 352–385.

Eagly, A. H. (1987). *Sex differences in social behavior: A social-role interpretation.* Hillsdale, NJ: Lawrence Erlbaum.

Emrich, E., Altmeyer, L., & Papathanassiou, V. (1994). Career counseling in an Olympic Center—A German experience. In D. Hackfort (Ed.). *Psycho-social issues and interventions in elite sport* (pp. 199–235). Frankfurt: Lang.

Gill, D. (1994). Psychological perspectives on women in sport and exercise. In D. M. Costa & S. R. Guthrie (Eds.), *Women and sport: Interdisciplinary perspectives* (pp. 253–284). Champaign, IL: Human Kinetics.

Greendorfer, S. (1992). Sport socialization. In T. S. Horn (Ed.), *Advances in sport psychology* (pp. 201–218). Champaign, IL: Human Kinetics.

Greendorfer, S. L., & Blinde, E. M. (1985). "Retirement" from intercollegiate sport: Theoretical and empirical considerations. *Sociology of Sport Journal, 2,* 101–110.

Grove, J. R., Lavallee, D., & Gordon, S. (1997). Coping with retirement from sport: The influence of athletic identity. *Journal of Applied Sport Psychology, 9,* 191–203.

Harris, D. (1987). The female athlete. In J. R. May & M. J. Asken (Eds.), *Sport psychology: The psychological health of the athlete* (pp. 99–116). New York: PMA.

Hastings, D. W., Kurth, S. B., & Meyer, J. (1989). Competitive swimming careers through the life course. *Sociology of Sport Journal, 6,* 278–284.

Holz, P., & Friedrich, E. (Eds.) (1988). *Spitzensportlerinnen und Spitzensportler der Bundesrepublik Deutschland 1986/87* [Elite athletes of the Federal Republic of Germany 1986/87]. Frankfurt: Stiftung Deutsche Sporthilfe.

Jackson, S. A., & Marsh, H. W. (1986). Athletic or antisocial? The female sport experience. *Journal of Sport Psychology, 8,* 198–211.

Janke, W., Erdmann, G., & Kallus, K.W. (1985). *Stressverarbeitungsfragebogen* [Inventory of Coping Strategies]. Göttingen: Hogrefe.

Koukouris, K. (1991). Quantitative aspects of the disengagement process of advanced and elite Greek male athletes from organized competitive sport. *Journal of Sport Behavior, 14,* 227–246.

Koukouris, K. (1994). Constructed case studies: Athletes' perspectives of disengaging from organized competitive sport. *Sociology of Sport Journal, 11,* 114–139.

Lerch, S. H. (1981). The adjustment to retirement of professional baseball players. In S. L. Greendorfer & A. Yiannakis (Eds.), *Sociology of sport: Diverse perspectives* (pp. 138–148). West Point, NY: Leisure Press.

Lindner, K. J., Johns, D. P., & Butcher, J. (1991). Factors in withdrawal from youth sport: A proposed model. *Journal of Sport Behavior, 14,* 3–18.

Ogilvie, B. (1987). Counseling for sports career termination. In J. R. May & M. J. Asken (Eds.), *Sport psychology: The psychological health of the athlete* (pp. 213–230). New York: PMA.

Ogilvie, B. C., & Howe, M. (1986). The trauma of termination from athletics. In J. M. Williams (Ed.), *Applied sport psychology* (pp. 365–382). Palo Alto, CA: Mayfield.

Ogilvie, B., & Taylor, J. (1993a). Career termination in sports: When the dream dies. In J. M. Williams (Ed.), *Applied sport psychology. Personal growth to peak performance* (2nd ed., pp. 356–365). Mountain View, CA: Mayfield.

Ogilvie, B., & Taylor, J. (1993b). Career termination issues among elite athletes. In R. N. Singer, M. Murphy, & L. K. Tennant (Eds.), *Handbook of research on sport psychology* (pp. 761–775). New York: Macmillan.

Parker, K. B. (1994). "Has-beens" and "wanna-bees": Transition experiences of former major college football players. *The Sport Psychologist, 8,* 287–304.

Pearson, R. E., & Petitpas, A. J. (1990). Transitions of athletes: Developmental and preventive perspectives. *Journal of Counseling and Development, 69,* 7–10.

Perna, F. M., Zaichkowsky, L., & Bockner, G. (1996). The association of mentoring with psychosocial development among male athletes at termination of college career. *Journal of Applied Sport Psychology, 8,* 76–88.

Reynolds, M. J. (1981). The effects of sports retirement on the job satisfaction of the former football player. In S. L. Greendorfer & A. Yiannakis (Eds.), *Sociology of sport: Diverse perspectives* (pp. 127–137). West Point, NY: Leisure Press.

Robinson, T. T., & Carron, A. V. (1982). Personal and situational factors associated with dropping out versus maintaining participation in competitive sport. *Journal of Sport Psychology, 4,* 364–378.

Rosenberg, E. (1981). Gerontological theory and athletic retirement. In S. L. Greendorfer & A. Yiannakis (Eds.), *Sociology of sport: Diverse perspectives* (pp. 118–126). West Point, NY: Leisure Press.

Sack, H. G. (1980). *Zur psychologie des jugendlichen leistungssportlers* [The psychology of the adolescent athlete]. Schorndorf: Hofmann.

Sands, R. (1978). A socio-psychological investigation of the affects of role discontinuity on outstanding high school athletes. *Journal of Sport Behavior, 1,* 174–185.

Seligman, M. E. P. (1991). *Learned optimism.* New York: Knopf.

Sinclair, D. A., & Orlick, T. (1994). The effects of transition on high performance sport. In D. Hackfort (Ed.), *Psycho-social issues and interventions in elite sport* (pp. 29–55). Frankfurt: Lang.

Singer, E. (1992). *Karriereabbruch im hallenhandball* [Dropout in handball]. Unpublished doctoral dissertation, University of Tuebingen, Germany.

Snyder, E. E., & Baber, L. L. (1979). A profile of former collegiate athletes and nonathletes: Leisure activities, attitudes toward work, and aspects of satisfaction with life. *Journal of Sport Behavior, 2,* 211–219.

Swain, D. A. (1991). Withdrawal from sport and Schlossberg's model of transitions. *Sociology of Sport Journal, 8,* 152–160.

Taylor, J., & Ogilvie, B. C. (1994). A conceptual model of adaptation to retirement among athletes. *Journal of Applied Sport Psychology, 6,* 1–20.

Thomas, C. E., & Ermler, K. L. (1988). Institutional obligations in the athletic retirement process. *Quest, 40,* 137–150.

Wann, D. L., & Hamlet, M. A. (1995). Author and subject gender in sports research. *International Journal of Sport Psychology, 26,* 225–232.

Webb, W. M., Nasco, S. A., Riley, S., & Headrick, B. (1998). Athlete identity and reactions to retirement from sports. *Journal of Sport Behavior, 21,* 338–362.

Werthner, P., & Orlick, T. (1986). Retirement experiences of successful Olympic athletes. *International Journal of Sport Psychology, 17,* 337–363.

Wheeler, G. D., Malone, L. A., VanVlack, S., Nelson, E. R., & Steadward, R. D. (1996). Retirement from disability sport: A pilot study. *Adapted Physical Activity Quarterly, 13,* 382–399.

Wylleman, P. (1995) (Chair). Career transitions of athletes. In R. Vanfraechem-Raway & Y. Vanden Auweele (Eds.), *Proceedings of the 9th European Congress of Sport Psychology* (pp. 827–873). Brussels: European Federation of Sports Psychology.

PART
II

Career
Transition
Intervention

4

Athlete Lifestyle Programs

Deidre Anderson
Athlete Career and Education Program
Australia

Tony Morris
Victoria University
Australia

Abstract

This chapter discusses life-skill programs for athletes, based on a tour of countries that had made progress in this area in the mid-1990s, contacts with colleagues working in the field, and the published literature. The chapter first presents the views of three eminent scholars in the field, whose pioneering work identified the need for life-skill programs in elite sport. These researchers reflected disappointment in the limited developments and a view that, whether in professional or Olympic sport, preparation for life after sport is not perceived as an attractive way to use limited resources. Examination of programs in Canada, the United Kingdom, and the United States suggested that efforts have largely been halfhearted. Programs have been located in the periphery of the infrastructure of elite sport, given limited funds, and not strongly promoted with athletes and coaches. The development of the Athlete Career and Education (ACE) Program in Australia is an exception. Its structure and development are described in detail. Implications are presented for the promotion of life-skill programs based on their immediate benefits and the long-term welfare of elite athletes.

Athlete Lifestyle Programs

To become elite athletes in the modern world, individuals must discipline themselves to train for many years. Usually, they need to dedicate most of every day to their sport, from their childhood years, in some sports even from infancy. More and more countries have developed systems to identify talent very early in life and to nurture that talent through local, regional, and national training programs that start during childhood. Having spent anything from 10 to 20 or more years maintaining an intense focus on their sport, elite athletes wake up one day to find that they are no longer involved in that sport at the elite level. It is only then that many realize that they still have most of their adult life in front of them, but they do not know how to do anything outside elite sport. Retirement from high-level sport can, thus, be a traumatic career transition for many athletes.

Research on the subject of the career transition out of elite sport, whether retirement occurs at the end of a natural competition career or is premature, resulting from injury or deselection, has been slow to emerge and even slower to be acted on. The limited early work in baseball in the United States (Lerch, 1981) and soccer in Yugoslavia (Mihovilovic, 1968) suggested that retirement was difficult for professional athletes, but had little impact on practices on professional clubs, let alone in sport more generally. The expansion of full-time sports performers in a wide range of Olympic sports that occurred in the 1970s and 1980s led to further research related to the impact of intensive, long-term preparation on broader personal development, in social and educational terms, and the implications of this for the transition out of elite sport (e.g., Baillie & Danish, 1992; Werthner & Orlick, 1986).

On the basis of this research, and the applied work with elite performers that stimulated much of it, sport psychologists began to develop schemes to prepare athletes for "life after sport." For example, Petitpas, Danish, McKelvain, and Murphy (1992) were involved in the development of the Career Assistance Program for Athletes (CAPA), based on extensive interviews with Olympic athletes in the United States. As will be described later in this chapter, this program was surprisingly terminated due to funding cuts before it had time to demonstrate its value. Blann and Zaichkowsky (1986, 1988) have also pointed out that the performance of athletes at any stage during their career could be affected by concerns about what they would do when they retired from elite sport.

It has been argued that the introduction of life-skill programs for athletes early in their careers can protect them from the anxiety about their futures that the one-eyed elite performers often experience, while preparing them for a smoother, less traumatic transition out of elite sport when that time comes.

The development of such programs in elite professional and Olympic sports around the world has been sporadic, to say the least. In this chapter, we review the major programs that have been developed in recent years. Before examining these programs themselves, we briefly consider the nature of life-skill programs and report the views of some of the sport psychologists who argued for their development and established them. This chapter cannot be comprehensive, and we apologize to those whose efforts are not included. The aim is to reflect the patterns of development and growth in athlete life-skill programs around the world. The final section assesses the current situation and makes recommendations for future development in the area of athlete life-skill programs.

What are Athlete Life-Skill Programs?

Athlete life-skill programs, also known as athlete career and education programs, are designed to develop social, educational, and work-related skills in elite athletes. They can include career counseling that helps athletes to identify an area of interest for a postsport career and directs the athletes to appropriate avenues of training for jobs in that field. Other services of such programs include the development of generic social and interpersonal skills that can help the athletes present themselves well in interviews and perform well in the job. Programs often emphasize the potential for athletes to transfer the skills they have developed in sport into other areas of life. Commitment, goal setting, time management, repeated practice, and disciplined preparations are only a few of the skills athletes have that can be transferred to many other spheres. Some programs also involve workshops on skills, such as relaxation, positive self-talk, and imagery, that will help the athlete to cope with the demands of elite sport and also have many uses beyond sport.

International Athlete Life-Skill Programs

Although published materials on career transitions and athlete education programs were beginning to appear in the early 1990s, detailed descriptions of the programs around the world were not available. In fact, even in 1998 this is still generally the case. For this reason, contact was made with the major researchers and applied practitioners working in this field, but correspondence with them did not give a full picture of the programs. Visits to some of these internationally recognized centers were therefore undertaken by the first author to examine their athlete lifestyle programs firsthand (D. Anderson, 1993). This chapter presents a description and analysis of the information collected during these visits to facilities and colleagues in the United Kingdom, United States, and Canada. These countries were selected on the basis of the level of research that had been undertaken and the fact that a support program had been in place or was being developed. The United Kingdom was chosen because athlete support personnel had identified a need for programs, although they had not taken steps to commence any implementation. Although it would have been useful, a visit to France was not possible due to budget and time constraints. However, Monsanson (1992) authorized an excellent document that provided an overview of the current status of life-skills programs in France. To facilitate comparison, discussions with leading researchers are considered first; then, international programs are presented and assessed.

Researchers

The main international researchers in the area of athlete support services were chosen, and as a result, interviews were conducted with Dr. Steve Danish of Virginia Commonwealth University, Dr. Albert Petitpas of Springfield College, and Dr. Wayne Blann of Ithaca College, all based in the United States.

Danish has written extensively on the need for life-skill programs for elite athletes and has developed numerous support programs that have been used within the college system in the United States. One of the more recent publications by Danish is *Going for Goal Handbook* (1993), which has been adopted for use by both high school and college students around the United States. This program was designed to assist young people achieve their sporting dreams by providing them with role models who facilitate a series of workshops. By 1995, some 3,000 students had been involved in the program. It was interesting to see that Danish, who has advocated life-skills programs for elite athletes for many years now, has turned his attention to the general population. The issue has become so important that a Life Skills Center has been established at Virginia Commonwealth University.

Danish described the Center as a multidisciplinary operation that assists students to develop "life skills." He defined life skills as those skills that enable us to master the tasks necessary to succeed in our social environment, for example, learning to transfer skills from one domain of life to another, in particular those skills learned in sport that can be applicable at home, at school, or in the workplace. Sport is used as a key component in the learning process, and Danish explained that the Center focused on sport because of the major role it plays in American society and its pervasiveness in that society. He felt that sport is a major influence in the development of identity and competence across the life span of many individuals. The Life Skill Center's mission statement is as follows:

- To develop, implement, and evaluate lifeskills programs for children, adolescents, and adults.
- To collaborate with our organizations seeking to develop and/or implement lifeskills programs.

- To conduct research on the effect of sport on the mental and physical fitness of participants.
- To advocate for programs emphasizing the value of both the mental and physical aspects of participation in sport. (Danish, 1993, p. 20)

In 1992–1993, the Going for Goal program was piloted in Atlanta, Boston, Los Angeles, and New York under the auspices of the Athletic Footwear Association. The program has also been conducted at the United States Olympic Training Center in Colorado Springs and at diving centers throughout the United States in conjunction with the U.S. Diving Federation. The program's financial support amounted to over two million dollars for 1992–1993, including a $15,000 grant from the United States Olympic Training Center in 1992.

It is not surprising that Danish diverted most of his energy away from elite sport. He was quite critical of the system of elite sport, particularly the nonacceptance of the need to support life-skill programs. Despite his extensive research over the years, he still believed that there was limited acceptance in sport, particularly in the United States, of the need for ongoing commitment to a life-skill program for elite athletes. Danish believed that if a life-skills program was to continually operate within sport, it would need clear policies and should be integrated with other athlete support programs. He also felt that within the United States, nothing of any depth was happening in the area despite the evidence from research that supported the need for introducing life-skills programs for elite athletes (e.g., Baillie & Danish, 1992; Danish, Petitpas, & Hale, 1993). He stated that this was because people in sports administration focus on the profile of the game, the coaches are concerned about their personal survival, and the college prioritizes the performance of the team; but "no one really cares about the athlete." Also, if a program were to be introduced, especially at the Olympic level, criticism and questions might be directed at the coaches and administrators for failing to address such issues earlier.

With respect to life-skills programs directed specifically at Olympic athletes, Danish was one of the original researchers who assisted in setting up the CAPA Program (Petitpas et al., 1992). This program was developed for the United States Olympic Committee to prepare athletes for the transition from elite competition. In an important and direct way, CAPA provided a forum where athletes could share concerns about disengaging from sport and learn the basics of the career development process. Danish and his colleagues quickly realized just how much the athletes valued the social support from other athletes involved in the forum. This was particularly noticeable for many athletes who expressed a sense of relief when they realized that others felt anger, confusion, and fear about disengaging from competition.

Despite the enormous success of the program, CAPA is not presently oper-ating, as a result of funding cuts. Danish pointed out that it is no wonder that researchers have become frustrated with the system of sport, when on a day-to-day basis they see the need for such programs. He believed that funding agencies do not perceive career preparation as an important area to fund. Dan-ish was, not surprisingly, now directing his energy more to young people in the general population, who, he believed would appreciate the value-added as-sistance emanating from life-skill-type programs.

Danish stated that part of the reason for CAPA's not continuing was that it was not promoted enough to the athletes and that coaches generally were ignorant of the important role of such a program. At the time of the interview, he was basically convinced that many elite athletes were not interested and that earlier educational intervention efforts should be directed at talented ath-letes during mid-junior high school. There was also a need to educate coaches that athletes are people who have lives outside and beyond sport.

In summary, although Danish's work has been the cornerstone for the de-velopment of the Australian Athlete Career and Education Program, the diffi-culties he faced in implementing the findings and recommendations of his re-search in the United States are an indication of the lack of integration presently taking place between sports administrators, coaches, support staff, and the athletes themselves.

Like Danish, Professor Albert Petitpas has become one of the most prolific writers on intervention programs for elite athletes (e.g., Danish, Petitpas, & Hale, 1990, 1993; Petitpas, Champagne, Chartrand, Danish, & Murphy, 1997; Petitpas et al., 1992). More recently, Petitpas and his colleagues from Spring-field College have been conducting research on the relationship between ath-letic identity and sports participation (e.g., Good, Brewer, Petitpas, Van Raalte, & Mahar, 1993; Murphy, Petitpas, & Brewer, 1996). This research has estab-lished the level of importance that athletes assign to their overall involvement in sport. The researchers felt that the findings might provide further insight into the career transition issues of elite athletes. Petitpas was also involved, on a daily basis, in counseling college-based athletes in the areas of education and career issues. The psychology department at Springfield College, in which Petitpas directs the graduate training program in athletic counseling, offered counseling to both college and Olympic athletes, and he believed that the provision of life-skill programs for elite athletes was an essential part of the services offered at the Center. Petitpas had gone through a torrid time trying to convince USA Sport that life-skill programs for elite athletes were necessary. He argued that although research supported the need, sport in general saw such areas as an adjunct to other services for athletes (e.g., sports science and medicine), rather than as essential to enhance both the current performance and the long-term psychological development of athletes.

Petitpas' research is continuing and is aimed at athletes, coaches, and organizations that see the need for life-skills programs. At the time of the interview, he felt that the United States was still a long way from introducing an integrated program. Since that time, he (together with Danish and their colleagues) has published the *Athlete's Guide to Career Planning: Keys to Success from the Playing Field to Professional Life* (Petitpas et al., 1997).

In summary, Petitpas' research has resulted in the development of a program focus that is based on individual counseling of athletes. His major focus is to assist athletes to establish their own identity and not just their athletic identity. His work is demonstrating the identity shift required for athletes upon retirement and the need to encourage the athlete to have a balanced view of their identity whilst competing.

Although a visit to Ithaca College was not possible, an interview was conducted with Professor Wayne Blann in New York to enable an introduction to be made to professional sporting bodies and to discuss his personal views of athlete life-skill programs. Blann and his colleagues have together researched career transition issues of professional athletes (e.g., Blann & Zaichkowsky, 1986, 1988; Hawkins & Blann, 1993). They have undertaken research in major league football, baseball, ice hockey, and basketball and have observed the postsporting career transition of professional athletes in general. Once again, despite the extensive research, Blann stated that some professional sports have totally ignored his findings, whereas others have introduced programs that still require ongoing development. When asked why this is the case, he described a system so tied up in billions of dollars that those involved found it hard to see the basic needs of athletes. Despite this environment, Blann was pleased with the introduction of some aspects of the program by the professional basketball and football organizations. In the college system, Blann noted that Ithaca College offered a subject to its sports studies students that looked at the importance of ensuring that life-skill education was encouraged.

Blann's approach to his work appeared to be different from that of Petitpas and Danish; that is, he seemed to be spending more time on promoting the needs for support programs within professional sporting bodies, rather than with Olympic or college athletes. When asked whether this was the case, Blann said that professional sport played an enormous role in the United States and the models that were often promoted to young people were not the most appropriate. If professional sport took a more responsible approach to developing athletes as people, young aspiring athletes might be more receptive to reconsider the need to maintain a well-balanced approach to their sport.

More recently, Blann and his associates have been looking at transitions in the career development of coaches (e.g., Blann, 1992; Hawkins, Blann, Zaichkowsky, & Kane, 1994). From their research undertakings in Australia, an interesting finding not previously documented was that coaches generally were reluctant to consider new careers outside of coaching; hence, their awareness of noncoaching occupations tended to be vague and general (Hawkins et al., 1994). What this indicated from Blann's point of view was that coaches cannot, and will not, encourage athletes to consider alternative career paths, as long as they do not understand the need to do so for themselves. Blann believed that the limited success of programs in the United States was due in part to the reluctance of administrators and coaches to understand, or fully appreciate, the need to assist athletes with life-skill programs. He also argued that this problem would remain as long as administrators and coaches perceived life-skill programs to be a peripheral need in developing athletic performance.

In summary, Blann's major focus has been to convince professional sporting bodies to develop support programs for athletes. Blann believes that as a consequence of the high profile of these sports in the United States, his challenge is to teach professional sport performers how they can combine their business needs with the individual needs of the athlete, a challenge he is yet to see become a reality.

Summary of Researchers

The majority of research that has been undertaken on life-skill programs for elite athletes has been carried out in the United States. Despite this extensive research, which has clearly indicated the need for such programs, the leading researchers all believed that the system of sport within the United States had not fully grasped the concept. Although it appeared that the college system of sport had developed successful programs, the researchers argued that they still had a long way to go before life-skill programs for elite athletes were entrenched in the system of sport in both amateur and professional elite sport. It is also ironic that Danish and Petitpas are now working mainly in nonelite sport, because their work in elite Olympic sport has been stifled by the lack of financial support. Blann argued that the large amount of money involved in professional sport is a key factor in explaining the lack of development of life-skills programs.

International Programs

The impact of research in the United States is currently being felt in the national sports organizations of the United Kingdom, Canada, and the United

States. This section highlights the information gathered from interviews about what existed in 1993, what organizational attitudes prevailed at that time, and what was being planned for the future. The scale of sport is greater in the United States than in Canada and the United Kingdom, as well as in Australia, because of a much larger population. In addition, the vast college system and the scale of professional football, baseball, basketball, and ice hockey mean that there is a greater need to consider a range of issues that affect highly committed athletes, including the impact of retirement from professional sport. The following section initially provides an overview of the Australian Athlete Career and Education (ACE) program. Life-skills education and programs in the United Kingdom, Canada, and United States are then reviewed (D. Anderson, 1993). The structure of elite sport in these countries is first discussed, and compared with Australia where appropriate, to provide a context to consider the development of life-skills programs for elite athletes.

Australia

The Australian ACE program has been coordinated on a national basis since 1995. It was as a result of a decision between the Australian Institute of Sport and Victorian Institute of Sport, whereby both programs were amalgamated (Fortunato, Anderson, Morris, & Seedsman, 1995). The Victorian Institute of Sport initiated the ACE program as part of its charter when the institute was first established in June 1990. The career assessment protocols developed during this time later formed the basis of the national ACE program. Whereas the personal development course established by the Life Skills for Elite Athletes program (SportsLEAP) provided an excellent platform for the competency-based training courses now offered to elite athletes, the integration of both programs has unified the delivery and enabled the skills and resources of all sports institutes to be more effectively used to assist the athletes. By 1996, athlete career and education advisors were appointed in each state institute/academy of sport, and in June 1996, a national manager was appointed to coordinate the program. Initially, the national ACE program offered only an athlete assessment service and a number of personal development courses. However, by 1997 it was delivering the most comprehensive athlete lifestyle program in the world.

The strategies of the national ACE program are as follows:

1. *Individual athlete assessment*: Provides a structured process in which to assess individual athletes' educational, vocational, financial and personal development needs.

2. *Personal development training courses*: Provides elite athletes with nationally accredited competency-based education programs.

3. *Nationally consistent career and education planning*: Utilizes a nationally consistent career and education process to enable elite athletes to manage their own individual vocational requirements.
4. *Community recognition*: Promotes community recognition of the program and its ideals.
5. *Transition program*: Provides career and education guidance for elite athletes who are undergoing a transition to a postsporting career.
6. *Program development*: Ensures athlete career and education personnel are appropriately trained to deliver the program services.
7. *Program integration*: Fosters the integration of ACE program personnel and services within the ongoing programs offered by state institutes and academies.
8. *Direct athlete needs-based assessment*: Provides a structured process to assess athletes' eligibility for needs-based support.
9. *Professional sports*: Provides a nationally consistent and coordinated athlete career and education program to professional sports.

The overall aim of the ACE program is to assist athletes to balance the demands of their sporting careers whilst enhancing their opportunities to also develop their educational and vocational skills. A major component of the program is to assist athletes to develop a career plan that integrates both sporting and nonsporting components. A practical package is then developed that is managed by the athlete and supported by the ACE advisor, coach and other significant people identified.

The program is coordinated by the Australian Institute of Sport and the state institutes/academies of sport. To be eligible for assistance, athletes must be a scholarship holder with the Australian Institute of Sport, state institute/academies of sport, or Olympic athlete program participants. The selected athletes are provided with ACE services as well as elite-level coaching, competition opportunities, and appropriate sports medicine support. The ACE program works in cooperation with the above areas to ensure an integrated approach so that Australia's elite athletes can achieve success in both sport and life.

The training of staff in this unique area has recently seen the development of a graduate certificate in athlete career and education management. There are presently 30 students undertaking the course with the first graduates expected in late 1998.

The service delivery has improved markedly in the past 3 years to a point where it is delivering a consistent and effective service to over 3,500 elite-level athletes throughout Australia. Although reaching this number of athletes would appear to be a strength of the program, it is also one of its main weaknesses, as the 20 staff who are employed in both full-time and part-time capacities attempt to service such a large number of athletes.

In order to reaffirm some of the identified strengths and weaknesses of the program, a national evaluation was undertaken by the University of Queensland (Gorely, Bruce, & Teale, 1998). The findings included lack of awareness of the program by athletes who live away from the major ACE service centers, need for a national ACE database to enable the movement of athlete information when athletes relocate to other states, need to develop flexible delivery materials for the athlete training courses, and modification of the athlete assessment procedures so they can be undertaken by telephone or in a group situation.

The ACE program has become the preeminent program of its kind in the world, an achievement that the staff do not rest upon as they strive to continually assist their athletes to achieve at the highest level. The philosophy of the program is clearly to create an environment where athletes can be encouraged to be independent and self-reliant and to have a capacity to meet the demands associated with elite sport. It is about a proactive approach rather than a reactive one resulting in nothing being left to chance.

United Kingdom

The structure of sport in the United Kingdom, as compared to Australia, was not too dissimilar; that is, professional sports existed, but not to the same diverse and/or large scale as in the United States. Thus, elite amateur or Olympic sport is the major context for nurturing full-time elite athletes. The state/regional sporting organizations were the main bodies representing sport, and they administered programs to encourage participation as well as elite performance. The coaching education program and accreditation procedures were also in line with the Australian National Coaching Council procedures, according to which coaches must participate and pass courses before being eligible to coach at club, state, and national levels. The United Kingdom, like Australia, had an excellent infrastructure of sport, but without the geographic difficulties that inevitably influence a country the size of Australia.

The United Kingdom had 16 coaching centers, which were similar to Australian regional sports assemblies. The coaching centers were the responsibility of the United Kingdom National Coaching Foundation (UKNCF). The United Kingdom Sports Council (UKSI), which was similar to the Australian Sports Commission, was moving quickly to encourage the introduction of a life-skills program for elite athletes. The idea was being driven by Sue Campbell, the Executive Director of the UKNCF at the time, who visited Australia in 1994 to see, firsthand, the Victorian Institute of Sport's ACE Program.

In 1997, the initial framework for the introduction of a British Sports Institute was developed, with plans to have a formal opening in 1998. The key organizations involved in developing such a program are the English Sports Council, and the British Olympic Committee. The structure of sport in the

United Kingdom should allow an easy introduction of a life-skills program, and until injections of funding from the lottery, it is likely that an athlete development program will be launched in 1999. Based formally on the Australian system, it will be coordinated by the UKSI and delivered through the home countries of Wales, Scotland, Northern Ireland, and England. Regional centers will assist in the delivery, and one coordinator will be working from each of the home countries. Approximately 2,000 athletes will have access to the program.

The United Kingdom did not offer a life-skills program for elite athletes in 1993, although the Professional Football Association (PFA) offered a basic program, which a very small number of players who had been identified as having the potential to play professionally were invited to attend. This was a residential program in which education and welfare issues of the players were monitored. The PFA program was an effort to produce outstanding professional players. To do this, it provided a rescheduled education and training program for 14- to 15-year-olds. Although the program has been operating since 1985, very few players have come through from it to the professional game. There were criticisms that this residential program did not produce excellence in sport and that there was a general lack of support given to young players who left as a result of not meeting the performance standards. In addition, although some time was given to education and life skills, the emphasis of this program was on intensive soccer training, not usually available to this age group. In 1998, the PFA reviewed its program and have instigated major changes including full education support and self-development courses for their residential players. It is, however, too early to review its effectiveness.

Another program in progress was the Goldstart program, introduced by the British Olympic Association in 1989. It was designed to assist Olympic athletes with education, career, and personal concerns, which had arisen as a result of competing at an elite level. Campbell felt that this program was not systematic in its approach and was problematic in its programming; that is, it introduced support to athletes in a reactive way rather than intervening in a proactive way. A further program recently introduced was the Planning for Success workshops, coordinated by the British Olympic Association. This program also involved life-skill and technical skills development in sports medicine, sports science, and career planning. The workshops were quite well received with over 150 athletes participating.

The career, education, and life-skill needs of elite athletes in the United Kingdom were not very different from those of athletes in Australia. Most athletes needed to work or establish a solid education base to enable them to make career choices. However, with the introduction of the lottery funding for

British elite athletes, it would appear that some might see this as an opportunity to forgo the need to develop alternative career and educational pathways. This could place some athletes at risk as they fully rely upon their sport for their total income, and should their performances diminish, may find themselves without any financial security. It will, therefore, be important to ensure that athlete career planning services be in place to assist with educating athletes, coaches, and their respective sports about the importance of a balanced lifestyle. It may also require instigating a similar strategy undertaken by Australia, where direct athlete funding is only provided on the provision that athletes are pursuing alternative vocational pathways. There was little to be learned from the United Kingdom system, which was itself learning from what existed in Australia. Perhaps this provided some confirmation that the ACE program was being seen as an innovative strategy aimed at fostering the overall welfare of the athlete.

Canada

The structure of sport in Canada and Australia is similar, in that the Canadian system was made up of the Olympic Council and Sports Federation and incorporated provincial or regional sporting associations. Sporting clubs were the major feeder group to sport rather than the college system, as in the United States, although Canadian colleges do offer sporting scholarships for major sports such as baseball and ice hockey. Volunteers played an integral role in administering sport at club level.

Canada created its first life-skills program for elite athletes in 1985, as part of its program for Olympic athletes. The program operated as part of the Canadian Olympic Association, and was organized as part of the Canadian Olympic Athlete Career Centre (COACC). Its main focus was to assist athletes with their career and educational needs. The services were available to all "carded" athletes, that is, athletes who had achieved approved rankings by way of their performances at Olympic, Commonwealth, and Pan Pacific Games.

The services of the COACC included résumé preparation, letters of support, job referrals, development of business cards, retirement assistance, career counseling, interview preparation, aptitude testing, and job-searching techniques. Sue Holloway managed the Centre's headquarters located in Ottawa. Since the approval by the Canadian Olympic Association Executive Committee for the COACC in 1988, several centers had been planned throughout Canada. The first, in Calgary, had been operating with a great deal of success, according to Holloway. By 1993, there were five centers operating at Toronto, Calgary, Montreal, Vancouver, and Ottawa, each one employing a consultant on a part-time basis, who became the contact for athletes living in or around that location. Ottawa was the exception, as Holloway was employed on a full-time basis. Budget constraints had delayed the development of further centers. In 1990, the COACC introduced a new program called the Shadow program, which was designed to give national team athletes the opportunity to explore career options in the field of their choice by "shadowing" professionals in that area for 2 to 5 days. At the time of the interview, more than 70 national seminars had been organized around the country. The COACC also coordinated countrywide sport-specific seminars for national teams every 2 years. Athletes were subsidized to attend the program by their respective sporting body. The total budget for 1990–1993 was in the vicinity of $800,000. Holloway believed the regionalization of athlete career and education services would provide a much-needed local resource for athletes.

The COACC was attempting to move towards an intervention program aimed at Olympic, Commonwealth, and Pan Pacific athletes. The introduction of the Centers in Montreal and Vancouver would lead to the service's taking on a decentralized approach. The only obvious criticism was the lack of service integration. Despite this, Canada had an athlete-driven program, based on a sound philosophy, which was seen as important to maintain. This was made evident in a report published in 1993 entitled *The Status of High Performance Athletes* (Ekos, 1993). It was suggested that an integration of athlete career and education programs with other support systems would be most beneficial. See chapter 8 for more information.

United States of America

The structure of sport in the United States in 1993 represented a fundamentally different system to that in Australia, Canada, and the United Kingdom, as most elite athletes came through college-based sports scholarship programs. Research has shown quite clearly that elite athletes in the United States face career transition problems when they attempt to combine elite sport with alternative education/career paths (Blann, 1992; Broom, 1982; Curtis & Ennis, 1988; Petitpas et al., 1992), yet there had been little attempt to address the issues. The research tour of the United States involved the Women's Sports Foundation, the National Football League, the National Basketball League, and the United States Olympic Education Center.

The Women's Sports Foundation. The Women's Sports Foundation (WSF) is a nonprofit educational organization that is dedicated to promoting and enhancing the sport and fitness experience for all girls and women. One of its founding members was the tennis player Billie Jean King, who in 1974, together with four other women, created the WSF. Its main programs at the time of the interview were Educational Opportunities and the Advocacy and

Recognition Program for Women in Sport. An advisory branch provided expertise in areas of sport psychology, sociology, administration, sports marketing, exercise physiology, and sports medicine.

The Director of Athlete Services, Yolanda Jackson, was investigating the introduction of an athlete career and education program as part of a trust that was set up in honor of the late Arthur Ashe. The philosophy behind this program was to promote the importance of education in the lives of African-American female athletes. One major area of consideration was how such an action would be received by the athletes' agents and coaches, who, it was thought, might not perceive the need for a life-skills training program. One of the main motives behind wanting to introduce a program was that African-American female athletes, like all other athletes, need support to assist them with life as elite athletes and with their transition from elite competition. The program operated by utilizing workshops and social functions; it did not offer individually designed support programs. According to Jackson, it was expected that this weakness in program delivery would be addressed in the future to gauge success of the program because there was no opportunity to speak with athletes. There was also great difficulty in accessing formal evaluation records and written material on programs held to date.

The National Football League. The Director of Player Programs for the National Football League (NFL), Dr. Len Burnham, believed the appointment of a Visionary Commissioner had resulted in a productive rethinking of player education/career programs within the NFL. In particular, he believed that this appointment was improving opportunities for retired players and assisting them with the transition from professional football. Since 1990, the NFL had introduced four new programs related to athlete career preparation, including a Continuing Education Program (CEP), Career Transition Program (CTP), Financial Education Program (FEP), and Family Assistance Program (FAP). The programs were facilitated by consultants and will now be briefly described.

The CEP was designed to assist athletes who were about to retire from the NFL, or who were trying to reenter educational institutions. By establishing the needs of each athlete, the CEP provided the financial and counseling support necessary for returning to study.

The CTP provided a preretirement seminar, career planning, and work experience program within selected business organizations. The aim of the program was to provide practical seminars that would assist the players to deal more effectively with their retirement from the NFL.

The FEP provided information to players on investment, insurance, and taxation, which were important issues as the average player's earnings were between $400,000 and $500,000 a season at the time, and according to Burnham, some players did not always understand the responsibility associated with earning this amount of money. Despite some initial problems, the NFL had a successful workshop, which all players attended.

The FAP was designed to provide services for players and their families in nonfootball matters, such as marriage counseling, parental care, and alcohol and drug counseling. More than 140 psychologists and social workers operated throughout the United States to assist in this area. According to Burnham, it was one of the most used services and indicated that many players had difficulties filling the role of a professional footballer or the combination of that role with the responsibilities to a partner and family.

Although the NFL should be commended for introducing such services, it can be criticized for offering the programs only in a workshop format, with the exception of the FAP. It must be recognized that some athletes deal totally with the present and pay little attention to needs other than those deemed to be immediate concerns, so they are unlikely to attend voluntary workshops. It is suggested that a more effective approach would be individual assessment of players before accessing workshop programs to sensitize them to future career and education issues. This approach should then be followed up with some form of action plan when the workshops have been completed. Most of the services offered by the NFL appeared to be reactive by nature.

Despite this criticism, the NFL had given a commitment to its players' association to provide an improved level of support, and although it would not be compulsory, Burnham was certain that promoting the findings of a recent unpublished research report to players would assist in educating them in the importance of career development. Burnham stated that the report found that players with a college degree, on average, played 50% longer than those who did not have a college degree. It was expected that these results would be used to "sell" career and education programs to coaches, as well as to athletes.

The United States Olympic Education Center. The United States Olympic Education Center (USOEC) was established in 1985 to assist elite athletes to combine a college degree with elite sport. Located at North Michigan University, the Center was the only Olympic residential program in the United States where athletes were able to combine college with training for top national and international competitions. The USOEC also offered the only national Olympic-bridging program in which "retired" Olympic athletes were able to finish their education with the same benefits as resident athletes. The USOEC was the home of Olympic badminton, boxing, cross-country skiing, ski jumping, speed skating, and luge. In 1992, the Center employed an education officer whose responsibilities included assisting the athletes with tutoring and other educational support programs as they arose. The number of athletes at the Center at the time of the visit was 80; however, it had a capacity to serve up to 300. Besides the USOEC in Michigan, there were three other Olympic-training centers that were located at Colorado Springs, Colorado; Lake Placid, New York; and San Diego, California. None of these centers offered educational programs, however.

To be eligible for the USOEC, athletes had to be qualified in the top 20 in the United States. Each resident was then provided with free room, board, and tutoring. The United States Olympic Committee supported the education center by providing $79,000 per year in funding. They also provided $27,750 to support tuition scholarships each year. The state government of Michigan provided an annual amount of $600,000 that funded the athletes' room, board, tutoring, transportation, and USOEC administration staff salaries. The remaining financial support came from governing bodies of sport that had residential programs located at the Center. This financial assistance also provided coaches' salaries and athletes' competition costs. The education officer spent a considerable amount of time attempting to deal with the day-to-day problems that student-athletes face, such as time scheduling and tutoring. The position did not appear to have a framework to enable athletes to be given counseling and education programs for their career/education and personal development at the time.

National Basketball League. The National Basketball League (NBL), in conjunction with the National Basketball Players' Association, introduced a career and education program in 1987. With a budget of $5 million, it provided services to some 320 athletes. The program included the following three areas: internship, degree completion/education training, and professional athlete career education.

The internship program provided opportunities for athletes to gain first-hand experience working in the business of their choice. It was an off-season work experience program in which players with clearer ideas about a postbasketball career could be exposed to areas of career interest.

The degree completion/education training program was developed to meet and support the needs of players who studied at university or who needed assistance with external study options. Assistance was provided in completing college degrees, enrolling in accredited home-study courses, participating in certificate programs, preparing for college entrance examinations, and obtaining remedial preparation for reentry into college programs. A private education consultant from the Professional Athlete Career and Education (PACE) organization provided this support.

PACE Sports Inc. was an organization specifically designed to provide career counseling and planning assistance to athletes (Stark, 1986). PACE offered services to athletes on a national basis and included career testing, counseling, education planning, and corporate internship programs. PACE also acted as a consultant to the NBL players in the above areas and also provided seminars for players and their wives. The seminars featured entrepreneurial opportunities, presentation skills, résumé development, and financial services.

Other programs the NBL had developed included The Rookie Transition Program, which provided the opportunity for new recruits to attend two half-day lectures, designed to assist players to prepare for the professional league. Also, the Legends Foundation provided past NBL players with financial grants to assist them when they experienced financial difficulties.

Observation and discussions revealed that, although a lot of money was being spent by the NBL, there was very little evidence of its effectiveness. No documentation was available on assessment procedures or, in fact, on the nature of the services at all; the information was gleaned from discussions only.

NCAA CHAMPS/Life Skills. The college athletics program in North America is a vast sports system that operates at a high level, demands a great deal of commitment from the athletes involved, but offers a career in professional or Olympic sport to only a relatively small proportion of them. In recognition of this, the National Collegiate Athletics Association (NCAA) Foundation and the NCAA Division I Athletic Directors Association recently introduced a new program called CHAMPS/Life Skills that offers life-skills education for college athletes. The program was piloted in 100 NCAA-affiliated colleges in 1994–96, before being offered to all NCAA member institutions. Carr and Bauman (1996) reported that the CHAMPS/Life Skills program is based on five general commitments, which are (a) academic excellence, (b) athletics excellence, (c) personal development, (d) service, and (e) career development. On the foundation of a holistic philosophy of college athletics, CHAMPS stresses developmental needs, including the development of personal, as well as athletic, skills. Beyond developing knowledge and skills, the program also emphasizes the development of a sense of belonging, the choice of informed attitudes, and the need to assume personal responsibility. Carr and Bauman described an eight-point learning program, including (a) fundamental values, (b) academic enhancement, (c) social enhancement, (d) emotional development, (e) physical development, (f) spiritual development, (g) financial instruction, and (h) career planning. They noted that the NCAA has established an annual conference on life-skills education to support this comprehensive program.

It was also pointed out by Carr and Bauman (1996) that an important aspect of the CHAMPS/Life Skills program is the recognition by NCAA that college student-athletes need life-skills education. Carr and Bauman indicated that it was expected that each participating institution would adapt the program to its own specific circumstances. It is also important for institutions to take into account the individual needs of each athlete. Carr and Bauman concluded that the CHAMPS program has great potential, but its effectiveness will depend on the degree of support provided by the colleges. They stated, rather starkly, that "life-skills programming is doomed to fail without complete support and recognition from university and athletic administration, coaching staffs, student-athlete support staffs, alumni, and, most important, the student-athletes" (p. 304). If this need for real commitment to life skills—as opposed to lip ser-vice—were accepted, the widespread adoption of the CHAMPS/Life Skills program or similar life-skills education support programs in North American college sport could have a powerful ripple effect across elite sport in that re-gion and, based on the influential position of North American elite sport prac-tices, on elite and subelite sport around the world. Thus, this development has the potential to be of great benefit to committed athletes, and we will follow its progress with great interest.

Summary. A common statement found in most of the interviews in the United States was that, with less than one percent of college athletes making professional sports teams, life-skills programs were urgently needed at the college level. This supports the viewpoints made by Danish and Petitpas, who were consistently advocating the need for college athletes to have access to an intervention program. Considering the intensive research that has been under-taken in the United States, the professional bodies had chosen to initiate only a limited number of programs that addressed some of the existing problems. Not one sporting body had asked the question: Where should such a program head in the future? It was all about "patching up" problems that existed rather than creating an environment to alleviate future problems. In that regard, such programs may be seen as a panacea by the sporting organizations.

Conclusion

The body of research on career transition out of elite sport has grown sub-stantially in recent years. Findings are relatively consistent. Primary among them is the conclusion that some elite athletes prepare for their retirement, especially when retirement is voluntary. For these performers, retirement is typically smooth, especially when they have met their sport career aspirations. This group is a minority, however. Most elite athletes do not prepare ade-quately for retirement from elite sport, lack the resources to be successful in postsport careers, and, thus, experience traumatic transition. Further, prema-ture retirement due to injury or deselection, as well as the feeling that aspira-tions were never met, typically exacerbates the negative aspects of retirement (e.g., Baillie & Danish, 1992; Fortunato, 1996). Much seems to be tied to the athletic identity the athlete holds at the time of retirement (Brewer, Van Raalte, & Linder, 1993). An identity that is highly focused on the self as athlete is likely to make retirement much harder. Fortunato, for example, found that voluntary retirees frequently reported that they no longer perceived themselves as elite athletes focused on goals in sport. Rather, their perceptions were that they had done that, and now their identities lay in other types of work and their families. Involuntary retirees frequently were still engrossed in their athletic identities and found it hard to let go of their lost dreams.

These conclusions have obvious implications for the early preparation of elite athletes for the end of their career and for life after sport. Despite this, many countries that have established large, full-time, elite athlete training programs during the last 20 years have been slow to develop life-skill programs for elite athletes that aim to address these issues. In addition, those countries that have developed programs have generally not implemented them with the conviction that is necessary to create the necessary impact. In the United States, the promising CAPA program at the start of the 1990s was prematurely terminated due to the lack of funding, just as it was starting to develop momentum and positive responses from athletes. Nothing significant has replaced it. The Canadian system has potential, but it has not been taken to the athletes with sufficient commitment to draw the most from it, and so the pattern goes on around the world. A similar story emerges for professional sport, typified in the United States, where a substantial amount of money has been invested in preparing for retirement, but the emotional aspects of the transition have been relatively neglected in the programs that have developed, which typically focus on financial issues.

Probably the most advanced program is the ACE program in Australia. Starting in a single state, this program has become national and now involves more than 3,500 athletes across Australia, with centers in every state and territory. The ACE program is the only formal life skill or career education program, of which we are aware, that has been examined by research (D. K. Anderson, 1998; Morris & Anderson, 1994). In a study by D. K. Anderson (1998), scholarship athletes from a number of sports were monitored for 12 months from their entry into the Victorian Institute of Sport ACE program in 1993. Their negative mood states reduced in the first few months and stayed low, whereas the mood of other scholarship athletes, not in the ACE program, fluctuated throughout the year, often peaking periodically at high levels. Self-reported performance indicators suggested more stable and consistent performance for the athletes in the program than for those not involved in ACE. This study suggests that comprehensive life-skill programs are likely to be of immediate benefit to elite athletes, a point that should be emphasized when talking to coaches and administrators perhaps. They often seem to think that life-skill programs will distract athletes from their present performance, so their support is halfhearted.

Strong conclusions cannot be drawn from the research by D. K. Anderson (1998), however. It was a relatively small, single study, with a specific group of athletes, and the design was influenced by the practical demands on those elite athletes. More cross-sectional studies are needed that examine the experience of athletes, while they are involved in life-skill programs and in sport. To enhance the richness of the data produced, qualitative as well as quantitative methods should be used. More important still, longitudinal studies should be conducted that follow athletes throughout their careers, especially focusing on the period prior to and following their retirement. This type of research is difficult to do, because of the timescale involved and the potential for attrition. Thus, original research designs must be created that examine the question of what aspects, if any, of life-skill programs do enhance the retirement experience.

Elite professional and Olympic athletes often dedicate themselves to many years of intensive work to give pleasure, excitement, and pride by association to millions of people. In doing this, the athletes are frequently digging a hole for themselves in terms of their adaptation to the rest of their lives. Although a few lucky, or well-organized, individuals make smooth transitions into other careers, for most, the more they dedicate themselves to their sport, the deeper their hole at retirement. It is the responsibility of sporting organizations to ensure that athletes develop a well-rounded approach to life, one that encourages them to expand their identity beyond sport. Athlete lifestyle programs can be the vehicle to assist sporting organizations particularly in setting the right environment well before athletes join the ranks of senior elite.

References

Anderson, D. (1993). *Research tour: Elite athlete education programs.* Melbourne: Victorian Institute of Sport.

Anderson, D. K. (1998). *Lifeskill intervention and elite performances.* Unpublished master's thesis, Victoria University, Melbourne, Australia.

Baillie, P. H. F., & Danish, S. J. (1992). Understanding the career transition of athletes. *The Sport Psychologist, 6,* 77–98.

Blann, F. W. (1992). Coaches' role in player development. *Journal of Applied Research in Coaching and Athletics, 7,* 62–76.

Blann, F. W., & Zaichkowsky, L. (1986). *Career/life transition needs of National Hockey League players.* Final report prepared for the National Hockey League Players' Association, USA.

Blann, F. W., & Zaichkowsky, L. (1988). *Major League Baseball players postsport career transition needs.* Preliminary report prepared for the Major League Baseball Players' Association, USA.

Brewer, B., Van Raalte, J. L., & Linder, D. E. (1993). Athletic identity: Hercules' muscles or Achilles' heel? *International Journal of Sport Psychology, 24,* 237–254.

Broom, E. F. (1982). Detraining and retirement from high level competition: A reaction to "Retirement from high level competition" and "Career crisis in sport". In T. Orlick, J. T. Partington, & J. H. Samela (Eds.), *Proceedings of the 5th World Congress of Sport Psychology* (pp. 183–187). Ottawa: Coaching Association of Canada.

Carr, C., & Bauman, N. J. (1996). Transitions of the student-athlete: Theoretical, empirical, and practical perspectives. In E. F. Etzel, A. P. Ferrante, & Pinkney, J. W. (Eds.), *Counseling college student-athletes: Issues and interventions* (2nd ed., pp. 281–307). Morgantown, WV: Fitness Information Technology.

Curtis, J., & Ennis, R. (1988). Negative consequences of leaving competitive sport? Comparative findings for former elite-level hockey players. *Sociology of Sport Journal, 5,* 87–106.

Danish, S. J. (1993). *Going for goal handbook.* Richmond: Virginia Commonwealth University.

Danish, S. J., Petitpas A. J., & Hale, B. D. (1993). Life development intervention for athletes: Life skills through sports. *The Counseling Psychologist, 21,* 352–385.

Ekos, N. (1993). *The status of high performance athletes.* Canada: Fitness and Amateur Sport.

Fortunato, V. (1996). *Role transitions in elite sports.* Unpublished doctoral dissertation, Victoria University of Technology, Melbourne, Australia.

Fortunato, V., Anderson, D., Morris, T, & Seedsman, T. (1995). Career transition research at Victoria University of Technology. In R. Vanfraechem-Raway & Y. Vanden Auweele (Eds.), *Proceedings of the 9th European Congress of Sport Psychology* (pp. 533–543). Brussels: European Federation of Sports Psychology.

Good, A. J., Brewer, B. W., Petitpas, A. J., Van Raalte, J. L., & Mahar, M. T. (1993). Athletic identity, identity foreclosure, and college sport participation. *Academic Athletic Journal, 8,* 1–12.

Gorely, T., Bruce, D., & Teale, B. (1998). *Athlete Career and Education Program 1997 evaluation.* Brisbane: The University of Queensland.

Hawkins, K., & Blann, F. W. (1993). *Athlete/coach career development and transition.* Canberra: Australian Sports Commission.

Hawkins, K., Blann, F. W., Zaichkowsky, L., & Kane, M. A. (1994). *Athlete/coach career development and transition: Coaches' report.* Canberra: Australian Sports Commission.

Lerch, S. H. (1981). The adjustment to retirement of professional baseball players. In S. L. Greendorfer, & A. Yiannakis (Eds.), *Sociology of sport: Diverse perspectives* (pp. 138–148). West Point, NY: Leisure Press.

Mihovilovic, M. A. (1968). The status of former sportsman. *International Review of Sport Sociology, 3,* 73–93.

Monsanson, N. (1992). *Counseling high performance athletes: A dynamic, interactive approach.* Paris: French National Olympic and Sports Committee.

Morris, T., & Anderson, D. (1994, October). *Career education, perceived performance and mood state in elite athletes.* Paper presented at the annual conference of the Association for the Advancement of Applied Sport Psychology, Lake Tahoe, NV, USA.

Murphy, G. M., Petitpas, A. J., & Brewer, B. W. (1996). Identity foreclosure, athletic identity, and career maturity in intercollegiate athletes. *The Sport Psychologist, 10,* 239–246.

Petitpas, A., Champagne, D., Chartrand, J., Danish, S., & Murphy, S. (1997).*Athlete's guide to career planning: Keys to success from the playing field to professional life.* Champaign, IL: Human Kinetics.

Petitpas, A., Danish, S., McKelvain, R., & Murphy, S. (1990, 1993). A career assistance program for elite athletes. *Journal of Counseling and Development, 70,* 383–386.

Stark, E. (1986). Life after sports. *Psychology Today, 19 (1),* 57.

Werthner, P., & Orlick, T. (1986). Retirement experiences of successful Olympic athletes. *International Journal of Sport Psychology, 17,* 337–363.

5

Practical Considerations in Implementing Sport Career Transition Programs

Albert J. Petitpas and Delight Champagne
Springfield College

Abstract

The authors discuss a number of the practical issues that often face sport psychologists and career development specialists when planning and implementing sport career transition programs for elite athletes. Logistical issues, such as timing, accessibility, and group membership, are considered in light of the unique nature of elite sport participation. In addition, suggestions for managing group diversity and for identifying and developing follow-up services are presented.

Practical Considerations in Implementing Sport Career Transition Programs

Although the sport psychology literature contains a number of articles that describe sport career transition programs (e.g., Petitpas, Danish, McKelvain, & Murphy, 1992; Werthner & Orlick, 1986), little has been written addressing practical considerations in providing such services. The goal of this chapter is to outline several of the practical issues that can surface when planning and implementing career transition programs for elite athletes. In particular, three main areas will be considered: (a) logistical concerns and program planning before the intervention, (b) group management and presentation issues during intervention programs, and (c) the need for planned follow-up and continuation of skill development.

Program Planning

In planning career transition programs for elite athletes, professionals must consider the complex nature of today's sport systems. Each sport has its own timelines, culture, governing body, and operating procedures. Each of these factors in turn influences players' availability, group makeup, program goals, and follow-up procedures. As a result, the first step in program planning is to become well versed in the idiosyncrasies of the targeted sport or sports groups.

A number of questions arise from logistical issues that are dependent upon the sport's organization, the type of sport, and the nature of the competitive events in which the players participate. For example, when should the program occur? Should it occur during the competitive season, before, or afterwards? To answer these questions, consideration has to be given to program timing in relation to playing season, convenience and access to program meetings, scheduling conflicts, program location, and selection of team or player subgroups.

Although it is normally advisable to run programs either before or after competition seasons, this is not always possible. With sports that do not have "home bases" where athletes come together for training on a regular basis, it may be necessary to offer career transition programs at competition sites during down periods in the athletes' practice or competition season. For example, in offering a career transition program for the Ladies Professional Golf Association (LPGA), the authors found it necessary to meet with the players at different tour stops over a 3-month period. Care had to be exercised in selecting the tour sites to target in order to provide adequate contact time (6 to 8 hours per site), continuity of program delivery (e.g., adequate time for self-exploration before moving into the career exploration phase of the program), and availability of resources (access to meeting rooms) without intruding on practice or sponsor-related commitments. If one factors in the need to avoid major tournaments and the fact that not all players choose to play each tour stop, the need for careful planning becomes quite obvious.

Contrast the LPGA example with athletes from other sports who play half of their contests in a "home" facility. In the latter cases, many of the athletes would have residences in the area and be available to attend programs outside of the normal competition schedule. In any event, it is important to get the athletes' input concerning scheduling prior to any program implementation. Our experiences suggest that just because management believes that a certain time period is best for their athletes, this does not guarantee that the athletes will feel the same way.

Another consideration in planning career transition programs for elite athletes is the makeup of the groups. Although it is possible to get considerable individual difference among athletes on one team, these differences are likely to become magnified if the program is open to multiple teams. For example, in countries such as Australia, Canada, or the United States that have regional Olympic Training Centers, it is possible to have open enrollment programs with participants ranging from teenagers to adults in their fifties. Although there are advantages and disadvantages inherent in different models based on the size and homogeneity of the group makeup, these factors will influence program delivery and should be considered carefully in program planning. Among the questions to consider:

- What is the existing relationship among the athlete-participants?
- Are they a close-knit group or people who barely know each other?
- Are there any tensions or competitive relationships already existing?
- Do some of the athletes come from sports that have high visibility and considerable financial support?
- Are some of the athletes well-paid professionals and others amateurs who are financially dependent on their national governing bodies for support?
- What are the educational and career backgrounds of the participants?
- Where are the participants in terms of their sport career (i.e., beginning, midcareer, or retired)?

There are both advantages and disadvantages to running career transition groups that include athletes from several different sports. Diversity among participants can enrich discussions and provide insights and information that can be useful to all participants. The sharing of life and work experience in a heterogeneous group can provide a rich source of career information and open up new areas of exploration. Participants may also feel less self-conscious in a group of strangers than they would if they are with only their teammates. These advantages are reinforced by research from the social support literature that suggests that the density of a group (i.e., how well everyone in the group knows each other) can inhibit exploration and the breadth of career information available (Pearson & Petitpas, 1990).

Unfortunately, there are also several potential disadvantages in running career transition programs with heterogeneous groups. At times, diversity issues based on factors such as age, life experiences, work histories, and educational backgrounds can be overwhelming for certain group members. For example, one open-enrollment career development group offered by the United States Olympic Committee contained participants ranging from middle-aged males competing in yachting to teenage female gymnasts. Participants in another group ranged from rowers who had earned doctoral degrees to boxers who had dropped out of high school (Petitpas et al., 1992). Without sufficient planning or skillful leadership, older participants can become frustrated with the lack of career and life knowledge of younger participants. On the other hand, those athletes with minimal education who need to explore entry-level jobs may be overwhelmed by the backgrounds and opportunities of their college-educated peers. Several of these diversity concerns warrant more discussion.

Age differences of workshop participants can be considerable and are typically dependent on the nature of the sports involved. Female gymnasts, for example, are quite young in comparison to athletes in most sports. Their retirement from sport happens at an earlier time period than for most other athletes, and their career needs are more likely to involve educational planning and the gathering of further knowledge about their values, needs, interests, and skills. Contrast the experience of most gymnasts to that of rowers, who tend to be older, have some work experiences, and be typically well educated.

Career programs that are offered to heterogeneous groups must be highly flexible in order to accommodate age and life-stage differences. In planning such programs, it may be necessary not only to have available a wide range of self- and career-exploration materials, but also to format the program to take advantage of the various life experiences of the participants. Structuring group activities to require older and more experienced participants to assume the role of mentor or coach for younger athletes is one example of how this can be accomplished.

Educational background is another diversity issue that requires planning. Depending on the sport, either the athletes may have had little formal education, or they may have reached the top of their sport career while completing a college degree. Some athletes have had to rely on private tutors, whereas others attended inner-city public schools. An academically mixed group requires considerable planning to accommodate the needs of participants from radically diverse educational backgrounds, particularly as these backgrounds relate to the breadth of the career exploration possibilities. In addition, athletes who have participated in sports that require intensive and primary focus from a very early age may have had limited opportunities to engage in normative exploratory behavior and find themselves considerably behind their age-mates in self-knowledge (Petitpas & Champagne, 1988).

Cultural and socioeconomic differences can also present challenges in program planning. Participants' ethnicity, financial status, and living situations (e.g., urban versus rural or developed versus underdeveloped region of the world) can have an impact on their overall level of career aspiration, perceptions about the world of work, and career self-efficacy. These factors, in turn, may influence attitudes toward other group members or the amount of information and knowledge one has about potential careers.

It should be pointed out that these diversity issues could also exist within same sport groups. For example, in some countries, jumpers or Nordic combined skiers receive very little sponsor or national governing body financial support when compared to their Alpine downhill teammates. Financial differences are also quite evident between male and female participants in several professional sports.

Another within-sport difference that is normative among all sports is the athletic career stage of the participants. Are the athletes at the beginning, midpoint, preretirement, or retired stage of their sports involvement? Athletes in the beginning or midphase of their athletic career may not be interested in exploring postretirement careers at this stage in their athletic life cycle. However, those athletes who are at a later stage in their athletic career can underscore the importance of career exploration and endorse the efficacy of early preparation that can take place concurrently with the sport career.

Competition or perceived status among participants can also be problematic in career transition groups. Underlying tension, jealousy, or other distractions can sometimes emerge when the notoriety, financial resources, or status of individual participants dominates a group's focus. Although some of these issues can be circumvented by a skillful group facilitator, status or subgrouping concerns often occur and require careful management.

Planning the Structure and Content of Programs

The specific structure and content of sport career transition programs will be dictated by all the factors above. Structural considerations include decisions about the type of intervention, group size, program format and scheduling, and whether participation will be required or voluntary. Many times career interventions with elite athletes may have to be delivered in less than ideal situations because of the nature of the sport and the needs of the participants. It is often the case that convenience and accessibility will supersede preferred workshop formats in terms of both contact time and depth of topic coverage offered. As a result, program planners who are unable to schedule workshops may need to utilize other options such as individual counseling, keynote speakers, and panel discussions.

There are advantages and disadvantages to each programming option. Whereas workshops may be the best format to convey large amounts of information in a short amount of time and to facilitate an exchange of career knowledge and social support among participants, workshops are often the

Programming Options for Sport Career Transition Programs

• Workshops
  • Three-day immersion programs
  • Workshop series over a period of weeks
  • Single full-day workshop with follow-up individual sessions
• Individual counseling and career development
• Keynote speakers
• Panel discussions

most difficult to schedule in terms of access and availability. Individual counseling is the easiest to schedule, but requires the greatest number of career development specialists and fails to provide peer support for the transition process. Keynote speakers and panel discussions can provide initial motivation for career exploration, but fail to provide the continuity of contact or social support necessary to maintain the self- and career-exploration process.

If a workshop program option is elected, the format of the workshop or the workshop series will be highly dependent upon the availability of the participants. Various workshop formats can be used, such as a 3-day immersion program, a series of workshops over a period of weeks, or a single full-day session with follow-up counseling or individual sessions. Three-day programs, which are sometimes the most difficult to schedule, allow for the development of group cohesion and synergy, intense focus on career issues, and increased rapport with the program presenters. Additionally, participants have more opportunities outside of the workshop hours to interact with spokespersons and other participants and share experiences in an informal atmosphere.

An easier format to schedule is a series of workshops that occur over a period of weeks. Such workshops enable participants to work intensely for a single day, digest and utilize the information gained from the session, and return for discussion and assistance. Additionally, program presenters can offer "homework" assignments in the areas of career exploration or job hunting, which will be followed up upon in later sessions. Disadvantages of the series approach include the loss of momentum if the series is not offered in a short span of time and the possibility that some participants may have to miss one or more of the workshops. In the latter case, program presenters will have to provide information to those who have missed sessions and reintroduce group members at each session.

With even more time restrictions, program planners may have to offer a single day workshop with follow-up counseling or individual sessions. Because single day sessions are so brief, presenters are often faced with the problem of having a great deal of information to convey in a short amount of time. Often, experiential and group work aspects of the program are sacrificed in order to accomplish the goals of the workshop. In some situations, however, it may be more important to sacrifice some program content, such as job-hunting techniques, for the sake of allowing time for group discussion about transition from sport or career exploration outside of the field of sport. Follow-up counseling or individual sessions are often an ideal adjunct to the single workshop format because they allow participants time to discuss their individual needs. Individual sessions can be expensive, however, and require the availability of counseling staff, private office space, and a means of scheduling individual appointments.

Regardless of the workshop format, group size will be an important aspect of the overall functioning of the session. Groups that are very small (i.e., 6 or fewer) provide a great deal of opportunity for interaction and personal attention, but they lack the synergy of the larger groups. Similarly, they do not provide diversity of experiences in discussions. Groups of 10 to 18 can be most easily managed by a single group facilitator and permit both discussion and individual attention. Larger groups of more than 25 may require two facilitators, additional discussion time, and more group management. A particular problem that occurs in the larger group situation is that some members dominate the discussion while others become silent, not wanting to take up too much of the group's valuable time.

The choice of program format and schedule may also depend on whether or not participation in the career transition program is required or voluntary. In some instances, coaches or team management will require their athletes to participate in activities together. If so, scheduling and format would be dependent on the availability of the entire team. A possible advantage of mandated participation is that management may be more accommodating if they know that all their athletes are participating. Also, in required programs, some athletes may have access to information and experiences related to their careers that they initially thought was not important to them. On the other hand, group facilitators may find negative attitudes, indifference, lack of readiness, and resistance to ideas and self-disclosure on the part of some participants to be difficult to manage in a group setting.

When programs are voluntary, enthusiasm and motivation are more likely to come from the athletes themselves. This is particularly true when the athletes collaborate with career development specialists in program planning and structuring. When this is the case, the athletes are typically more committed to achieving program goals and often contribute energy and positive attitudes that can become motivational for all participants. In voluntary situations, however, some athletes who might benefit the most from career development information may choose not to participate.

Although determining the structure of the intervention is a critical aspect of program development, deciding on the content of the program is also important. In planning career transitions programs for elite athletes, the authors have found that a blend of traditional career development content and athlete-specific content is useful. Beyond the traditional career development content areas of self-exploration, career exploration, and job acquisition, elite athletes in transition typically need to manage the emotional aspects of separating from sport and begin the process of accepting sport as their first career (Petitpas, Champagne, Chartrand, Danish, & Murphy, 1997). Many athletes report feeling behind their age-mates in career skills and job experience. By reframing sport participation as a first career, athletes are often able to mollify their need to catch up with their age-peers and focus their attention on making sure that they have enough information to select a career path that is consistent with their interests, needs, values, and skills.

Program Content for Sport Career Transition Programs

- Management of emotions related to separation from sport
- Reframing of sport participation as a first career
- Self-exploration including issues of athletic identity
- Career exploration within and outside of sport
- Job acquisition

As with other aspects of program planning, the determination of program content should be based upon the needs of a particular group. "Canned programs" have not proven successful with many athletic groups. Teams, individual players, and circumstances are all unique. Information from team coaches and managers, informal surveys, and collaboration with team athletes prior to program planning are helpful in determining the special needs of each group. Diversity issues, discussed earlier, would be important considerations in all decisions about program content. For example, a group of college-educated athletes may need content areas that help them integrate their sports careers with their academic degrees. Younger athletes may need more self-exploration information and activities that help them in the selection of college majors or training programs.

Regardless of the content areas covered in the program, technology can be used to enhance the content and range of information available. In addition to the usual slides, computer-generated graphics, and other media, Internet resources can be integrated into the program content. The use of on-line inventories, job search resources, and Internet career information during the program not only enhances workshop offerings, but also provides information to participants about how to access career information at other sites after the career transition program is over. Lists of Internet resources and information for novices using the Internet would be essential items to hand out to participants.

Facilitating Sport Career Transition Programs

Although careful planning can go a long way to ensure that sports career transition programs run smoothly, it is inevitable that group management concerns will arise during the selected intervention. Understanding the makeup of the group and the unique dynamics of the sport career transition process is an important first step in group management for career development practitioners and group facilitators. This information can prove invaluable in anticipating potential problems and having planned activities or resources available. Emotional reactions, self-image, entitlement, and diversity are several of the most common issues that require skillful management.

Although many athletes choose to attend career transition programs to acquire the knowledge necessary to position themselves to get a job or start a new career, they often have to deal with the emotional meaning of leaving elite sport competition. Our experience suggests that many athletes, particularly those in the midst of disengaging from competition, experience emotions such as fear, sadness, and anger during their transition out of elite sport participation. Without getting into a lengthy discourse about the causes of these emotional reactions, there are often political, identity, and support system issues that must be addressed before these individuals are ready to engage in self-exploration activities. This does not imply that all these issues have to be resolved, but only that many athletes will need a safe forum in which to share their feelings.

Unfortunately, many transitioning athletes believe that few people understand what they are going through. As a result, the first task in any sport career transition intervention is to give the participants opportunities to express their feelings in a forum in which they feel understood. This can be accomplished through activities in which athlete spokespersons or those who have gone through the disengagement process self-disclose their experiences and encourage participants to do the same.

A related issue is what has been called the Olympic self-image (Petitpas et al., 1992). Athletes at elite levels are often revered by fans and placed on pedestals. As a result, it is sometimes difficult for these athletes to imagine themselves in anything but high-paying and high-visibility careers that will give them the same types of exciting and compelling experiences that they had during their athletic careers. It is often necessary to ask athletes to recall what it took for them to become elite performers. This will set the stage for looking at sports participation as a first career and for introducing the notion of transferable skills in order to accelerate their rate of advancement within a new career.

Some athletes, because of their celebrity status, may have developed a sense of entitlement. They assume that they will be given a great job because of their athletic achievements, and they may not be willing to start at the bottom level of a new career progression. If this kind of negative attitude surfaces, it can be destructive to group cohesion, and it requires immediate attention. Ironically, this expression of entitlement may be covering up feelings of fear or insecurities about lacking the skills necessary to become an elite performer in another career. Discussions about the strength and exclusivity of the athletic identity and self-disclosures by other elite athletes on how they used their transferable skills to jumpstart their new career can begin to foster a better sense of career self-efficacy for all participants.

The most common practical problem confronting sport career transition group facilitators is managing diversity among group participants. As discussed earlier, differences in age, education, socioeconomic background, and status among participants can be disadvantageous if not managed correctly. Five strategies that have proven helpful in managing diverse career groups are:

1. Review all instruments and activities planned to ensure that they do not contain material that could be insulting or condescending to any of the participants.
2. Come prepared with a wide range of examples and case studies in order to take advantage of teachable moments.
3. Divide larger group discussions into smaller subgroups or pairs based on clearly defined roles (e.g., older participants serve as mentors to younger participants) or individuals' ability to relate to one another.
4. Supplement the information distributed during the workshop with take-home materials that are individualized for the participant's specific career and personal situations.
5. Integrate some individual counseling and private consultation as part of the intervention or have such services available to supplement group work done during the workshops.

It is beyond the scope of this chapter to address all the challenging situations that can arise during a sport career transition workshop. Whether managing threats between participants or controlling sarcasm, group facilitators must not only be skillful group leaders, but also have credibility with the participants. At a minimum, group leaders must have a basic knowledge of the sport experience and a good sense of what athletes typically face during the process of disengagement from their sport. Credibility with the participants is earned by demonstrating a sincere interest in their unique experiences. It is not something that can be assumed or forced. Leaders must understand that their role is likely to be perceived as less important than that of the athlete spokespersons. In fact, during a series of transition programs offered by the United States Olympic Committee, retiring athletes rated the self-disclosures by athlete spokespersons about their emotional reactions to leaving sport and their use of transferable skills as far more important than any career development information presented by professional workshop facilitators (Petitpas, et al., 1992).

Postintervention Issues and Strategies

A common problem with most intervention programs is that there is not enough attention paid to the follow-up programs that are necessary to keep the career development process moving forward. Workshops and brief individual career consultations are typically effective in challenging attitudes, but they may not go far enough to ensure that participants continue to try new behaviors or put forth the effort necessary to result in an optimal transition to a new career.

Kelman (1958) provides a helpful framework for looking at the role of motivation in the change or skill acquisition process that underscores the importance of follow-up programming. This framework assumes that for behavior change to be lasting, individuals must move from an external to an internal locus of motivation. Athletes who attend career transition programs because attendance is mandated or who seek to gain external rewards or to avoid punishment are in a *compliance* level of motivation. Those athletes who attend programs simply because their peers are participating are conforming to peer expectations and exemplify an *identification* level of motivation. In both compliance and identification, the motivation to participate is externally based and quickly abandoned if social support or organizational affiliations change. For behavior change to occur, individuals must experience the benefits of the new behavior over a period of time. By so doing, the new behavior becomes functionally autonomous and intrinsically motivated. When this occurs, the person has reached the highest level of motivation, *internalization*.

Extrapolating from Kelman's (1958) framework, sport career transition programs are likely to be most effective if strategies are in place that will keep the career development momentum moving after the workshops or individual consultations have ended. Research from the counseling literature supports the belief that the longer individuals stay connected to a counselor or support group, the greater the likelihood of achieving the stated counseling goals (Sexton & Whiston, 1994). Therefore, in situations in which the sponsoring organization does not have an easily accessible career resource available, alternative support provisions have to be identified and integrated into the career program intervention. These resources can come from the local community, area colleges or universities, planned organization sponsored follow-up meetings, or even the Internet.

Career program participants should be encouraged to identify local resources and establish linkages that will provide them with the ongoing support necessary to achieve their career goals. Those athletes with college affiliations can typically use their college career center resources at no cost. These services can be accessed in person or via the Internet and provide athletes with a wide array of assessment and job-hunting services, as well as access to extensive alumni networks. Those individuals without college affiliations can typically tap into community college, adult education, or nonprofit organizations' career development resources at minimal costs.

Another effective method for keeping the career development momentum moving is the creation of local support groups among participants or local retired athletes. Exchanging contact information and arranging for periodic meetings to share experiences and resources promote continued attention to the career development process. Support-group membership can be expanded to include present or former Olympic and professional athletes who reside in the area, as well as key contacts from the business and professional community. In addition, the support network can be expanded further by establishing Web sites and Internet interest groups.

Whatever the vehicle, it is important to ensure that workshop participants have or create a means to follow up on the knowledge and strategies acquired during the career transition workshop or individual consultations. When discussing the possibility of implementing career transition workshops with sport governing-body officials, it is advantageous to build in planned organization-sponsored follow-up activities. If this is not logistically feasible, then linkages with community resources should be investigated prior to program implementation.

Conclusion

The purpose of this chapter was to introduce practitioners to some of the practical considerations involved in planning and implementing sport career transition programs for elite athletes. These practical considerations included logistical and planning concerns that need to be taken into consideration prior to the program, issues that are often encountered during the program, and recommendations for follow-up activities after the program has ended. A major conclusion that can be drawn from all of the information provided in this chapter is that career transition program planning and implementation for elite athletes must be tailored to the unique needs and circumstances of the specific team or participant group. Athletes have a variety of experiences and come from diverse educational, cultural, and socioeconomic backgrounds. As a result, career development and sport psychology practitioners are often required to use creative and adaptive approaches when working with this highly specialized population. Guidelines and recommendations for program development can be gleaned from this chapter, but the skills and abilities of the program planners and facilitators will ultimately determine the success of any sport career transition program.

References

Kelman, H. C. (1958). Compliance, identification, and internalization: Three processes of opinion change. *Journal of Conflict Resolution, 2,* 51–60.

Pearson, R., & Petitpas, A. (1990). Transitions of athletes: Developmental and preventive perspectives. *Journal of Counseling and Development, 69,* 7–10.

Petitpas, A., & Champagne, D. (1988). Developmental programming for intercollegiate athletes. *Journal of College Student Personnel, 29,* 454–460.

Petitpas, A., Champagne, D., Chartrand, J., Danish, S., & Murphy, S. (1997). *Athlete's guide to career planning: Keys to success from the playing field to professional life.* Champaign, IL: Human Kinetics.

Petitpas, A., Danish, S., McKelvain, R., & Murphy, S. (1992). A career assistance program for elite athletes. *Journal of Counseling and Development, 70,* 383–386.

Sexton, & Whiston (1994). The status of the counseling relationship: An empirical review, theoretical implications, and research directions. *The Counseling Psychologist, 22,* 6–78.

Werthner, P., & Orlick, T. (1986). Retirement experiences of successful Olympic athletes. *International Journal of Sport Psychology, 17,* 337–363.

6

Transferable Skills for Career Change

Lisa Mayocchi
Stephanie J. Hanrahan
The University of Queensland
Australia

Abstract

In promoting the positive and beneficial aspects of athletics, it is often claimed that sport experiences help athletes to develop qualities or skills that are important for athletic achievement, as well as for success outside of the sporting domain (Petitpas & Schwartz, 1989). Skills that may be applied to various domains are described as transferable skills and have recently been considered by counselors who conduct career assistance programs for athletes and dancers. This chapter explores the concept of transferable skills, discusses in detail the types of skills that athletes may transfer from sport to work, and draws upon research and literature from the field of organizational psychology to examine the factors that may help or hinder transfer of skills. Finally, implications for practitioners, researchers, athletes, coaches, parents, and employers are highlighted.

Transferable Skills for Career Change

Transferable skills, also known as life skills, are skills that are potentially transferable to any field or career, regardless of where they were first learned or developed (Bolles, 1996). Most transferable skills are context and content free and contain little, if any, suggestion of their specific or intended application (Wiant, 1977). According to Wiant, the more specific the description of the skill, the more limited its usefulness and applicability. When the difference between two occupations is large, the skills that are transferred from one to the other tend to be abstract. To illustrate this point, consider the example of a baseball player whose second career is as a salesperson. A specific skill such as being able to throw a ball hard is considered to be critical for success for the athlete who plays baseball, but is not necessary for effective performance in that person's nonathletic career as a salesperson. The skill of throwing a ball hard has a specific, intended application for the person involved in baseball. In contrast, concentration skills may be important for effective performance in a variety of settings, including competing in a javelin event, chairing a corporate board meeting, or performing in dance.

Figure 1 depicts the skill transfer process (adapted from Alliger, Bennett, & Tannenbaum, 1995) for an athlete moving from a sporting career to a nonathletic career. As can be seen in the figure, skill transfer involves individuals' applying the same skill—in this case goal setting—in the sporting environment, as well as in their nonathletic careers.

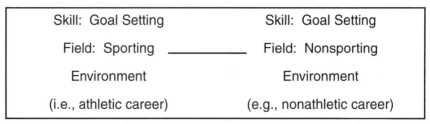

Figure 1. The skill transfer process.

Why Examine Transferable Skills in the Career Change Setting?

Research findings indicate that athletes are interested in learning how to transfer their mental skills from sport to their new career or interest (Sinclair & Orlick, 1993), and they become concerned about the transferability of their knowledge and skills when considering retirement from sport (Swain, 1991). It has also been demonstrated that athletes respond positively to being taught about transferable skills (Petitpas, Danish, McKelvain, & Murphy, 1992). Finally, it has been stated that in today's ever changing work environment, those employees who have flexible work attitudes and transferable skills (or who are able to attain them) are likely to be the ones who succeed (Hesketh, 1997). The above statements highlight several key reasons why researchers and practitioners have discussed and investigated the role of transferable skills for career change.

In a survey designed to determine the career assistance needs of athletes who had participated in the Olympics or Pan American Games, respondents indicated a preference for identifying transferable skills and preparing for the transition out of active sport competition over and above workshops related to résumé preparation or job interview strategies (Petitpas et al., 1992). The resulting workshop focused on three main topics: managing the impact of transitions, increasing understanding/awareness of personal qualities relevant to coping with transitions or career development, and introducing information about the world of work. Upon completion of the program, the transferable-skills presentation was rated as the most useful content area. It appeared to increase athletes' confidence that their skills could be used in other settings and challenged some of the athletes' doubts about their ability to begin a new career (Petitpas et al., 1992). Given these findings, a greater understanding of the process of skill transfer is likely to be of value and interest to practitioners who work with athletes as they undergo career change.

What Skills Transfer From Sport to Work?

Within the career transition literature, several lists that contain examples of life skills/transferable skills have been compiled (e.g., Danish, Petitpas & Hale, 1993; United States Olympic Committee, 1993). Table 1 presents a selection of these skills.

Table 1
Examples of Commonly Cited Transferable Skills or Life Skills

1. Ability to perform under pressure

2. Problem-solving skills

3. Organizational skills

4. Ability to meet deadlines/challenges

5. Ability to set and attain goals

6. Dedication and perseverance

7. Self-motivation

8. Patience

9. Adaptability/flexibility

10. Ability to recognize one's limitations

A recent investigation (Mayocchi, 1999) involving in-depth interviews with 50 elite athletes who had made the transition from a sporting career to a nonathletic career supported the notion that athletes possess a wide variety of transferable skills. There was a high level of similarity between the skills typically cited in lists of transferable skills (e.g., see Table 1) and those described by the athletes interviewed in the study. Interestingly, the study revealed several types of knowledge, skills, abilities, and personal characteristics not traditionally included in lists of transferable skills for athletes. These are listed in Table 2 and are described in more detail below.

Table 2
Transferable Skills Identified During In-Depth Interviews With Athletes (Mayocchi, 1998)

Type of transferable skill	The skill as described by athletes
Interpersonal	People skills; social skills; ability to mix with people; ability to get along with people; ability to deal with people (e.g., media, tv, sponsors)
Team related	Ability to contribute in a team to work toward a common goal; knowing how to be a team player; knowing how to work as a team to reach the final goal
Supervisory/leadership	Coaching skills; leadership skills; managerial ability; people management skills; ability to motivate people to work well; ability to provide regular feedback on performance
Management and administrative skills	Administrative skills; financial management skills
Understanding and comprehension	Understanding of skills development; understanding of teamwork; understanding of individual differences
Self-assurance	Assertiveness; ability to say what one thinks; confidence; willingness to do things one's own way
Ambition	Will to win; will to succeed; competitiveness; desire to be the best
Will	Determination; single-mindedness

Athletes developed their interpersonal skills through contact with coaches and teammates in competition and training. They also developed these skills through their interaction with politicians, journalists, and sponsors. One athlete believed his "people skills" were put to good use during the job interview for his current place of employment. Through their experience in a variety of sports, and particularly for athletes who were in the role of "captain" of their team, athletes developed a better understanding of certain elements that are critical to a supervisory or leadership role. These included knowing how far you can push people and knowing what motivates people as well as having the ability to get people to work as a team and an ability to persuade.

Financial management and general administrative skills were also developed by some athletes as a result of involvement in high-performance sport, not directly from training and competition but rather through other activities associated with their sport. Sporting experiences also helped heighten athletes' understanding of topics such as skill development, job requirements, and teamwork, as well as a better appreciation of individual differences. Being self-assured (i.e., confident, assertive), ambitious (i.e., having a competitive spirit, wanting to be the best), and willful (i.e., determined and single-minded) were characteristics mentioned by athletes from a variety of sports, such as rifle shooting, decathlon, and cricket, as being useful in both their sport and the workplace.

In addition to identifying some transferable skills not traditionally cited in lists of transferable skills, the data collected during the interviews (Mayocchi, 1999) provided some specific, real-life examples that may assist practitioners and researchers to better understand how athletes have transferred skills from the sporting domain to the nonsports domain. Three quotes taken directly from the interviews conducted with the retired elite athletes (Mayocchi) are shown in the examples (Examples 1a-1c) below.

Example 1a. Goal setting and planning.

At the start of a cricket season or a sporting season you set yourself certain goals. If you're a batsman, you set yourself to score so many runs. Or if you're a bowler, wickets. I suppose another characteristic is planning. You've got to plan. There's no doubt about that. You know if you're setting goals, you can't just expect to turn up and let it happen. You've got to plan it . . . Just like I plan my work situation. As you can see from the plan on the wall, I plan 6 to 8 months, sometimes 12 months ahead. And I used to do that while I was playing cricket. —(From cricket to public relations officer)

Example 1b. Perseverance.

. . . this job . . . it's been really tough. Lots of times I've felt like walking away from it, but I've kept at it because I've wanted to succeed. I didn't want it to beat me. So, yeah, a real perseverance and . . . setting my mind to be there for the long run because . . . the Olympics were 4 years apart . . . everything was on a really long time scale where you're training now, but the event is 12 months away. So you set yourself for a long effort.

—(From track and field to architect)

Example 1c. Supervisory skills.

If you get too far apart, you know, the us and them thing, you don't get very good work results . . . They'll work when you're there but when you turn around they'll stop . . . if you can get them all to work, and that probably comes back to the bowling thing, if you can get them to work as a team and they can all feel a part of the one group, it works a lot better.

—(From ten-pin bowling to foreperson in a factory)

What Skills Do Not Transfer?

If athletes fear that certain skills or characteristics will be viewed as unacceptable or undesirable in the workplace, it is unlikely these skills will be transferred to the work setting. Single-mindedness, selfishness, and aggression have been described by retired elite athletes in this light (Mayocchi, 1999). In a similar vein, Parker (1994) reported that former football players regarded behaviors such as aggression to be tolerated and in some cases encouraged in sport, but found that these behaviors were not positively transferable to life outside of sport.

What Influences Skill Transfer?

As noted earlier in this chapter, transferable skills are defined as being *potentially* transferable to any field or career. Given that skill transfer is never guaranteed, the following section draws upon research and literature from the field of industrial/organizational psychology to help examine some of the reasons that athletes do or do not transfer their skills from sport to other areas of their life.

In recent years, an increasing number of researchers have begun to forge links between industrial/organizational psychology, which is concerned with behavior in work situations (Muchinsky, 1993), and sport psychology. For example, Locke and Latham's (1985) article in the *Journal of Sport Psychol-*

ogy brought together some of the findings of research conducted in organizational settings on goal setting and considered its application to sports. Similarly, this section of the chapter describes some of the key findings of research on organizational transfer of training and discusses the implications of these findings for career transitions and, in particular, the transfer of skills from sport to the nonsport setting.

For many years, researchers and practitioners within the field of organizational and industrial psychology have puzzled over one of the key dilemmas of training. That is, skills learned in the training setting do not automatically transfer to the workplace. Factors related to the individual and to the work environment can enhance or stand in the way of transfer of training (Baldwin & Ford, 1988; Foxon, 1993, 1994; Mathieu, Tannenbaum, & Salas, 1992; Mayocchi, 1999; Mayocchi & Hanrahan, 1997). Individual characteristics include levels of skill awareness, motivation to transfer skills, motivation to do well in the new occupation, and self-efficacy. Factors within the work environment include job clarity, job control, rules and restrictions, and support from supervisors and coworkers. The impact of these factors on skill transfer is highlighted below. To assist the reader's understanding of how these factors enhance or inhibit the transfer of skills, where relevant, direct quotes from interviews with athletes who have made the transition to a nonsporting career have been included (Mayocchi, 1999, see Examples 2a-2d).

Individual Characteristics

Perceived value and levels of skill awareness. A common concern heard from athletes at Career Assistance Program for Athletes' seminars is "I'm just an athlete, I don't know how to do anything else" (Murphy, 1995, p. 341). Without an understanding of the value of the types of skills that they possess, and an awareness of when certain skills may be applicable in different settings (Yelon, 1992), it is likely that skill transfer will occur by chance or unintentionally, if at all. Therefore, the challenge is to help athletes realize and identify what physical and psychological skills they have developed through sport, so that where relevant, these skills will be applied in different settings. The Career Assistance Program for Athletes seminars devote a large segment of the program to helping athletes realize the variety of skills they have learned through sports participation, and the ways in which these skills can be targeted at potential employers in new career areas. The importance of believing in the value of the skills learned or knowledge gained is highlighted in the research findings of Baumgartel, Reynolds, and Pathan (1984). They found that managers who believed in the value of their training for their job were more likely to apply the skills learned in training.

Motivation and job enthusiasm. If athletes are to apply their skills to their nonathletic careers, they must have the motivation to do so. Research findings in organizational training suggest that individuals will be more likely to transfer their skills when they are motivated to put those skills into practice (Martineau, 1996). In two separate studies conducted by Mayocchi and Hanrahan (1997)—the first with 242 retired athletes from a variety of sports and the second involving 135 retired professional Australian Rules football players—athletes who reported that they found their job interesting and challenging, and who were motivated to do well in their job, were more likely to apply transferable skills in their nonathletic careers. These skills included determination, persistence, and goal setting. Conversely, those who were not interested in their job, and were not motivated to do well in their job, were less likely to transfer their skills from sport to the work setting.

Example 2a. High motivation facilitating skill transfer.
It's really come to the fore just recently. There wasn't an immediate follow-on . . . when I finished my sports career and was getting into my working career I was . . . a bit lost and was probably really slow starting off, but now I think the skills I learnt as an athlete have really come to the fore and that's like determination to succeed . . . because things have been pretty tough in this job, and that probably needs a bit of explanation, but this was my first civil design job, and there's a lot more responsibility and a lot more onus on the designs I come up with in engineering whereas the jobs I had before weren't.

Example 2b. Low motivation hindering skill transfer.
I didn't really set any goals [at work] because that wasn't my ultimate goal.

Self-efficacy. Self-efficacy is defined as "people's judgments of their capabilities to organize and execute courses of action required to attain designated types of performance" (Bandura, 1986, p. 391). As noted by Bandura (1977), people fear and tend to avoid a situation if they believe that it will exceed their coping skills, whereas they will become involved in activities and behave confidently if they perceive they are capable of handling the situation. If individuals perceive a lack of support from others at work or a lack of resources to do the job, they may persist in trying to transfer their skills if they possess high levels of self-efficacy, but they may cease all transfer attempts if they are less certain of their abilities. Recent research findings (Mayocchi & Hanrahan, 1997) support this claim. In a study involving 242 individuals who had competed in sport at an elite level, the relationship between athletes' use of skills in sport and use of those same skills at work was most evident for those individuals with high levels of self-efficacy.

Example 2c. Low confidence in ability to do the job leading to low levels of skill transfer.

I'm not inhibited at all when it comes to a soccer ball, and I'm always confident with soccer and stuff. Sometimes with nursing it's a bit iffy, and I don't always feel confident.

Characteristics Related to the Work Environment

Level of job autonomy. Job autonomy refers to the degree to which a job provides substantial freedom, independence, and discretion to the employee in scheduling his or her work and in determining the procedures to carry it out (Hackman & Oldham, 1976, 1980). Interviews with 50 athletes who had retired from elite-level sporting competition (Mayocchi, 1999) indicated that a lack of control over the way they performed their work was a particular hindrance to skill transfer. In contrast, having a supervisor who allowed them a great deal of autonomy and the ability to self-plan was viewed as a positive feature of the workplace. Three athletes believed that being self-employed, and as a result having no supervisor, provided them with the freedom to be able to apply skills they believed were relevant, from sport to their workplace. Interestingly, this finding was not supported in later empirical studies by Mayocchi and Hanrahan (1997), which included measures of job control.

Rules and restrictions in the work environment have been described by athletes as a hindrance to skill transfer (Mayocchi, 1999). Specifically, these factors include organizational politics, the policies and procedures to be followed, and corporation ethos. In organizations that contained many rules and restrictions, several athletes found it difficult to apply skills such as goal setting, evaluative skills, and a general use of initiative.

Example 2d. High levels of rules and restrictions inhibiting skill transfer.

I know that in a corporation I personally feel closed in and restricted. That's because I'm one of those sorts of people who like to . . . plan and get things done and then say let's evaluate. Did we do it or didn't we do it, and if we didn't, what went wrong? So I guess I'm more practical oriented in as much as getting results which you think the corporations would appreciate. But there are certain ways of doing things.

Relations with supervisors and coworkers. Depending on the workplace, supervisors and coworkers have been described by athletes as either a help or a hindrance to skill transfer. Some athletes found that support and help from others at work, as well as recognition and encouragement from supervisors, assisted with skill transfer. In contrast, poor supervisory relations, a lack of openness by others to new ideas, negative reactions in general by others to the athlete being in the workplace, and a lack of a team environment were all features of the work environment that hindered skill transfer. In a study involving 242 athletes from a variety of sports, the relationship between use of skills in sport and use of those same skills at work was more marked for individuals who reported high, rather than low, levels of encouragement and recognition for good performance from their supervisors (Mayocchi & Hanrahan, 1997). Thus, feedback from supervisors was found to have a significant impact on skill transfer.

Strategies for Enhancing the Likelihood of Skill Transfer

Methods for enhancing skill transfer have been described by researchers and practitioners from fields such as human performance technology, industrial/organizational psychology, cognitive psychology, sport psychology and counseling psychology (Danish, Petitpas & Hale, 1993; Foxon, 1994; Garavaglia, 1993; Hesketh, Chandler & Andrews, 1988; Nisbet & Shucksmith, 1986; Reber & Wallin, 1984; Sternberg, 1987; Yelon, 1992). A variety of these methods are listed in Table 3. As shown in the table, motivating trainees to use their skills effectively, increasing individuals' awareness that they actually possess transferable skills, and providing both physical and psychological support during attempts at skill transfer have been suggested as possible ways to create a good environment for transfer to occur. Suggestions for the specific application of three of the methods listed in Table 2 (i.e., goal setting, feedback, and action planning) are described in more detail below. For a more detailed description of the other methods listed in Table 2, the reader is directed to the above-cited sources.

Goal Setting and Feedback

Goal setting is an effective motivational strategy for assisting behavioural change in a variety of settings (Locke &·Latham,), and has recently been considered in terms of its ability to help individuals with the process of skill transfer. Goal setting is specifically recommended for use in combination with feedback, to enhance skill transfer (Reber & Wallin, 1984). Within the career counseling setting, counselors may wish to encourage athletes to discuss the

Table 3
Methods to Enhance Skill Transfer

1. Motivate trainees to use their skills

2. Increase awareness of learners that they possess transferable skills

3. Increase awareness of when to use skills

4. Enable trainees to master and apply their skills

5. Provide psychological and physical support

6. Illustrate the underlying principles

7. Teach and model the skills of learning

8. Teach skills with transfer in mind

9. Teach how and in what context the skills are/were learned

10. Provide domain-specific information: Place it in context

11. Deal with the fear of trying and failing a new task

12. Encourage athletes to set some specific goals for skill transfer

13. Provide feedback to athletes about their attempts/efforts to transfer their skills

14. Develop action plans to help trainees anticipate and resolve possible transfer problems

various ways in which they could apply their skills and to set some specific goals for skill transfer that are challenging, yet realistic and achievable. An assessment of the level of situational constraints that exist in the individual's work environment should also occur during the goal-setting phase, because, if severe, situational constraints may act as a barrier to the individual's reaching his or her goals.

Action Plans

Yelon (1992) and Foxon (1994) advocated the use of action plans to help trainees anticipate and resolve possible transfer problems. Action planning results in written commitments to action that are determined by the individual. In the case of the career counselor teaching athletes about transferable skills, the following questions (based on the general approach outlined by Foxon) may be useful to consider within the action planning context:

1. What skills, knowledge or characteristics would be relevant for you to apply to your new career?
2. What specifically will you need to do in order to apply your skills, knowledge or characteristics in your new career? That is, what steps will you need to take to be able to apply these skills?
3. How will you know if you have successfully applied your skills? (Write down some observable behaviors that will give you evidence of application.)
4. What difficulties might you encounter in applying these skills, and what strategies will you employ to overcome these difficulties?

Implications

For Athletes

As noted by Danish et al. (1993), one of the barriers to skill transfer may be that athletes are not aware of the skills they have developed through sport that are transferable to other areas of their life. By increasing athletes' awareness of the skills that they possess, they may be more likely to try to use those skills that are relevant in their nonsport setting. Teaching athletes about transferable skills can increase athletes' confidence that their skills can be used in a variety of settings (not just in their nonathletic careers), and can challenge athletes' doubts about their ability to begin a new career (Petitpas et al., 1992). Increased awareness of the skills they possess may also help athletes improve their performance in their athletic career, through heightened awareness of the role that certain skills can play in their sporting performance. In developing a better understanding of the skills they possess, athletes place themselves in a better position of being able to explain what skills they have to potential employers and to describe how these skills are important for high performance on the job.

Research findings suggest that a number of factors influence athletes' motivation and ability to transfer their skills from sport to the workplace. Before athletes make the decision to embark upon a particular nonathletic career or to accept a job in a certain workplace, they may wish to consider the following questions of themselves, their potential employer and/or place of employment:

- Am I interested in this type of work?
- Will I find it challenging? That is, will there be opportunities and cause for me to apply my skills?
- Am I motivated to do well in the job? Am I motivated to progress/advance further in the position?

- Do I personally believe I have the ability to carry out the tasks/activities I will be required to do as part of the job?
- Are there any formal qualifications I need to perform in this job effectively? Do I have them? If not, how do I go about acquiring them?
- What skills do I have that I may be able to apply in this new occupation and/or job?
- What sorts of opportunities are there for training and career development?
- Can my employer clearly convey to me what I will be required to do in the job? Do others in the organization clearly understand their job requirements?
- How much control will I have over the way I perform my work? Will I have the freedom to apply skills from sport to work that I think are relevant?
- Does my supervisor understand what skills I will bring to the workplace? Will my supervisor be supportive of me attempting to apply skills from sport to the workplace? Will my supervisor be supportive of new ideas and new ways of doing things? What about my coworkers?
- Will the job meet my personal needs in terms of encouragement and recognition?
- Will there be strict rules, regulations, and procedures to follow?
- What are the links between the skills I applied in my sport and those that will be required of me in this job?

For Coaches and Parents

Coaches and parents have a role to play in helping increase athletes' awareness of the skills they possess and in encouraging athletes to consider how and when these skills could be applied to other settings. These other areas of their life may be career related, social, or even financial. For example, skills such as goal setting and planning may be useful for athletes in terms of day-to-day performance on the job, as well as for long-term career planning. These skills may also be useful in terms of athletes setting longer-term goals for the personal or social side of their life, such as travelling, buying a car, or learning a new language.

For Career Transition Program Facilitators

As discussed earlier in this chapter, a number of career assistance programs already contain components that focus upon helping athletes learn about transferable skills. The additional knowledge, skills, abilities and personal characteristics that emerged from analysis of 50 interviews with retired athletes (Mayocchi, 1999) may provide some additional ideas for counselors working with athletes, in terms of the types of skills that transfer. In addition, there is potential for counselors to move beyond exploring what types of skills are transferable, to exploring the potential barriers to skill transfer. By doing so, athletes may be better prepared to cope with these hindrances to skill transfer if they do arise. In particular, teaching athletes to use strategies such as goal setting and action planning may help them prepare for and work out ways to counter the possible barriers to skill transfer.

For Employers

Within the field of organizational training transfer, there is a growing body of literature that emphasizes the importance of the work environment for effective and enduring skill transfer. As discussed, characteristics in the work environment such as job clarity, job control, relations with coworkers and supervisors, and the number of rules and restrictions operating in the work environment can all affect athletes' attempts to transfer their skills. There is great potential for employers to facilitate the skill transfer process for athletes who are beginning a new career or job. Research evidence suggests that recognition and encouragement from supervisors can have a positive effect on skill transfer (e.g., Mayocchi & Hanrahan, 1997). If employers are genuinely interested in helping athletes to transfer their skills, it is suggested that they meet individually with athletes to discuss the types of skills they believe could usefully be brought to the job.

For Researchers

Research findings in the area of transferable skills and their application by athletes in nonsporting careers must be regarded as preliminary. It is recommended that future research be conducted in this area. Specifically, researchers may wish to examine the following questions:

- When and how do athletes develop the skills regarded as transferable?
- Is effective skill transfer related to adjustment to the transition out of elite sporting competition?
- How do individual characteristics and work-environment characteristics affect skill transfer? That is, what is the nature of the relationship?
- For athletes who engage in a second nonathletic career while they are still pursuing their sporting career, what is the potential for skills learned at work to be transferred back to the sport setting?

Conclusion

This chapter has examined career change and skill transfer within the context of athletes undergoing retirement from sport. Drawing upon recent research and literature within the field of sport psychology, a variety of transferable skills were described, including goal setting and problem solving, as well as some skills not traditionally listed in the sport psychology literature, such as supervisory/leadership skills. The chapter then turned to consider a key question asked by practitioners and researchers within the field of retirement from sport: What factors help or hinder athletes' attempts to transfer their skills from sport to the nonsporting domain? It was noted that characteristics related to the individual and the work environment may influence the skill transfer process, either positively or negatively. It is hoped that through a greater understanding of transferable skills, and of the factors that can influence skill transfer, researchers and practitioners may better facilitate athletes' adjustment process to their second or postathletic careers.

References

Alliger, G. M., Bennett, W., & Tannenbaum, S. I. (1995). *Transfer of training: Comparison of paradigms.* Paper presented at the annual conference of the Society for Industrial and Organizational Psychology, Orlando, FL.

Baldwin, T. T., & Ford, J. K. (1988). Transfer of training: A review and directions for future research. *Personnel Psychology, 41,* 63–105.

Bandura, A. (1977). Self-efficacy: Toward a unifying theory of behavioral change. *Psychological Review, 84,* 191–215.

Bandura, A. (1986). *Social foundations of thought and action.* Englewood Cliffs, NJ: Prentice-Hall.

Baumgartel, H., Reynolds, M., & Pathan, R. (1984). How personality and organizational-climate variables moderate the effectiveness of management development programmes: A review and some recent research findings. *Management and Labor Studies, 9,* 1–16.

Bolles, R. N. (1996). *What color is your parachute: A practical manual for job-hunters and career-changers.* Berkeley, CA: Ten Speed Press.

Danish, S. J., Petitpas, A. J., & Hale, B. D. (1993). Life development intervention for athletes: Life skills through sports. *The Counseling Psychologist, 21,* 352–385.

Foxon, M. (1993). A process approach to the transfer of training: I. The impact of motivation and supervisor support on transfer maintenance, *Australian Journal of Educational Technology, 9,* 130–143.

Foxon, M. (1994). A process approach to the transfer of training: II. Using action planning to facilitate the transfer of training. *Australian Journal of Educational Technology, 10,* 1–18.

Garavaglia, P. L. (1993). How to ensure transfer of training. *Training and Development,* 63–68.

Hackman, J. R., & Oldham, G. R. (1976). Motivation through the design of work: Test of a theory. *Organizational Behavior and Human Performance, 21,* 289–304.

Hackman, J. R., & Oldham, G. R. (1980). *Work redesign.* Reading, MA: Addison-Wesley.

Hesketh, B. (1997). Dilemmas in training for transfer and retention. *Applied Psychology, 46,* 317–386.

Hesketh, B., Chandler, P., & Andrews, S. (1988). Training for transfer: Developing learning skills. *The Australian TAFE Teacher,* 51–56.

Locke, E. A., & Latham, G. P. (1984). *Goal setting: A motivational tool that works.* Englewood Cliffs, NJ.: Prentice-Hall.

Locke, E. A., & Latham, G. P. (1985). The application of goal setting to sports. *Journal of Sport Psychology, 7,* 205–222.

Martineau, J. W. (1996, April). *A contextual examination of the effectiveness of a supervisory skills training program.* Paper presented at the annual conference of the Society for Industrial and Organizational Psychology, San Diego, CA.

Mathieu, J. E., Tannenbaum, S. I., & Salas, E. (1992). Influences of individual and situational characteristics on measures of training effectiveness. *Academy of Management Journal, 35,* 828–847.

Mayocchi, L. (1999). *Transferable skills and the process of skill transfer: The athlete's experience.* Unpublished doctoral dissertation, The University of Queensland, Brisbane, Australia.

Mayocchi, L., & Hanrahan, S. J. (1997). *Adaptation to a post-athletic career: The role of transferable skills.* Belconnen, ACT: Australian Sports Commission.

Murphy, S. M. (1995). Transitions in competitive sport: Maximizing individual potential. In S. M. Murphy (Ed.), *Sport psychology interventions* (pp. 331–346). Champaign, IL: Human Kinetics.

Nisbet, J., & Shucksmith, J. (1986). *Learning strategies.* London: Routledge.

Parker, K. B. (1994). "Has-beens" and "wanna-bes": Transition experiences of former major college football players. *The Sport Psychologist, 8,* 287–304.

Petitpas, A., Danish, S., McKelvain, R., & Murphy, S. (1992). A career assistance program for elite athletes. *Journal of Counseling and Development, 70,* 383–386.

Petitpas, A., & Schwartz, H. (1989). Assisting student athletes in understanding and identifying transferable skills. *The Academic Athletic Journal, 6,* 37–42.

Reber, R. A., & Wallin, J. A. (1984). The effects of training, goal setting, and knowledge of results on safe behavior: A component analysis. *Academy of Management Journal, 27,* 544–560.

Sinclair, D. A., & Orlick, T. (1993). Positive transitions from high-performance sport. *The Sport Psychologist, 7,* 138–150.

Sternberg, R. J. (1987). Questions and answers about the nature and teaching of thinking skills. In J. B. Baron and R. J. Sternberg (Eds.), *Teaching thinking skills: Theory and practice* (pp. 251–260). New York: Freeman and Company.

Swain, D. A. (1991). Withdrawal from sport and Schlossberg's model of transitions. *Sociology of Sport Journal, 8,* 152–160.

United States Olympic Committee (1993). *Positioning yourself for success: An employment counseling handbook for athletes.* Colorado Springs: Author.

Wiant, A. A. (1977). *Transferable skills: The employer's viewpoint.* Columbus, OH: National Center for Research in Vocational Education.

Yelon, S. (1992). M.A.S.S.: A model for producing transfer. *Performance Improvement Quarterly, 5 (2),* 13–23.

Author Note

Funding for the research described in this chapter (Mayocchi & Hanrahan, 1997) was provided in part by a grant from The Applied Sports Research Program and the Australian Sports Commission.

7

Intervention Strategies for Athletes in Transition

David Lavallee
University of Teesside
England

Mark Nesti and Erika Borkoles
Leeds Metropolitan University
England

Ian Cockerill and Amanda Edge
The University of Birmingham
England

Abstract

Research reveals that a population of athletes exists who require(d) considerable personal adjustment to career transitions from sport. In this chapter, the authors present three intervention strategies for practitioners working with athletes in transition. These approaches include an information processing approach, mentoring, and an existential psychology approach.

Intervention Strategies for Athletes in Transition

A growing body of empirical research is emerging on psychological adjustment difficulties experienced by athletes in transition (Lavallee, Sinclair, & Wylleman, 1998; Lavallee, Wylleman, & Sinclair, 1998). Notwithstanding this increase in research, there exists considerable debate regarding the number of athletes who experience distressful reactions to retirement from sport. Numerous empirical studies have suggested that a significant number of elite athletes experience transition-related distress (e.g., Allison & Meyer, 1988; Werthner & Orlick, 1986). At the same time, several contrasting studies have revealed minimal or no evidence of adjustment difficulties associated with athletic career transition (e.g., Curtis & Ennis, 1988; Greendorfer & Blinde, 1985). An issue that has been overlooked in this debate, however, is how to assist the population of athletes who require treatment of transitional-related difficulties.

A review of the literature indicates that 14 studies have specifically examined and documented adjustment difficulties associated with career transitions in sport (Aflermann & Gross, 1997; Allison & Meyer, 1988; Blinde & Stratta, 1992; Curtis & Ennis, 1988; Greendorfer & Blinde, 1985; Lavallee, Gordon, & Grove, 1997; McInnally, Cavin-Stice, & Knoth, 1992; Parker, 1994; Sinclair & Orlick, 1993; Svoboda & Vanek, 1982; Webb, Nasco, Riley, & Headrick, 1998; Werthner & Orlick, 1986; Wylleman, De Knop, Menkehorst, Theeboom, & Annerel, 1993; Zaichkowsky, Lipton, & Tucci1997). The athletes in these studies (N = 2,665) represented a wide range of sports and participation levels. As outlined in Table 1, a synthesis of results revealed that 20.1% (n = 535) of the individuals surveyed required considerable career transition adjustment.

A number of traditional therapeutic approaches, including cognitive restructuring, stress management, and emotional expression, have been proposed in the career transition literature as intervention strategies for athletes suffering from distress associated with athletic career termination (Gordon, 1995; Ogilvie & Taylor, 1993; Taylor & Ogilvie, 1994). Although the application of these interventions has been largely supported with a broad range of populations outside of sport, and Wolff and Lester (1989) have outlined a postretirement intervention package for athletes that incorporates various components of cognitive therapy and emotional expression, the utility of these interventions has received little attention in the literature. In this chapter, we present three interventions for practitioners working with athletes in transition, including an information processing approach, mentoring, and an existential psychology approach.

Information Processing

In this section, Harvey, Weber, and Orbuch's (1990) theoretical conception of account-making in response to stress is proposed as an intervention strategy for athletes in transition. In an article published in the *Annual Review of Psychology*, Berscheid (1994) suggested that Harvey et al.'s coping approach that involves account-making is one of the most effective interventions in social psychology. Researchers have found there to be considerable efficacy in this

Table 1
Studies Measuring Psychological Adjustment Difficulties Associated with Career Transitions in Sport

Research Study	Total sample		Sample who experienced psychological adjustment difficulties		
	N	Level	n	%	Description
Svoboda & Vanek (1982)	163	Olympic	29	17.7	had yet to recover psychologically (p. 171)
Greendorfer & Blinde (1985)	1124	Collegiate	191	17.0	indicated some/extreme dissatisfaction with self (p. 107)
Werthner & Orlick (1986)	28	Olympic	9	32.1	had a very difficult time in the transition (p. 344)
Allison & Meyer (1988)	20	Professional	6	30.0	had feelings of isolation and loss of identity (p. 218)
Curtis & Ennis (1988)	96	Amateur	14	14.6	experienced quite a feeling of loss (p. 95)
Blinde & Stratta (1992)	20	Collegiate	16	80.0	indicated the feelings often paralleled to death and dying (p. 8)
McInnally et al. (1992)	367	Professional	96	26.2	experienced moderate to severe emotional adjustment (p. 4)
Sinclair & Orlick (1993)	199	Amateur	22	11.1	felt generally dissatisfied about life (p. 143)
Wylleman et al. (1993)	44	Olympic	3	6.8	were confronted with severe emotional problems (p. 904)
Parker (1994)	7	Collegiate	6	85.7	reflected negative expressions and experiences (p. 299)
Alfermann & Gross (1997)	90	Amateur	11	12.2	reported feelings of depression, helplessness, and other psychological disturbances (p. 66)
Lavallee et al. (1997)	48	Amateur	18	37.5	experienced highly distressful reactions to retirement (p. 7)
Zaichkowsky et al. (1997)	354	Collegiate	71	20.0	reported experiencing distress upon leaving their sport (p. 784)
Webb et al. (1998)	93	Collegiate	43	46.2	reported that a difficult retirement was characteristic (p. 355)
Total	2653		535	20.1	

Note: This table has been modified from the one presented in Grove, Lavallee, Gordon, and Harvey (1998).

information processing approach (e.g., Harvey, 1996; Meichenbaum & Fitz-patrick, 1993) and, in particular, with athletes experiencing adjustment diffi-culties during a career transition (e.g., Grove, Lavallee, Gordon, & Harvey, 1998; Lavallee et al., 1997; Sparkes, 1998). Grove et al. and Sparkes, for ex-ample, have illustrated the beneficial role of account-making in the career transition process for Olympic athletes who experienced distressful reactions to retirement from sport. Lavallee et al. have also assessed the benefits of account-making among a sample of elite athletes who experienced extreme psychological adjustment to athletic career termination.

Account-making has been defined as the act of explaining, describing, and emotionally reacting to problematic or influential life events, with the resul-tant narratives being story-like constructions developed for situations in which a relatively in-depth understanding is required or desired (Harvey, Orbuch, Weber, Merbach, & Alt, 1992). Theorists have proposed that accounts and narratives are psychosocial phenomena that are often initiated in private reflection and later refined and modified through the process of confiding (Harvey et al., 1990). Confiding is the act of disclosing one's narratives to a significant other or others (i.e., confidants), and investigations have suggested that this activity is pivotal in movement towards recovery from a distressful reaction (e.g., Frank, 1995; Harvey, 1996; Harvey, Orbuch, Chwalisz, & Gar-wood, 1991). In addition to the social-communicative method of confiding, writing has been identified as a way to help people make better sense of dis-tressful reactions (e.g., Pennebaker, 1990; Sparkes, 1998; Uematsu, 1996). Regardless of whether people write about or discuss their experiences, how-ever, developing an account in some form is pivotal in coping with the cogni-tive-emotional-behavioral aspects of a career transition (Denison, 1996; Grove et al., 1998; Harvey, 1996) and assists in movement through the steps to adaptation, recovery, and closure (i.e., an important Gestalt principle signi-fying completeness). Therefore, Harvey et al.'s (1990) model of account-mak-ing addresses Taylor and Ogilvie's (1994) call for a theoretical model applied to retirement from sport that indicated which factors lead to the traumatic re-sponse and that enabled individuals to progress through the respective stages of adjustment to reach closure (p. 4).

In order to facilitate the development of theory and research in the area, Harvey et al. (1990) developed a model of account-making in response to stress. This conceptualization has been grafted onto Horowitz's (1986) model of coping, which suggests that people react to stress in a series of steps that may be linear or may involve back and forth movements over time. Grove et al. (1998) have argued that, upon the earliest recognition of a stressful reac-tion, an athlete in transition may show panic and experience an emotional cry for help. Evidence has demonstrated that some athletes have experienced this reaction upon career termination (see Table 1), and as outlined by Taylor and Ogilvie (1998), the initial reaction varies as a function of several interrelated factors (viz., causal factors, developmental influences, and coping resources). When the athletes feel ready, Grove et al. contended that they will be best served by confronting their career transition experiences mentally by thinking about them, putting them aside, cognitively constructing the various components of the transition (i.e., its nature, why it happened, how the athletes feel about it, and what it means for the future), and then coming back again and renewing the analysis. This 'account' is then partially confided to close others, whose reaction may help or hinder the individual in dealing with career transition experience. If the confidants react to the account with empathy, the athlete may move with dispatch to confront what has happened and deal with it rationally and constructively (Lavallee et al., 1997). However, if confidants do not react with empathy (e.g., by lending an 'ear', being there to listen; or offering advice, encouragement, and/or feedback when desired), the negative impact of the career transition may grow, and the individual may become discouraged in trying to engage in this confiding-social interaction activity that appears to be so vital to positive psychological adaptation (Grove et al., 1998; Harvey et al., 1991). Sparkes (1998) has also added that an additional concern for retired athletes is that they often do not have alternative narratives available to them in times of crisis.

Following these early experiences, the account-making model suggests that transitional athletes may show signs of denial. As suggested by Baillie and Danish (1992), denial is often used as a coping strategy by athletes during the career transition process. According to Carver, Scheier, and Weintraub (1989), however, denial has the potential to make the transition even more stressful, and thus, athletes need to move beyond it and confront the often uncontrolled experience of intrusive thoughts, emotions, and images. As Harvey et al. (1990) have argued, the greatest efficacy-conveying benefits of account-making occur when problematic situations are recalled, reviewed, and reexperienced in detail in some capacity. Moreover, overcoming these intrusions facilitates the development of a more coherent account and, thus, prepares the individual for the important working-through phase of account-making (Harvey, 1996).

Working through is critical in the recovery process because it is at this point that career transition difficulties are often confronted directly through the process of confiding (Lavallee et al., 1997). Whereas account-making is theoretically most coherent, refined, and intense during the working-through phase, the effects may be long-term and quite debilitating if the working-through process is negative (Harvey et al., 1990). Harvey et al. (1991) have found account-making and confiding activity to be significantly related to successful coping and the perceived reaction of the confidant to be especially critical in stress reduction. Confiding attempts that involved feedback from caring, close confidants have also been found to be significantly related to positive psychological adaptation (Harvey et al., 1991; Staudacher, 1987; Stroebe & Stroebe, 1987). In addition, researchers have suggested that failure to engage in confiding activity following a traumatic event is associated with measures of subjective distress (e.g., Pennebaker, 1985, 1990) and that this can lead to further negative consequences, such as prolonged despair and hopelessness, continued maladjustment, and difficulty in coping with current and future stressful experiences (e.g., Horowitz, Field, & Classen, 1993). Psychologists, therefore, have adopted information processing approaches such as account-making in numerous counseling settings (e.g., Frank, 1995; Gergen & Gergen, 1988; Harvey et al., 1990).

Although little research has been conducted in this area with athletes in transition (e.g., Lavallee et al., 1997), several sport psychologists have suggested the benefits of working through and confiding. For example, Werthner and Orlick (1986) have stated that for many retiring athletes, "simply having someone to talk to was very important" (p. 357). "Talking about problems regarding career termination" (Wylleman et al., 1993, p. 904) and "clarifying feelings about sport careers" (Parker, 1994, p. 301) have also been recommended as ways for athletes to rhetorically work-through any retirement-related difficulties. Because athletes often lose their primary social support group upon career termination (Kane, 1995; Murphy, 1995), they may not have the opportunity to work through any issues that require resolution. As Parkes (1988) has suggested, a distressful reaction may be aggravated if the person to whom one turns to as a confidant is no longer there as a result of the experience itself.

When athletes finalize their account and, hence, have completed the account-making process, it is hypothesized that they will have developed a better sense of their career transition experience. As Harvey and colleagues (Harvey, 1996; Harvey et al., 1990; Harvey et al., 1992) have suggested, account-making often plays a critical role in helping people achieve an enhanced sense of psychological control over thoughts and feelings regarding stressful events. Although not every individual will be able to work through all feelings of distress and reach a state of closure, account-making often assists in transforming the experience into something meaningful. Moreover, people often reach a point when they become motivated to impart to others what they have learned from their adjustment experiences (i.e., their account). This culmination of the account-making process is known as *generativity* (i.e., an active concern for the welfare of future generations; Erikson, 1963), and it has been suggested that this can help people forge a new identity in their lives (Harvey, 1996). Indeed, several notable athletes have engaged in generative behavior by relating their traumatic stories to others (e.g., Louganis, 1995; Seles, 1995). It appears likely, therefore, that the process of account-making can serve as a pathway for the restoration of identity for athletes in transition (Lavallee, Grove, Gordon, & Ford, 1998; Sparkes, 1998).

As previously noted in a critique of thanatological research in chapter 1, the psychological effects of severe stress are varied and, at times, even contradictory. For this reason, the account-making model represents an idealized scheme and hypothesizes at what points account-making is most likely to occur. It is not contended that all individuals who suffer distressful reactions to career transition go through a series of stages. Rather, an emphasis is placed on the course of account-making activity in the recovery process and its utility, as opposed to the exclusive cognitive appraisal of the event. Indeed, models that postulate cognitive appraisal are invaluable in identifying the way athletes assess their emotional response to career transition (cf. Brewer, 1994).

By providing an environment that facilitates account-making, practitioners may be able to assist athletes in coping with problems associated with their career transition. Because individuals vary in their abilities to understand their own experiences and articulate their stories to appropriate confidants (Harvey, 1996; Sparkes, 1998), such an intervention needs to provide athletes with sufficient opportunities to develop their account. Encouraging athletes to talk and/or write about their career transition experience may help in the construction of an account that they feel comfortable with (Grove et al., 1998). Although it does not matter whether the sharing of an account first occurs with professionals or peers, what is essential is that the sharing occurs at a time when the athlete feels most ready and with an individual who fosters positive account-making.

Once sufficient information is assessed from the athlete at the outset, practitioners may also want to determine to what extent the transitional athlete has engaged in the cognitive-emotional work associated with account-making up to that point, as well as the quality of the individual's confiding experiences. An account could then be developed that raises awareness of unresolved emotional issues and encourages the athlete to discuss them with others. Whereas this process could provide therapeutic benefits to the individual, valuable information may also be provided about the degree to which the athlete has acknowledged and/or dealt with stress-related phenomena such as denial, feelings of hopelessness/despair, and obsessive rumination (Grove et al., 1998). Insight may also be offered into the extent to which the athlete's self-concept has evolved to include more than the athlete role, an awareness that appears to be an important step in the transition process (Lavallee et al., 1997). As Petitpas, Champagne, Chartrand, Danish, and Murphy (1997) have suggested, any intervention when working with athletes must be multidimensional and involve enhancement, support, and counseling because the timing and duration of career transition adjustment varies considerably. Last, the benefits of account-making might also extend beyond athletes in transition if they were given the opportunity to present and discuss their account with athletes in the midst of the careers (Grove et al., 1998). We would recommend that such an approach be incorporated into career mentoring programs for athletes (Cockerill & Edge, 1998; Perna, Zaichkowsky, & Bocknek, 1996), which are described in the following section.

Mentoring

Mentoring has been referred to as a close relationship in which a mentor counsels, supports, and guides a protégé (Hardy, 1994; Kram, 1992). Research in a number of settings outside sport has documented the benefits of such a paradigm (Burke, McKeen, & McKenna, 1993; Chao, Walz, & Gardner, 1992; Noe, 1988; Pollock, 1995), and several sport psychologists have suggested mentoring as a possible way to assist athletes to cope with the career transition process (Danish, Petitpas, & Hale, 1993; Jackson, Mayocchi, & Dover, 1998; Perna et al., 1996). In addition, Perna et al. (1996) have assessed levels of mentoring among a sample of athletes and a matched group of nonathletes at the end of a college career. In this study it was demonstrated that student-athletes benefited from being more "vocationally mature" if they had a mentor to guide them through the crucial stage of transition.

In this section, the efficacy of a mentoring approach to facilitate the adjustment process for athletes in transitions is further explored in a study by Cockerill and Edge (1998). This study incorporates both qualitative and quantitative procedures to determine the nature of mentoring, its extent, and also the perceived benefits among four former Olympic-level athletes. "John" retired involuntarily because of long-term injuries. "David" retired from competition involuntarily because he was unable to train at the level expected of him. "Mike" retired voluntarily, choosing to devote more time to his family, although he suggested that a persistent injury had contributed to his decision to stop competing. Last, "Paul" retired because he had been considered to be too old for international athletics and was unable to maintain the standard he had previously reached. It was hypothesized that those who found adjusting to retirement from competition difficult and upsetting would not have experienced mentoring, whereas those who had received support from a mentor during their career transition would cope satisfactorily.

Initially, each participant completed a personal data questionnaire to generate basic information about his highest level of performance, when and why he retired, and to whom he felt closest through the career transition process. An individual interview followed, which was not tape-recorded to encourage informality and honest responses during questions and discussion. A personal-construct format was employed during the interviews according to the following four stages outlined by Banister, Burman, Parker, Taylor, and Tindall (1994) to produce a repertory grid (Jones & Harris, 1996):

1. Identifying the area for discussion (i.e., retirement from competitive sport).
2. Nominating the elements that define the area of construing (i.e., roles of personal relevance to the participant and representative of the topic under consideration). The six elements used were: "myself when competing," "myself near to retirement," "myself ideally," "myself now," "myself 6 months after retirement," and "myself one year after retirement."
3. Creating constructs using the triadic method. Initially, each element was written on a card, and three cards were selected randomly and shown to the athlete, who was then asked: "Please say how two of the elements are similar and different from the third." This procedure was repeated until an appropriate number of triads was elicited. According to Button (1993), no fewer than 10 and not more than 50 triads are necessary.
4. Placing constructs in a grid and having the participant rate each element for all constructs on a scale from 0 (*never*) to 6 (*always*).

Button's (1993) self-grid analysis technique was used to interpret the data. This hand-scoring procedure focuses on self-esteem, and a mean self-esteem score was calculated by determining mean differences between ratings for "self" and "ideal self" over all constructs. According to Button, this procedure considers subjective experience and provides a global self-esteem measure, together with a profile of particular constructs to highlight that individual's particular strengths and weaknesses. As outlined in the personal-construct data shown in Table 2, the difference between John's actual and ideal self was smallest when

Table 2
Mean Personal Construct Discrepancies

	When competing	Near to retirement	Six months post-retirement	One year post-retirement	Now
John	0.79	2.11	2.16	2.05	2.58
Mike	1.07	1.29	0.14	0.21	0.14
David	0.61	1.28	0.50	0.78	0.50
Paul	1.37	1.26	1.37	1.11	0.74

competing and greatest now, which suggests that his self-esteem was relatively low when interviewed. By contrast, Mike appears to have adjusted well after competition with a relatively high current self-esteem.

During the second part of the interview, the participants completed the Mentoring Functions Scale (Noe, 1988), an instrument that measures the extent of vocational and psychosocial mentoring received by an individual. The vocational mentoring section assesses the amount of feedback on personal attributes, introductions to useful contacts, and provision of opportunities for career advancement, whereas psychosocial mentoring items determine the extent to which the mentor serves as a confidant and counselor. Each participant was asked: "Please consider as your mentor the person that was closest to you through your retirement from competition. Now read each of these sentences carefully, and for each of them circle which of the five descriptions is most applicable to you." For example, for the item "I agreed with my mentor's attitudes and values regarding sport and retirement," if the response was "to a very large extent," the athlete circled the maximum score of 5. Scores for all statements were summed to produce a combined total score for psychosocial and career development mentoring with a range from 21 to 105. Scores greater than 41 on each individual scale indicated that the athlete had experienced satisfactory mentoring (Noe, 1988). These data are presented in Table 3.

Results revealed that John and Mike had been closest to their coach during retirement; David, to his wife; and Paul, to a friend. Table 3 shows that John had received a good deal of support for both components of the scale, whereas Mike's mentoring had been very limited, with little psychosocial or career development support. The personal-construct grids of both these athletes also contrasted. While competing, John had been excited, free, fulfilled, goal driven, and certain of the future. At the time of this study, however, he rarely felt free, and most of the time he was under pressure and apprehensive. Although this athlete received support and career guidance during the transition period from competitive sport, he had not adjusted to his present life especially suc-

Table 3
Aggregate Scores for Mentoring Functions Scale

	Psychosocial	Career development
John	52	46
Mike	13	10
David	47	32
Paul	55	14

cessfully. He commented that although he had every aspect of a mentor in his coach, a similar level of support from others would have made things easier in terms of both the quality and quantity of support. John was enthusiastic about the need to implement a mentoring system for elite athletes who had invariably devoted much of their formative years to the sport, but often with little prospect of progressing within it afterwards.

By contrast, Mike was much closer to his ideal self now than when competing. His mentoring scores showed that he had received little support during the retirement process. When competing he described himself as contemplative, often "suffocated" and, although happy most of the time, only occasionally "comfortable." Mike said that he was able to make decisions about his future when in hospital being treated for an injury. He had considered what he wanted from life and recognized that it was time to finish competing and to begin a new stage in his life. Such a positive attitude is probably rare among elite performers, and Mike was able to use the contemplative aspect of his personality expressed while competing to greater advantage at a later stage in his life. A key feature of his career transition from sport was that he chose to do so, and the outcome was positive, despite a lack of mentoring. Leaving sport involuntarily, as many do, suggests that mentoring is especially important for those denying that they are past their best as athletes.

It was notable that all the constructs used by the four participants in the study were emotional descriptions, rather than physical states, when referring to their career transition experiences. Issues such as physical condition, financial concerns, and employment difficulties were rarely mentioned. It was felt that by adopting a two-stage approach to mentoring, and employing both qualitative and quantitative methods, it was possible to explore a richer source of material than would have been the case had individual perceptions not been taken into account. It can be seen that each of the four athletes perceived his career transition differently, eliciting diverse responses and constructs. Although three of the four mentors provided satisfactory psychosocial support, only one was adequate in respect of career guidance. It is suggested that the latter is especially important for those whose personal presentation and communication skills may be underdeveloped.

Although this study remains limited in scope, it has generated much that is of interest and with implications for practitioners. It has also contributed to the growing research on mentoring in sport settings (e.g., Bloom, Durand-Bush, Schinke, & Salmela, 1998; Perna et al., 1996). Taylor and Ogilvie (1994) have argued that the effects of financial, social, psychological, and physical change can be manifested in trauma for the athlete in transition, especially when two or more stressors are combined. However, Cockerill and Edge (1998) have suggested that terms such as mentoring and counseling do not often sit easily alongside the extroverted, aggressive, ambitious, and positive images that are synonymous with contemporary elite athletes and the publicity that surrounds them. Nonetheless, these data have indicated that mentoring for transitional athletes can be an important service that sport should provide. Although a variety of research approaches are possible, the present methodology was found to be successful in providing sufficiently detailed information for the development of intervention strategies.

Existential Psychology

This section considers the contribution that existential psychology can make to an understanding of career development and transition in sport. A brief outline of the major theoretical propositions of existential psychology is initially provided, specifically focusing on some of the key features of existential counseling. This will be further illuminated by a discussion of case studies involving elite-level athletes, which additionally will begin to examine some of the practical issues facing practitioners who adopt an existential approach in their work.

Existential psychology has its roots in the metaphysical speculations of St. Thomas Aquinas, an Italian university professor and Dominican in the 13th century, and in the writings of Soren Kierkegaard, a 19th-century Danish philosopher and Christian apologist. Subsequent developments witnessed a major fracture during the latter part of the 19th century and the 20th century. Existentialists divided into two different traditions with, Nietzsche, Sartre and Camus denying the possibility of God, whereas others such as Buber, Marcel, Tillich, and Maritain affirmed their belief in an absolute being. This brief historical account clearly reveals several important aspects of existential psychology that may begin to explain why it has been so largely ignored by much of modern mainstream psychology and sport psychology until recently (e.g., Dale, 1996; Nesti & Sewell, 1999). First, existentialism and existential psychology have European rather than North American foundations and have always considered the question surrounding belief in a supreme being or God as of fundamental importance. Second, and perhaps even more problematic for the modern mind, existential psychology has dared to declare its clear link with a school of philosophy and, by doing so, exposes other psychologies in their refusal to examine their own philosophical roots and metaphysical assumptions (Valle, King, & Halling, 1989). Existential psychology differs most radically from other approaches by its focus on four key existential concerns: death, freedom, isolation, and meaninglessness (Schneider & May, 1995). In addition, the concept of anxiety holds a central place, following Kierkegaard's earlier writings on the *Concept of Dread* (1844/1944), and May's (1977) work on the meaning of anxiety.

In terms of sport and exercise psychology, few studies have adopted an existential psychology perspective. Fahlberg, Fahlberg, and Gates (1992) provided a comprehensive introduction to existential phenomenological psychology as part of their work on exercise dependency. Continuing along similar lines, Dale (1996) has attempted to introduce applied researchers in sport psychology to the phenomenological interview, an important method frequently used in existential psychology. From a professional practice perspective, the work of Corlett (1996) and Salter (1997), although not focusing exclusively on existential psychology, has alluded to important existential concerns such as meaning, spirit, and values. Interestingly, both Corlett and Salter have warned that applied sport psychology in the United States and the United Kingdom is in danger of becoming almost synonymous with mental skills training. This tendency, according to Corlett, has led sport psychologists to rely excessively on "technique based symptomatic relief" (p. 88) when often athletes should really be encouraged to focus on knowledge of self.

The value of adopting an approach to counseling based on existential psychology in dealing with athletic retirement and career development will be discussed in relation to the experiences of two elite-level athletes. In each of the two illustrative cases, specific existential concerns will be considered, and attention will be drawn to how these themes helped provide a framework of meaning, for both the athlete and the sport psychologist.

The first case involved a national-level racquet sport player who approached the sports psychologist for help with a severe and long-term decline in competitive performance. The athlete had experienced rapid and extraordinary success in the sport at the junior level and had apparently quite suddenly experienced an almost complete reversal of this earlier level of achievement. Unable to discern a technical or physical explanation for this situation, the athlete, against the coach's wishes, contacted the sports psychologist for help aimed at restoring self-confidence, motivation, and self-belief. It very quickly became apparent that without a rapid resolution of the difficulties faced by the player, early retirement from high level competitive sport would be the most likely outcome. The player used the term *retirement* when describing feelings towards competitive play. However, the player refused to consider dropping out of the sport altogether. Although the retirement literature in sport has tended to focus on a total cessation of activity, athletic retirement could be better understood as a process that may involve a more gradual reduction in activity, rather than complete termination.

A central theme that emerged from an initial series of meetings with the

athlete centered on the existential concerns of isolation and freedom. It became clear that the athlete-coach relationship was maladaptive and involved a
psychologically abusive cycle where the coach altered his approach to a more
supportive style whenever there was an indication that the player intended to
move on, only to revert to the former domineering and aggressive pattern of
behavior as the player remained under his care. At the player's insistence, a
mental skills training program was initially taught, because in the player's
words, "sport psychologists can teach you how to relax and give you targets to
aim for." Alongside this, a more existentially focused series of meetings were
held between the athlete and the sport psychologist; at these meetings the
issues of fear at being isolated from other members of the squad and anxiety
related to leaving the coach and going at it alone came into sharp focus. As
this level of analysis continued, the mental skills program was abandoned by
the player. More in-depth work revealed in clear terms the paralyzing effect of
what May (1977) has called neurotic anxiety. The player's words expressed
this in the following statement: "I know that I need to get away from it all and
maybe even work with another coach, although much less than I've been used
to, but I feel like I'm cornered and just can't make a move."

The consideration of retirement from high competitive sport was mentioned repeatedly by the athlete, particularly where frequent losses to players
ranked much lower became commonplace. Retirement was seen as a way
around the problem and a solution to the suffocating and manipulative relationship with the coach. However, from an existential psychological perspective, neurotic anxiety is a direct result of a repeated failure to face up to normal
anxiety (May, 1977). Another way of expressing this is that, taking responsibility, at least in part, for one's own actions, and the act of choosing itself,
almost always is accompanied by feelings of anxiety. This 'normal' anxiety
should be welcomed and confronted creatively because, according to existential counseling, it is a natural part of the human condition. It is this dimension
to which Kierkegaard (1844/1944) referred when he claimed that anxiety is
the great teacher and that, contrary to the pronouncements of modern sport
psychology, the greater the self, the greater the anxiety. Quite clearly, an existential sport psychology would have no interest in using techniques to wash
away anxiety, given that it considers the experience of normal anxiety as fundamental to personal growth and the development of inner fortitude.

After almost 2 years of work, the athlete had discarded any notions of early
retirement and, without regular coaching support, had begun to win again and
move up the national rankings. A further 2 years later the player, had progressed to the collegiate level and returned the best win-loss statistics of anyone on the player's team. Although this case study reveals how retirement can

be used inappropriately by an athlete to avoid responsibilities for growth, or to evade the anxiety associated with freedom and choice, sometimes an athlete will avoid thoughts about retirement because it signifies symbolic death and a movement into the meaningless.

A second case study with an international professional soccer player demonstrated how important existential concerns are even in sports where the highest earners are financially secure for life. Again, for this player, sport retirement can be understood better as an ongoing event, involving periods both of gradual disengagement and more abrupt and unplanned incidents. In attempting to make sense of the increasingly volatile and unpredictable world of international professional soccer, the player had met on a regular basis with the sport psychologist over a 3-year period. Yalom (1980) has claimed that an existential approach is particularly useful when clients face boundary situations, such as those involving personal and work transitions. Meetings between the player and sport psychologist explored a myriad of issues, some directly related to performance and others less so. An interesting existential concern frequently raised by the player related to the question of life goals. The player described how he had come to view success as "related to achieving as a player and a person in life, and that these two persona were not really separate, and in a deeper sense were actually impossible to divide." Through these encounters with the sport psychologist, the player was able to express his anger at the media, club owners, and managers. This emotional behavior was avoided initially by the player; however, as May (1995) has stated, the existential approach to counseling requires that the therapist fully immerse him- or herself in the client's lived world. The world as lived is to be distinguished from the artificial world of abstract concepts and theories found in most other approaches (Caruso, 1964). May (1995) has advocated that the counselor choose to express rage on behalf of the client at something that has happened in the client's life. This controversial approach appears less so when it is understood that existential psychology demands of its practitioners their full emotional involvement in the encounter. In addition, this approach represents a recognition that value-free counseling, therapy, and psychology as a whole, are an impossibility, and even if they were possible, such treatments would represent a degeneration and lessen effectiveness. Using this approach allowed the player to increasingly express his anger at particular injustices that he had faced and continued to confront in his athletic career and allowed him to begin to reflect on his retirement with a clearer focus.

Interestingly, the player began to construct new meaning for himself by recognizing that each time he had progressed in his career he had (in his own words) "striven for immortality over death!" Salter (1997), from a different perspective, has described the sports psychologist as "a purveyor of immortality" (p.259) whereby the client and psychologist work creatively to confront the anxiety being faced by athletes in an increasingly impermanent sports world. This recognition that a type of death (i.e., retirement) was in some way necessary before growth could continue was expressed in profound terms by the player when talking about his new understanding of the retirement process: "It feels like I have to make a leap out into the dark; it's hard to see why everything should be this way, but it's like a flower, I suppose. It dies so that the new bulb can build up its strength and bloom again next year."

In terms of a meaningful framework for understanding the retirement process of athletes, it can be argued that compared to other approaches, existential psychology offers a very different perspective, one that requires a radical outlook. Existential counseling demands a considerable level of personal commitment and emotional involvement throughout each individual case. It requires the sport psychologist to fully immerse him- or herself in a relationship or encounter with the client-athlete that focuses on the discovery of sound values and highlights the importance of recognizing the universal human situation, where in Sartre's terms, we find ourselves "condemned to freedom." Fromm (1994) has claimed that a fear of freedom, which involves the personal refusal to accept some responsibility for one's own life, and at a societal level, the associated conformity of the mass of people, is the greatest source of anxiety and psychological problems facing modern man. When we turn more fully to the implications of this approach for practitioners specifically dealing with the career transition process, the following key issues emerge:

1. The "lived world" provides the only data upon which the athlete and psychologist can work together. Another way of expressing this is that the psychologist will avoid the use of abstract concepts and theories and instead will work directly only with the descriptions of events, feelings, and emotions provided by the athletes themselves.
2. Athletic career transition may be associated with feelings of isolation and even death, symbolically speaking, and it frequently results in a greater awareness by athletes that they must exercise a choice regarding their future. Failure to confront the anxiety that accompanies the act of choosing may lead to regressive behaviors, such as a refusal to accept that retirement is an unavoidable juncture in competitive sport. The practitioner must help athletes in the career transition process to understand these feelings and must consistently challenge the athletes to face up to these important existential concerns.
3. According to both Fromm (1994) and May (1995), the personality of the counselor is an extremely important component in the effectiveness of this approach. Both have stressed that a deep knowledge of the arts and

humanities through academic study and/or exposure to the great literary masterpieces should form a major part of the education and training of existential psychologists and therapists. This has been supported by Corlett (1996) within sport psychology.

4. This approach would, except in the most extreme cases, avoid use of specific anxiety-control techniques. Focus would be directed at encouraging the athlete to use the anxiety associated with the career transition process creatively to help develop a deeper level of self-knowledge and to grow towards new configurations of meaning. To begin to achieve this, the sport psychologist needs to adopt a sincere and empathic approach and remain present to the person with whom the psychologist is working. Put another way, the career transition practitioner must attempt to truly see the other as a person, not as a collection of habits, traits and environmental histories, but as a unique, sovereign, and living human being.

Conclusion

It is clear that some athletes experience personal adjustment difficulties during the career transition process. Indeed, assisting athletes to make a successful transition to a postathletic career may be one of the most commonly encountered issues for sport psychology practitioners (Murphy, 1995; Ogilvie & Taylor, 1993). It is, therefore, surprising that intervention strategies for athletes in transition have not, for the most part, been delineated or investigated (Grove et al., 1998).

In this chapter, three intervention strategies for athletes in transitions have been reviewed. Although quite different in their theoretical foundations, each of these approaches highlight several common themes that confront athletes in the career transition process. The most important of these are concerned with the need for empathy and attentive listening on the part of the career transition practitioner. In addition, although using different methods, each approach recognizes the positive outcomes associated with encouraging athletes to become actively involved in making sense of their experiences. Given the expanding literature in this area and developments in professional practice, we believe that further attention should be devoted to the development of additional interventions from different psychological perspectives for athletes in transition.

References

Alfermann, D., & Gross, A. (1997). Coping with career termination: It all depends on freedom of choice. In R. Lidor & M. Bar-Eli (Eds.), *Proceedings of the IX World Congress on Sport Psychology* (pp. 65–67). Netanya, Israel: International Society of Sport Psychology.

Allison, M. T., & Meyer, C. (1988). Career problems and retirement among elite athletes: The female tennis professional. *Sociology of Sport Journal, 5,* 212–222.

Baillie, P. H. F., & Danish, S. J. (1992). Understanding the career transition of athletes. *The Sport Psychologist, 6,* 77–98.

Banister, D., Burman, E., Parker, I., Taylor, M., & Tindall, C. (1994). *Qualitative methods in psychology: A research guide.* Buckingham, England: Open University Press.

Berscheid, E. (1994). Interpersonal relationships. *Annual Review of Psychology, 45,* 79–129.

Blinde, E., & Stratta, T. (1992). The "sport career death" of college athletes: Involuntary and unanticipated sports exits. *Journal of Sport Behavior, 15,* 3–20.

Bloom, G. A., Durand-Bush, N., Schinke, R. J., & Salmela, J. H. (1998). The importance of mentoring in the development of coaches and athletes. *International Journal of Sport Psychology, 29,* 267–281.

Brewer, B. W. (1994). Review and critique of models of psychological adjustment to athletic injury. *Journal of Applied Sport Psychology, 6,* 87–100.

Burke, R. J., McKeen, C. A., & McKenna, C. (1993). Correlates of mentoring in organizations: The mentor's perspective. *Psychological Reports, 72,* 883–896.

Button, E. (1993). *Eating disorders: Personal construct therapy and change.* New York: Wiley.

Caruso, I. A., (1964). *Existential psychology: From analysis to synthesis.* London: Darton, Longman & Todd.

Carver, C. S., Scheier, M. F., & Weintraub, J. K. (1989). Assessing coping strategies: A theoretically based approach. *Journal of Personality and Social Psychology, 56,* 267–283.

Chao, G. T., Walz, P. M., & Gardner, P. D. (1992). Formal and informal mentorships: A comparison on mentoring functions and contrast with nonmentored counterparts. *Personnel Psychology, 45,* 619–636.

Cockerill, I., & Edge, A. (1998). *A two-stage approach to examining the effects of mentoring on disengagement from elite competition in sport.* Unpublished manuscript, School of Sport and Exercise Sciences, The University of Birmingham, England.

Corlett, J. (1996). Sophistry, Socrates and sport psychology. *The Sport Psychologist, 10,* 84–94.

Curtis, J., & Ennis, R. (1988). Negative consequences of leaving competitive sport? Comparative findings for former elite-level hockey players. *Sociology of Sport Journal, 5,* 87–106.

Dale, G. A. (1996) Existential phenomenology: Emphasizing the experience of the athlete in sport psychology research. *The Sport Psychologist, 10,* 307–321.

Danish, S. J., Petitpas, A. J., & Hale, B. D. (1993). Life development intervention for athletes: Life skills through sports. *The Counseling Psychologist, 21,* 352–385.

Denison, J. (1996). Sport narratives. *Qualitative Inquiry, 2,* 351–362.

Erikson. E. (1963). *Childhood and society* (2nd ed.). New York: Norton.

Fahlberg, L. L., Fahlberg, L. A., & Gates, W. K. (1992). Exercise and existence: Exercise behavior from an existential phenomenological perspective. *The Sport Psychologist, 6,* 172–191.

Frank, A. (1995). *The wounded storyteller.* Chicago: University of Chicago Press.

Fromm, E. (1994). *The art of listening.* London: Constable.

Gergen, K. J., & Gergen, M. M. (1988). Narrative and the self as relationship. *Advances in Experimental Social Psychology, 21,* 17–56.

Gordon, S. (1995). Career transitions in competitive sport. In T. Morris & J. Summers (Eds.), *Sport psychology: Theory, applications and issues* (pp. 474–501). Brisbane: Jacaranda Wiley.

Greendorfer, S. L., & Blinde, E. M. (1985). "Retirement" from intercollegiate sport: Theoretical and empirical considerations. *Sociology of Sport Journal, 2,* 101–110.

Grove, J. R., Lavallee, D., Gordon, S., & Harvey, J. H. (1998). Account-making: A model for understanding and resolving distressful reactions to retirement from sport. *The Sport Psychologist, 12,* 52–67.

Hardy, C. J. (1994). Nurturing our future through effective mentoring: Developing roots as well as wings. *Journal of Applied Sport Psychology, 6,* 196–204.

Harvey, J. H., Orbuch, T. L., Chwalisz, K., & Garwood, G. (1991). Coping with sexual assault: The roles of account-making and confiding. *Journal of Traumatic Stress, 4,* 515–531.

Harvey, J. H. (1996). *Embracing their memory: Loss and the social psychology of story-telling.* Needham Heights, MA: Allyn & Bacon.

Harvey, J. H., Weber, A. L., & Orbuch, T. L. (1990). *Interpersonal accounts: A social psychological perspective.* Oxford: Blackwell.

Harvey, J. H., Orbuch, T. L., Weber, A. L., Merbach, N., & Alt, R. (1992). House of pain and hope: Accounts of loss. *Death Studies, 16,* 99–124.

Horowitz, M. J. (1986). *Stress response syndromes* (2nd ed.). Northvale, NJ: Jason Aronson.

Horowitz, M. J., Field, N. P., & Classen, C. C. (1993). Stress response syndromes and their treatment. In L. Goldberger & S. Breznitz (Eds.), *Handbook of stress: Theoretical and clinical aspects* (pp. 757–773). New York: Free Press.

Jackson, S., Mayocchi, L., & Dover, J. (1998). Life after winning gold: II. Coping with change as an Olympic gold medallist. *The Sport Psychologist, 12,* 137–155.

Jones, F., & Harris, P. (1996). The repertory grid technique in exercise psychology. In C. Robson, B. Cripps, & H. Steinberg (Eds.), *Qualitative and quantitative research methods in sport and exercise psychology.* Leicester: The British Psychological Society.

Kane, M. A. (1995). The transition out of sport: A paradigm from the United States. In R. Vanfraechem-Raway & Y. Vanden Auweele (Eds.), *Proceedings of the 9th European Congress of Sport Psychology* (pp. 849–856). Brussels: European Federation of Sports Psychology.

Kierkegaard, S. (1944). *The concept of dread* (W. Lowrie, Trans.). Princeton, NJ: Princeton University Press. (Original work published 1844)

Kram, K. E. (1992). *Mentoring at work.* London: Scott, Foreman, and Company.

Lavallee, D., Gordon, S., & Grove, J. R. (1997). Retirement from sport and the loss of athletic identity. *Journal of Personal and Interpersonal Loss, 2,* 129–147.

Lavallee, D., Grove, J. R., Gordon, S., & Ford, I. W. (1998). The experience of loss in sport. In J. H. Harvey (Ed.), *Perspectives on loss: A sourcebook* (pp. 241–252). Philadelphia: Brunner/Mazel.

Lavallee, D., Sinclair, D. A., & Wylleman, P. (1998). An annotated bibliography on career transitions in sport: I. Counselling-based references. *Australian Journal of Career Development, 7 (2),* 34–42.

Lavallee, D., Wylleman, P., & Sinclair, D. A. (1998). An annotated bibliography on career transitions in sport: II. Empirical references. *Australian Journal of Career Development, 7 (3),* 32–44.

Louganis, G. (with Marcus, E.) (1995). *Breaking the surface.* New York: Orion.

May, R. (1977). *The meaning of anxiety.* New York: Ronald Press.

May, R. (1995). Origins and significance of existential psychology. In K. Schneider & R. May (Eds.), *The psychology of existence: An integrative, clinical perspective* (pp. 82–88). New York: McGraw Hill.

McInnally, L. J., Cavin-Stice, J., & Knoth, R. L. (1992). *Adjustment following retirement from professional football.* Paper presented at the annual meeting of the American Psychological Association, Washington DC.

Meichenbaum, D., & Fitzpatrick, D. (1993). A constructive narrative perspective on stress and coping: Stress inoculation applications. In L. Goldberger & S. Breznitz (Eds.), *Handbook of stress: Theoretical and clinical aspects* (pp. 706–723). New York: Free Press.

Murphy, S. M. (1995). Transition in competitive sport: Maximizing individual potential. In S. M. Murphy (Ed.), *Sport psychology interventions* (pp. 331–346). Champaign, IL: Human Kinetics.

Nesti, M., & Sewell, D. (in press). Losing it: The importance of anxiety and mood stability in sport. *Journal of Personal and Interpersonal Loss.*

Noe, R. A. (1988). An investigation of the determinants of successful assigned mentoring relationships. *Personnel Psychology, 41,* 457–479.

Ogilvie, B. C., & Taylor, J. (1993). Career termination issues among elite athletes. In R. N. Singer, M. Murphey, & L. K. Tennant (Eds.), *Handbook of research on sport psychology* (pp. 761–775). New York: Macmillan.

Parker, K. B. (1994). "Has-beens" and "wanna-bes": Transition experiences of former major college football players. *The Sport Psychologist, 8,* 287–304.

Parkes, C. M. (1988). Bereavement as a psychosocial transition: Processes of adaptation to change. *Journal of Social Issues, 44* (3), 53–66.

Pennebaker, J. W. (1985). Traumatic experience and psychosomatic disease: Exploring the roles of behavioral inhibition, obsession, and confining. *Canadian Psychology, 26,* 82–95.

Pennebaker, J. W. (1990). *Opening up.* New York: Morrow.

Perna, F. M., Zaichkowsky, L., & Bocknek, G. (1996). The association of mentoring with psychosocial development among male athletes at termination of college career. *Journal of Applied Sport Psychology, 8,* 76–88.

Petitpas, A., Champagne, D., Chartrand, J., Danish, S., & Murphy, S. (1997). *Athlete's guide to career planning: Keys to success from the playing field to professional life.* Champaign, IL: Human Kinetics.

Pollock, R. (1995). A test of conceptual models depicting the developmental course of informal mentor-protégé relationships in the work place. *Journal of Vocational Behavior, 46,* 144–162.

Salter, D. (1997). Measure, analyze and stagnate: Towards a radical psychology of sport. In R. J. Butler (Ed.), *Sports psychology in performance* (pp. 248–260). Oxford: Butterworth-Heinemann.

Schneider, K. J. & May, R. (1995). *The psychology of existence: An integrative, clinical perspective.* New York: McGraw Hill.

Seles, M. (with Richardson, N. A.) (1996). *Monica: From fear to victory.* London: Harper Collins.

Sinclair, D. A., & Orlick, T. (1993). Positive transitions from high-performance sport. *The Sport Psychologist, 7,* 138–150.

Sparkes, A. C. (1998). Athletic identity: An Achilles' heel to the survival of self' *Qualitative Health Research, 8,* 644–664.

Staudacher, C. (1987). *Beyond grief.* Oakland, CA: New Harbinger.

Stroebe, W., & Stroebe, M. (1987). *Bereavement and health: The psychological and physical consequences of partner loss.* New York: Cambridge University Press.

Svoboda, B., & Vanek, M. (1982). Retirement from high level competition. In T. Orlick, J. T. Partington, & J. H. Salmela (Eds.), *Proceedings of the 5th World Congress of Sport Psychology* (pp. 166–175). Ottawa: Coaching Association of Canada.

Taylor, J., & Ogilvie, B. C. (1994). A conceptual model of adaptation to retirement among athletes. *Journal of Applied Sport Psychology, 6,* 1–20.

Taylor, J., & Ogilvie, B. C. (1998). Career transition among elite athletes: Is there life after sports? In J. M. Williams (Ed.), *Applied sport psychology: Personal growth to peak performance* (3rd ed., pp. 429–444). Mountain View, CA: Mayfield.

Uematsu, M. A. (1996). Giving voice to the account: The healing power of writing about loss. *Journal of Personal and Interpersonal Loss, 1,* 17–28.

Valle, R., King, M., & Halling, S. (1989). An introduction to existential phenomenological thought in psychology. In R. V. Halling & A. S. Halling (Eds.), *Existential phenomenological perspectives in psychology* (pp. 3–16) New York: Plenum Press.

Webb, W. M., Nasco, S. A., Riley, S., & Headrick, B. (1998). Athlete identity and reactions to retirement from sports. *Journal of Sport Behavior, 21,* 338–362.

Werthner, P., & Orlick, T. (1986). Retirement experiences of successful Olympic athletes. *International Journal of Sport Psychology, 17,* 337–363.

Wolff, R., & Lester, D. (1989). A theoretical basis for counseling the retired professional athlete. *Psychological Reports, 64,* 1043–1046.

Wylleman, P., De Knop, P., Menkehorst, H., Theeboom, M., & Annerel, J. (1993). Career termination and social integration among elite athletes. In S. Serpa, J. Alves, V. Ferreira, & A. Paula-Brito (Eds.), *Proceedings of the VIII World Congress of Sport Psychology* (pp. 902–906). Lisbon: International Society of Sport Psychology.

Yalom, I. (1980). *Existential psychotherapy.* New York: Basic Books.

Zaichkowsky, L., Lipton, G., & Tucci, G. (1997). Factors affecting transition from intercollegiate sport. In R. Lidor & M. Bar-Eli (Eds.), *Proceedings of the IX World Congress of Sport Psychology* (pp. 782–784). Netanya, Israel: International Society of Sport Psychology.

8

The Role of the Sport Organization in the Career Transition Process

Dana A. Sinclair
Human Performance International
Canada

Dieter Hackfort
Universitat Der Bundeswehr
Germany

Abstract

Previous chapters have elucidated the theoretical perspectives underlying the career transition process. The focus of this chapter is not to debate the philosophical underpinnings of whether sport organizations should or should not provide transitional services to athletes. The intention is to briefly explore the factors associated with the adjustment process, outline the services currently available to high-performance athletes in Canada, and suggest potential methods for improving the contribution of transition services in general.

The Role of the Sport Organization in the Career Transition Process

In this world of constant change, transitions are inevitable and often unpredictable. Human life is characterized by these various life changes, discontinuities, or turning points (George, 1980; Schlossberg, 1984; Schlossberg,

Lynch, & Chickering, 1989), and all transitions are followed by a period of disruption in which old routines, assumptions, and relationships change and new ones evolve (Schlossberg et al.). Furthermore, every transitional event has the potential to be a crisis, a relief, or a combination of both, depending on the individual's perception of the situation. The retirement from high-performance sport is a type of transition that has the potential to illuminate the complex patterns of change and stability.

In the case of the elite athlete, even though the timing may be uncertain, the transitional event of a career change will definitely occur. The event of retirement is a normal consequence of elite participation as a career in sport is much shorter than most other careers or occupations as the majority of athletes retire, voluntarily or involuntarily, during their mid to late 20s (Sinclair, 1990; Sinclair & Orlick, 1993). This "second" career often requires entirely different skills than those learned and perfected as an athlete and is one in which the individual rarely has the same competencies. Consequently, this transition, at a relatively young age, is often said to engender identity crises and coping difficulties. As Baillie (1993) and others (Baillie & Danish, 1992; Lerch, 1981; McPherson, 1980; Ogilvie & Howe, 1982; Sinclair, 1990; Werthner & Orlick, 1986) have noted, few athletes make sufficient preparations for this major life event, and many struggle with their adjustment to retirement.

National sport organizations in several countries have responded to the transitional difficulties experienced by their athletes by implementing programs designed to make the adaptation process to life after sport a more positive experience for those in need. Historically, sport organizations have not paid the same attention to helping athletes exit from the organizational structure as they have to helping them enter. Now that more countries are recognizing the humanistic need to assist athletes in moving smoothly and quickly through the transition process, more effective transition programs are emerging.

In an effort to gain a better understanding of the athletic career-transition phenomenon, sport theorists have proposed a variety of explanatory conceptual models. As outlined in chapter 1 of this volume, these models have contributed to the efforts to define and explain those factors specifically related to career transition and the ways in which these factors influence the overall quality of adjustment.

Despite great research and practical interest, the literature has not identified a consolidating theoretical framework from which to study athletic transition. Empirical testing of these models is critical to furthering the conceptual development of the transition process and will positively inform the services and interventions proposed by high-performance transition programs. Preliminary findings from a project testing Charner and Schlossberg's (1986) model (modified by Sinclair & Orlick, 1993) in the context of the transitional experiences of 199 Canadian high-performance athletes have revealed significant results. The study found that athletes high in assets relating to transition characteristics (e.g., minimal life change, minimal degree of stress, and fewer difficulties encountered in transition) were more satisfied about their lives in retirement and felt more in control of their progress through the transition than did those athletes who were high in liabilities related to transition characteristics.

Factors Associated With the Transition Process

The overall quality of adjustment to career termination is influenced by a variety of factors (Lavallee, Wylleman, & Sinclair, 1998). Both positive and negative factors will have an impact on the transition process and on the specific paths or trajectories taken by different individuals as they negotiate their changing biographies (Grove, Lavallee, & Gordon, 1997; Lavallee, Grove, & Gordon, 1997; Murphy, 1995; Petitpas, Brewer, & Van Raalte, 1996; Sinclair & Orlick, 1994; Taylor & Ogilvie, 1994; Webb, Nasco, Riley, & Headrick, 1998).

Negative Adjustment Factors

- unplanned (e.g., deselection from the Olympic team or program for failing to make a performance standard)
- forced out (e.g., injury; political or subjective selection process)
- poor performance (e.g., at the World Championships, leading the slalom with five gates to go, catching an edge, and skiing out)
- strong athletic identity (e.g., an athlete who derives self-identity primarily from his or her role in sport)
- little assistance (e.g., lack of interpersonal support from family, friends, intimate relationships, and/or coach)
- lack of options (e.g., not having a high school diploma; lack of vision regarding new career choice; no coaching positions available within the sport organization or exclusion by the sport organization from coaching opportunities)
- lack of coping resources (e.g., capable of using very few coping strategies rather than being able to use a wide range of available coping strategies)
- financial difficulties (e.g., insufficient resources to résumé education)

Positive Adjustment Factors

- planned (e.g., making the decision to retire after performing in the Olympic games)
- voluntary (e.g., deciding to retire next year after the World Championships)
- achieved goals (e.g., ran a personal best time in the Olympic final)

- low athletic identity (e.g., self-identity is derived primarily from areas that are not associated with the athlete role)
- balance and options (e.g., using one's education to gain employment; having the prospect of employment as an assistant national team coach; entering a training program to prepare for a new type of job or career)
- coping resources (e.g., using multiple strategies to deal with life's circumstances)
- support (e.g., having a social support network, especially interpersonal support systems such as intimates, family, and friends, as well as institutional support from sport organizations)

Any practical and effective transition program must not only be aware of the factors that will positively or negatively influence one's adjustment profile, but also must use these factors to formulate and design the intervention services to be offered through the sport organization. The Canadian Olympic Association's (COA) Athlete Services transition program is continually modifying its services to reflect their athletes' needs.

Athlete Transition Services in Canada

The COA first funded the Olympic Athlete Career Centre (now under the COA umbrella term of Athlete Services) in 1985. The mandate of the program was to assist athletes through the transition process from high-performance athlete status to a second career, primarily through a career and educational planning process. Similar transition programs offered to high-performance athletes in other countries, most notably Australia and the United States, are referred to as athlete life-skill programs (Anderson & Morris, this volume).

The following career and educational planning services were those originally offered to athletes by the COA:

- Individual career planning: Clarification of career planning needs, self-assessment, identification of suitable options, career research, decision making, and action-planning skills.
- Retirement guide: Booklet outlining the transition process and what athletes should expect during the adjustment period.
- Transition workshop and peer support group: Individual or group meetings to help athletes deal effectively with the transition process.
- Aptitude/Interest assessment: Availability of career interest inventories to assist in identification of a specific vocation or occupation of interest.
- Résumé preparation: Booklet and consultation available to assist in effective résumé preparation.
- Interview preparation: Booklet and consultation available to assist in developing effective interviewing skills.

- Job-search techniques: Booklet and consultation available to assist in developing effective job search skills.
- Informational interviewing: Booklet and consultation available to assist in obtaining meaningful information regarding jobs/careers of interest.
- Letters of support: Reference letters provided by the Canadian Olympic Association.
- Business cards: Personalized business cards bearing the Canadian Olympic Association logo for networking.
- Shadow program: Linking athletes with individuals currently established in specific career areas and allowing the athlete to "shadow" the individual for a workday.

In recent years, Athlete Services has initiated a reorganization process that has resulted in not only additions to the services offered but also an increase in the number of centers operating within the country. Six centers are currently providing services to athletes who are competing, or who have competed, for Canada at the international level. The standardization of service provision across centers is ongoing and is influenced by the need and utility of the services for the athlete population in each region. The additional services include the following:

- Personal counseling referrals: Confidential individual counseling services regarding interpersonal relationships, family issues, stress, marital concerns, career decisions, transition issues, and referral for legal questions.
- Athlete resource center: Computer workstations, email and Internet access, telephone and printing services, job and special event postings, access to sport information resources.
- Employability skills portfolio development: Development of an individual and unique portfolio that demonstrates participants' skills.
- Injured athlete education and support seminar: Seminars and peer support meetings to share information on how coaches and peers can support athletes throughout the injury period.
- Financial management workshop: Group seminars that help athletes manage finances by building a financial plan, preparing a personal budget and taking control of their spending.
- Public speaking workshop: Training seminars to enhance the athletes' ability to speak clearly and effectively in presentations.
- Media relations workshop: Training seminar related to developing one's ability to deal with the media in a positive, stress-free manner.
- Job opportunities program: Program placing athletes in salary-subsidized jobs (i.e., athletes received full-time payment for part-time work).

Athlete Transition Programs: Future Considerations

The transition program currently in place for Canadian athletes has, over the past decade, been well received by a specific group of elite athletes. It is important to recognize that a significant number of high-performance athletes do not utilize the services either because they have been self-regulatory in their career development behavior and do not perceive a need for such services or because the services offered do not meet their specific needs. It is this second group of athletes that sport organizations must consider if their programs are to be comprehensive and truly effective. If sport organizations are to move beyond the basic career services currently offered to provide the athlete with professional, individualized information related to their emotional and career well-being, then program enhancements are necessary. Specific areas to consider are psychological assessment and professional job profiling, as well as a variety of other intervention strategies.

Psychological Assessment

Transition research indicates that some athletes are profoundly affected by retirement and experience emotional and psychological distress. Both anecdotal and empirical articles make the case that the transition process can pose a significant problem for many athletes and cite cases of emotional turmoil, depression, and even attempts of suicide. Although it is well-known that athletes may experience depressive symptomatology and anxiety as they negotiate the transition process, most, if not all, transition programs consistently fail to screen athletes for clinical disorders or potential risk.

Research has also noted that individuals possessing a high, rather than a low, athletic identity tend to find the adjustment to retirement more problematic. Perfectionism may also contribute to a more arduous adjustment, yet sport organizations do not attempt to prophylactically identify or treat these individuals. Either the organizations do not see such difficulties as part of their service domain, or they expect athletes to recognize their psychological symptoms and to have the personal resources to take action in such a compromised state thereby finding the appropriate treatment on their own. Based on the clinical observations of the personnel working within their transition program, the COA has recently recognized this need and now has a network of professionals in place to provide personal counseling. Transition programs may provide the opportunity for personal counseling; however, the bridging of the gap from individual symptom identification to treatment has not yet been recognized or attended to.

All effective transition programs have an intake process in place. That is, when an athlete contacts the program for assistance, pertinent background and other descriptive information is gathered from that individual. The athlete is advised of the services offered and guided through the appropriate options. Extending this procedure to include psychodiagnostic assessment to identify at-risk individuals would be quick, simple, and nonintrusive.

There are several effective and efficient tools available to assess clinical disorders (e.g., major depression or panic disorder), depressive or anxious symptomatology, athletic identity, and perfectionism (see Table 1). A screening procedure to identify individuals at risk for transitional adjustment difficulties could occur while the athlete is an active member of the national team, or is at the point of retirement or at intake into the transition program. It is important to note that those individuals administering and interpreting any screening or assessment instruments should be appropriately qualified and trained to do so. To permit individuals not trained in the appropriate areas of psychology and psychiatry to collect data or take action on processed data would be irresponsible and potentially be an ethical and/or legal liability.

Table 1
Tools for the Early Detection of At-Risk Athletes

Depression symptoms Anxiety symptoms	The Symptom Questionnaire (Kellner, 1987) —screening tool
Major depression Panic disorder	Mini-International Neuropsychiatric Interview (MINI; Sheehan et al., 1996) —structured interview
Athletic identity	Athletic Identity Measurement Scale (AIMS; Brewer, Van Raalte, & Linder (1993)
Perfectionism	Activity Vector Analysis System (AVA; Goldberg, Sweeney, Merenda, & Hughes 1996) —requires a certified analyst to interpret results

If an athlete is identified as high risk, he or she could be referred to one of the regional specialists (e.g., sport psychologist, clinical psychologist, clinical counselor, or psychiatrist) identified by the transition program. The early detection of at-risk individuals would permit the sport organization to decrease the prevalence of emotional distress or disorder and reduce the severity and duration of an individual's condition through appropriate intervention strategies that are specific to the high-performance athlete population.

Job Profiling

Current transition programs are very effective in providing athletes with career interest inventories (e.g., Self-Directed Search; Holland, 1990). That is, athletes have access to instruments that will assist them in identifying a specific vocation or occupation of interest (e.g., chemist, silversmith, tractor operator). Although these tools can be important for self-discovery and personal development, they are not sufficient for determining a good career fit or for predicting successful job performance.

Professional behavioral profiling, through such procedures as the Activity Vector Analysis System (AVA) or the Myers-Briggs Type Indicator System, is needed to help the athlete in effective job placement. It is well documented that the majority of people are hired for their technical abilities and knowledge, and between 70 and 90% of those who are terminated are released as the result of behavioral mismatches between the person and the job (Beatty, 1994). For example, in a sales position an individual may have very good knowledge of the product to be sold, but not be appropriately risk taking, decisive, or fast paced enough to be successful, long-term, at that sales job. In this instance, the person's behavioral competencies do not match the job and will decrease his or her job performance and chances for success.

Behavioral assessments, developed for the workplace to measure specific characteristics that have been linked to the actual demands of the job, significantly increase the likelihood of both job performance success and job satisfaction (McIntosh-Fletcher, 1996; Robbins & Finley, 1995). The direct and proactive assessment of one's strengths, weaknesses, and motivations and the determination of the environments and types of organizational cultures in which one would function most effectively would assist the athlete in identifying the type of occupation that holds the most potential for job success and satisfaction.

Interest tests are useful for career and vocational counseling and are satisfactory for predicting job choice. Behavioral assessments based on specific job-related factors are utilized by many organizations to assist in selection and placement and are considered to be powerful predictors of job performance and satisfaction (Robertson & Kinder, 1993). If they intend to provide their athletes with effective services for a smooth adjustment, sport organizations should approach this aspect of their athlete services program with the same professional demeanor as the organizations that will be hiring their "graduates."

Education Regarding the Need for Options

The distribution of materials designed to inform and educate athletes about the transition process and what to expect during this time has proved to be useful to them. In addition, further education regarding the importance of maintaining a balanced lifestyle while competing or of having other options to move toward once one retires is a critical variable that significantly affects the speed and satisfaction of transition adjustment.

Maintaining Contact With Transitional Athletes

A significant, yet often neglected issue in the transition process is the frequency of contact between the organization and the athlete once he or she has left the program. A recurring research finding is that athletes tend to feel isolated and "used" once they are no longer an official part of the elite team. Whether a person is on long-term injury status or is newly retired, simple contacts such as telephone calls, email, or regular mailings from the organization can ease the path to a second career.

Providing Opportunities to Contribute to the Sport System

Former athletes are a valuable resource in terms of their specific sport knowledge with respect to skill, technique, and strategy. They represent a substantial investment of time and money, and their expertise is invaluable to continued coaching depth or administrative continuity. Sport organizations could facilitate a system for communication between athletes and involvement in the various coaching positions, developmental programs or other roles available within the sport structure.

Needs Assessment

An ongoing, systematic process for determining the changing needs of high-performance athletes as they move out of sport and into another career is of utmost importance. Too often, the services provided to transitional athletes are added to or deleted from a program based on the intuitive feel of the service providers rather than on a demonstrated need. A needs assessment is an organized and objective way of measuring athlete opinions, attitudes, behaviors, feelings, and beliefs relative to an initiative, in this case, the transitional program and its services. Such an assessment focuses on how the athletes feel about the services or on what they need, rather than on what they want. An effective needs-assessment, which has gathered multiple perceptions, thoughts, and beliefs, will ensure an accurate analysis of what services are appropriate.

Program Evaluation Versus Client Satisfaction Surveys

The concept of evaluation as a one-time effort is nonproductive (Geis & Smith, 1992). Program evaluation is critical to determining which services are working well, why they are working well, and what can be done to improve the existing program. Often, asking athletes who have experienced the transition program about their level of satisfaction with the available services is regarded as an evaluation of the utility of the program as a whole. That is, if the athletes who use the services are happy, then the program's utility is substantiated and justified. Knowing that athletes like a service is different from knowing if the service is actually assisting the athlete in the transition process. Periodical evaluation of the program, through a database monitoring system, would permit the regular and minimally disruptive collection of appropriate program data.

Database Development for Research and Intervention Generation

Transition programs provide a rich and accessible environment for gaining insight into how athletes adjust to retirement. Prospective, versus retrospective, data are not yet available for the high-performance athlete population. Observing athletes as they adapt to life after sport is critical to the provision of appropriate, effective interventions.

One strategy for facilitating such observation would be to focus on the development of a database to standardize critical research questions as well as to provide a cost- and time-effective data entry and analysis procedure. The creation of an Internet solution is currently being developed within the COA's Athlete Services. This database will be used to simplify the management of the database across athlete services centers, will enable global accessibility (e.g., sharing of data), and will easily permit any expansion/revision of the information to be obtained from the athlete at the time of intake into the transition program. In addition, it will increase the frequency with which the information can be collected throughout the adjustment phase. This Internet database will allow for more in-depth and meaningful investigations that will positively inform the services provided by the transition program and maximize the benefits to the athlete.

Conclusion

As the demands associated with competitive sport have increased over the years, so has the interest regarding career transition issues among athletes (Grove, Lavallee, Gordon, & Harvey, 1998). As a result, the sport organizations of several countries have developed transition programs designed to assist athletes through the adjustment phase from high-performance athlete to former high-performance athlete.

This chapter has provided a summary of the negative and positive factors associated with the quality of one's adjustment to life after elite sport and has outlined the services currently available to high-performance athletes in Canada. To be effective, transition programs must ensure that they provide services based on athlete needs rather than on athlete wants—a distinction that may often be overlooked. Future considerations for enhancing the sport organization's contribution to an athlete's adjustment include a screening procedure for the early identification of at-risk athletes, professional job profiling from a behavioral perspective (e.g., the AVA system), systematic needs assessments, and formal program evaluation. Finally, the incorporation of an Internet solution, not only to obtain prospective data on the athlete's transition as it unfolds but also to monitor the athlete's progress for early intervention purposes, would be a meaningful contribution from any sport organization.

References

Baillie, P. H. F. (1993). Understanding retirement from sports: Therapeutic ideas for helping athletes in transition. *The Counseling Psychologist, 21,* 399–410.

Baillie, P. H. F., & Danish, S. J. (1992). Understanding the career transition of athletes. *The Sport Psychologist, 6,* 77–98.

Beatty, R. H. (1994). *Interviewing and selecting high performers.* Toronto: Wiley & Sons.

Brewer, B. W., Van Raalte, J. L., & Linder, D. E. (1993). Athletic identity: Hercules' muscles or Achilles' heel? *International Journal of Sport Psychology, 24,* 237–254.

Charner, I., & Schlossberg, N. K. (1986, June). Variations by theme: The life transitions of clerical workers. *The Vocational Guidance Quarterly,* 212–224.

Geis, G. L., & Smith, M. E. (1992). The function of evaluation. In H. D. Stolovitch & E. J. Keeps (Eds.), *Handbook of human performance technology* (pp. 130–150). San Francisco, CA: Jossey-Bass.

George, L. K. (1980). *Role transitions in later life.* Monterey, CA: Brooks/Cole.

Goldberg, L. R., Sweeney, D. C., Merenda, P. F., & Hughes, J. E. (1996). The big-give factor structure as an integrative framework: An analysis of Clarke's AVA model. *Journal of Personality Assessment, 66,* 441–471.

Grove, J. R., Lavallee, D., & Gordon, S. (1997). Coping with retirement from sport: The influence of athletic identity. *Journal of Applied Sport Psychology, 9,* 191–203.

Grove, J. R., Lavallee, D., Gordon, S., & Harvey, J. H. (1998). Account-making: A model for understanding and resolving distressful reactions to retirement from sport. *The Sport Psychologist, 12,* 52–67.

Holland, J. L. (1990). *Self-Directed Search.* Odessa, FL: Psychological Assessment Resources.

Kellner, R. (1987). A symptom questionnaire. *Journal of Clinical Psychiatry, 48,* 268–274.

Lavallee, D., Grove, J. R., & Gordon, S. (1997). The causes of career termination from sport and their relationship to post-retirement adjustment among elite-amateur athletes in Australia. *Australian Psychologist, 32,* 131–135.

Lavallee, D., Wylleman, P., & Sinclair, D. A. (1998). An annotated bibliography on career transitions in sport: II. Empirical references. *Australian Journal of Career Development, 7 (3),* 32–44.

Lerch, S. H. (1981). The adjustment to retirement of professional baseball players. In S. L. Greendorfer & A. Yiannakis (Eds.), *Sociology of sport: Diverse perspectives* (pp. 138–148). West Point, NY: Leisure Press.

McIntosh-Fletcher, D. (1996). *Teaming by design.* Toronto: Irwin.

McPherson, B. D. (1980). Retirement from professional sport: The process and problems of occupational and psychological adjustment. *Sociological Symposium, 30,* 126–143.

Murphy, S. M. (1995). Transition in competitive sport: Maximizing individual potential. In S. M. Murphy (Ed.), *Sport psychology interventions* (pp. 331–346). Champaign, IL: Human Kinetics.

Ogilvie, B. C., & Howe, M. (1982). Career crisis in sport. In T. Orlick, J. Y. Partington, & J. H. Salmela (Eds.), *Proceedings of the 5th World Congress of Sport Psychology* (pp. 176–183). Ottawa: Coaching Association of Canada.

Petitpas, A. J., Brewer, B. W., & Van Raalte, J. L. (1996). Transitions of the student-athlete: Theoretical, empirical, and practical perspectives. In E. F. Etzel, A. P. Ferrante, & J. W. Pinkney (Eds.), *Counseling college student-athletes: Issues and interventions* (2nd ed., pp. 137–156). Morgantown, WV: Fitness Information Technology.

Robbins, H., & Finley, M. (1995). *Why teams don't work.* Princeton, NJ: Peterson's/Pacesetter Books.

Robertson, I. T., & Kinder, A. (1993). Personality and job competencies: The criterion-related validity of some personality variables. *Journal of Occupational and Organizational Psychology, 66,* 225–244.

Schlossberg, N. K. (1984). *Counseling adults in transition: Linking practice with theory.* New York: Springer.

Schlossberg, N. K., Lynch, A. Q., & Chickering, A. W. (1989). *Improving higher education environments for adults.* San Francisco: Jossey-Bass.

Sheehan, D. V., Janavs, J., Knapp, E., Sheehan, M., Baker, R. & Sheehan, K. H. (1995). *Mini International Neuropsychiatric Interview, Clinician Rated (Version 4.4).* Tampa: University of South Florida.

Sinclair, D. A. (1990). *The dynamics of transition from high-performance sport.* Unpublished doctoral dissertation, University of Ottawa, Canada.

Sinclair D. A., & Orlick, T. (1993). Positive transitions from high-performance sport. *The Sport Psychologist, 7,* 138–150.

Sinclair, D. A., & Orlick, T. (1994). The effects of transition on high-performance sport. In D. Hackfort (Ed.), *Psycho-social issues and interventions in elite sports* (pp. 29–55). Frankfurt: Lang.

Taylor, J., & Ogilvie, B. C. (1994). A conceptual model of adaptation to retirement among athletes. *Journal of Applied Sport Psychology, 6,* 1–20.

Webb, W. M., Nasco, S. A., Riley, S., & Headrick, B. (1998). Athlete identity and reactions to retirement from sports. *Journal of Sport Behavior, 21,* 338–362.

Werthner P., & Orlick, T. (1986). Retirement experiences of successful Olympic athletes. *International Journal of Sport Psychology, 17,* 337–363.

PART
III

Special
Populations

9

Transitions in Youth Sport: A Developmental Perspective on Parental Involvement

Paul Wylleman and Paul De Knop
Vrije Universiteit Brussel
Belgium

Martha E. Ewing and Sean P. Cumming
Michigan State University

Abstract

Transitions in competitive sports have generally been looked at from an adult point of view. However, young athletes are also confronted with specific transitions and transitional periods throughout their athletic career. This chapter describes four transitions with which young athletes are often confronted in competitive youth sport. Taking into account the influential role parents play in young athletes' lives, an emphasis is put on how parents may support their daughters or sons in coping with the demands and consequences of these transitions. Strategies are presented that may enable parents to optimize involvement in their young athletes' sporting careers. Finally, attention is drawn to transitions with which young athletes are confronted that may affect their involvement in competitive sports, namely, transitions occurring in academic careers.

Transitions in Youth Sport: A Developmental Perspective on Parental Involvement

Although an athletic career may seem to develop in a smooth and continuous way from beginning to end, it has been shown that the athletes themselves describe the development of their athletic career in terms of specific moments or situations that occurred or will occur throughout their career (Wylleman & De Knop, 1997a,b). Not only do these moments or situations require athletes to cope with specific changes, but they are also perceived to influence the quality of athletes' participation in organized sport and may be denominated as being transitions. As each sport has a life cycle of similar expected moments or situations, it is possible to delineate those transitions that are predictable in character. For young and adolescent athletes, these moments may include, among others, starting out in organized sport, initially participating in competition, and making the national team. Young athletes may also face transitions that have a low degree of predictability and do occur unexpectedly (e.g., dropping out due to a physical injury), as well as transitions that were expected to take place, but that, due to circumstances, do not occur (e.g., making the team; A. Petitpas, Champagne, Chartrand, Danish, & Murphy, 1997). Although these transitions may differ in degree of predictability or in origin (e.g., physical, psychological, social), research has revealed that social support is an important key to an optimal athletic career transition (Murphy, 1995; Schlossberg, 1981). The availability of social support (i.e., the exchange of resources between individuals intended to enhance the well-being of the recipient) and social support networks (e.g., friends, family, teammates) has been shown to play a strong mediating role in the occurrence of transitions, as well as to influence athletes' adjustment to athletic transitions (Alfermann, 1995; Pearson & Petitpas, 1990; Reynolds, 1981; Sinclair & Orlick, 1994; Stambulova, 1994; Swain, 1991; Werthner & Orlick, 1986; Wylleman & De Knop, 1998). In the setting of competitive youth sport, characterized by its adult-dominated structure and organization, young athletes are provided with social support especially by parents and coaches (DeFrancesco & Johnson, 1997; Hellstedt, 1995; Kirk et al., 1997; Michigan Joint Legislative Study on Youth Sports, 1987; Smith, Smoll, & Smith, 1989). In fact, the importance of this support system has been coined in expressions, such as the "primary family of sport" (Scanlan, 1988), or the "athletic triangle" (Hellstedt, 1987; Smith et al.).

Notwithstanding the importance awarded to this support system in talented young athletes' sports career, researchers (e.g., Bloom, 1985; Régnier, Salmela, & Russell, 1993; Salmela, 1994) have focused primarily on the role of the coach and less on the way in which parents may be involved in this triangle.

In this chapter we will take a closer look at how parents may provide young athletes with the support required to cope with some of the transitions that athletes may face throughout their athletic career. Following an introductory overview of parental involvement in organized youth sport, four transitions will be described, which have been shown to occur in different sporting cultures (Stambulova, 1998; Wylleman & De Knop, 1998). These will include the transition into organized sport, the transition into intensive-level training and participation in competitions, the transition into high-level competitive sport, and the transition out of competitive sport. These transitions concur with the onset of the career phases of talented performers, as described by Salmela, Young, and Kallio in this volume. Combining research data with the counseling experience of the authors in working in youth sport, specific recommendations will be made on how parents may provide support to young athletes in order to cope as best as possible with the demands and consequences of these transitions. A final transition that will also be highlighted and that strongly influences young athletes' involvement in competitive sport is related to their scholastic/academic career. With each transition, strategies will be presented on how parents may support young athletes in coping with these transitions.

Parental Involvement in Youth Sport

Research into the interactions between young athletes and their parents has been limited, notwithstanding the emphasis put on the need for a better recognition of parents' roles in youth sport (American Sport Education Program, 1994; Rotella & Bunker, 1987). The limited amount of empirical research on the relationships between young athletes and their parents has been linked to the fact that "research on family influences is complex and difficult, and that a quantitative methodology is often unable to explore the intricacies of the family processes that exist in athlete families" (Hellstedt, 1995, p. 119). Youth sport researchers have only recently focused their attention on the role parents play in shaping the quality of children's sport involvement (Brustad, 1996).

In reviewing the research on parental involvement in competitive youth sports, two related, yet diverse perspectives can be acknowledged. In a first perspective, sport psychologists have been looking at the way in which parents influence the young athletes, as related to the athletic setting itself. The second perspective focuses on the involvement of parents within the family setting. The ecological validity of both perspectives has been underlined in recent research with talented young athletes (Wylleman, Vanden Auweele, De Knop, Sloore, & De Martelaer, 1995). Using the *Sport Interpersonal Relationship Questionnaire* to assess 265 talented young athletes' perceptions of the quality of their relationships with their parents, Wylleman et al. found athletes' interpersonal perceptions to be context specific: In a first context, parents were perceived to be a part of the athletic setting, focused on the coach, and with limited athlete-parents interactions; a second context situated the athlete-parent interactions in the home setting, without interactions with other significant others. It could be concluded that young athletes perceived their parents to be involved in their sport participation indirectly in the actual athletic setting, and directly in the home setting. Ewing and Weisner (1996) interviewed parents of regionally ranked tennis players, ages 12 to 15, about their involvement in their children's tennis careers. Parents consistently reported that they took their children as infants to the tennis courts while they played tennis, and as children grew, they tossed balls for children to hit in the driveway and, finally, played tennis with them as they worked on stroke development and strategies. All of the parents reported a direct involvement with their children's development as competitive tennis players, even though each child had a coach from one of the local clubs. This diversity in parental involvement can be illustrated with a quote from Claudine Merckx (wife of the world-famous, five-time winner of the Tour de France, Eddy Merckx, and mother of Axel Merckx, rising star in the world of professional cycling), when questioned on her most important role as "cyclist-mom":

> What another mother does for her child: daily householding. And in times of trouble, I need to be there for him. If he cycles well, he won't feel alone. If he doesn't feel up to par, if he's sick, or if he's not performing as expected, he'll need my support. (qtd. in Heylen, 1995, p. 22).

Researchers have up until now generally focused upon the involvement of parents within the athletic setting and, more particularly, on how parents may influence their children cognitions, emotions, and behaviors. Findings have shown that parental encouragement and support not only enhance athletes' level of enjoyment and perceived competence (Brustad, 1988, 1993; Ommundsen & Vaglum, 1993; Power & Woolger, 1994; Scanlan & Lewthwaite, 1986), but may also create a special bond between young elite athletes and their parents (Bakker, De Koning, Van Ingen Schenau, & De Groot, 1993; Carlson, 1988). For example, talented athletes' level of athletic achievement was shown to be linked to the quality of their relationship with their father (Wylleman et al., 1995). On the other hand, parents can be a source of stress or discouragement to young athletes, by worrying about physical injuries, by formulating unrealistic expectations, or by overt "pushing" (Hellstedt, 1995; Lee & MacLean, 1997). Young athletes' competitive trait anxiety has also found to be related to parental expectations and evaluations of performance (Brustad, 1988; Gould, Horn, & Spreeman, 1983; Scanlan & Lewthwaite,

1984). Overzealousness, parental stress, intrusiveness, and extreme and/or maladaptive behavior were some of the negative parental behaviors leading young athletes away from active involvement in competitive sport (Iso-Ahola, 1995; Martens, 1993; Rowley, 1986).

Although youth sport researchers eventually turned their focus to the athlete-parents relationships, the parents-coach relationships have remained largely undiscovered. This is surprising, as the need for more research into the parents-coach relationships was stressed more than a decade ago (e.g., Hellstedt, 1990; Rowley, 1986; Smoll, 1993), more particularly in order to promote effective coach-parents relationships so to improve the quality of the athlete's sport experience (Smoll). Youth sport researchers reported, generally on the basis of their clinical experience, that parents-coach relationships could have a distinct influence on young athletes. For example, Hellstedt (1987) reported that "coaches often have difficulty working with the parents of their athletes. Communication problems, conflict, and sometimes power struggles over who has control over the child's training occasionally develop" (p. 151). Although specific interpersonal behaviors related to the parents-coach relationships were identified as influencing young athletes' involvement in sport (e.g., coaches' scapegoating, excluding, or distancing themselves from parents; parents behaving in a jealous way, making unrealistic demands of, or challenging the coach; Byrne, 1993; Hellstedt, 1995; Rowley), few empirical studies have focused on this relationship specifically. In their study of parent and coach perceptions of their mutual relationships in a competitive youth sport setting, Vanden Auweele and Wylleman (1993) found that coaches' age and gender and parents' involvement in sport were related to the quality of their interactions. Wylleman et al. (1995) have also showed that qualitative parents-coach relationships consisted of mutual consultative and, to some extent, independent interactions between parents and coach, whereas reciprocal negative attitudes and feelings of inferiority were associated with negative parents-coach relationships.

A second perspective on the role of parents in young athletes' participation in competitive sport has drawn the attention to the family setting. Parental pressure influences athletes' enjoyment level over the course of the season (Brustad, 1988). Additionally, Scanlan and Lewthwaite (1986) reported that youth wrestlers' enjoyment was predicted by high parental satisfaction with the athletes' performance, positive adult involvement and interactions, and a low frequency of negative maternal interactions, plus a high level of perceived ability. From a different perspective, parents report that having one child who is more successful in sport than the other child(ren) creates a significant amount of tension within the family as parents balance family time and financial resources with attempts to make each child feel special (Ewing & Weisner, 1996). These findings have prompted sport psychologists to stress the need to address the role of parents, not only within the athletic setting, but also within the family setting (Wylleman & De Knop, 1999).

As specified earlier, talented athletes have been shown to perceive this setting also to be related to their sport involvement. Although athletes report that parents are generally supportive, Scanlan, Stein, and Ravizza (1989) found that a few former elite figure skaters continued their involvement in skating as a way to avoid unpleasant or dysfunctional family experiences. Taking a broader perspective, Hellstedt (1995) has provided a developmental model of the athlete family in which he proposes not only that the athlete family undergoes a constantly changing developmental process, but also that family members need to cope successfully with different major transitional tasks, which may be unique to the athlete family, in order to proceed developmentally.

Transitions in the Athletic Career of Young Athletes

In the following paragraphs, four transitions will be described that have been shown to influence strongly the development of young athletes' sport careers. Whereas the first three transitions reflect a progress in athletes' level of athletic proficiency, the fourth transition relates to the athletes' discontinuing competitive sports. Although the different transitions are described separately, providing young athletes with support needs to be a continuous process for parents. Quotes from press releases from talented young athletes and from their parents are used to illustrate aspects relevant to a particular transitional period. Major players in these quotes are Sebastien Godefroid (vice-Olympic champion sailing Finn-class, 1996), Vanina Ickx (daughter of Jacky Ickx, Belgium's foremost formula one pilot during the 1960s and 1970s), and Kim Hannes (World University ladies squash champion, 1996).

Transitions Into Organized Sport

The introduction into organized sport (approximately from 6 to 8 years of age) can be seen as one of the first transitions young athletes face. It constitutes the start of the initiation phase in which youngsters evolve from their initial contacts with organized sport to a level of specialization into one particular type of sport (e.g., soccer, track and field), specialty (e.g., shot-putter), or role (e.g., goal keeper). This transition requires young athletes to adapt to the demands of organized sport in general, and to the chosen discipline or specialty, to the coach, and to the team members in particular (Stambulova, 1994). Confronted with a largely adult-dominated world, organized in function of training sessions, and (small-scale) competitions at weekends or during holiday periods, young-sters are required to adapt to different changes at both the individual (e.g., higher level of physical exertion) and psychosocial level (e.g., leadership of the coach, play with peers, development of new friendships). It is a transition that is generally savored by athletes later in life. For example, Sebastien Godefroid remembers his first steps into the world of sailing:

> In fact, when I was eight . . . I sailed for the first time alone in my own boat. But I had already many hours of sailing behind me. My parents took me almost every weekend sailing . . . I imagine that they gave me the love for sailing. ("Sebastien Godefroid," 1996).

Youngsters need to be able, among other tasks, to make participation choices, to be ready for participation and competition, to form an "athlete identity" within the context of a particular group of sport participants, to adhere to the organization and rules of organized sport activities, to work under the guid-ance of a youth sport coach, and so forth. As young athletes try to master the new social role of being an "athlete," they may find themselves confronted with the need to shift from "playfulness" to sometimes hard and rigid training sessions, from competing for fun to competing to achieve.

The way in which young athletes may cope with these transitions will be determined by their readiness for participation as well as by the support pro-vided by their parents. This readiness implies that the youngster has reached a level of maturity and skill development that allows for sport involvement and for the opportunity to succeed (Malina, 1996). Although generally age-related standards for youth sport participation have included physical and motor char-acteristics, the most important factor in this transitional period consists of youngsters' psychological readiness for participation. Such psychological readiness occurs when a youngster has sufficient psychological maturation and/or experience to derive benefits from sport participation (Brustad, 1993). An important determinant of psychological readiness is the young athletes' motivation to become and stay involved in organized sport. These, primarily intrinsic, motives include (a combination of) learning and improving skills (competence), being with and making friends (affiliation), being part of a group (team identification), getting and staying in shape (health and fitness), taking part in competitions, and having fun (Weiss, 1995). Youngsters must also have the ability to learn and demonstrate competence in the requisite sport skills. This ability is dependent upon their cognitive (e.g., perceptual) and physical (e.g., coordination, size) maturation.

Once young athletes are introduced to the competitive aspects of their sport participation, they need a psychological readiness to compete. This readiness includes, among other qualities, a need for empathy, a comprehension of each other's roles in the competitive situation, and an understanding of the need for cooperative behaviors (Brustad, 1993). When young athletes evolve toward a higher level of involvement and specialization, they are required to develop different psychological skills that facilitate optimal performance or that are needed to maintain a positive attitude toward enjoyment of participation (Scanlan, 1988; Weiss, 1995). These include positive self-perceptions, intrinsic motivation, interpersonal skills, coping with competitive stress, sportspersonship, and positive affect. As young athletes' abilities to cope with the requirements of this transition are generally developmental in nature, they need to be supported and enhanced by significant others in the athletes' close environment. For example, parents can, via (verbal and nonverbal) modeling, feedback, and reinforcement, influence directly youngsters' perceived physical competence, affect, and motivation (Weiss, 1993). Parents need to provide their children with the opportunity to participate in different sports and encourage them to experience a variety of skills. Parents also have to be supportive toward this varied form of participation and, consequently, avoid directing their children toward early specialization. As young athletes' interest, motivation, and athletic proficiency increase, parents may help to secure a safe and supportive sporting environment, in which appropriate coaching is provided on the way toward participation in competitions. Sometimes, parents who have been closely involved in competitive sport themselves may be able to provide their children with information and support this initial competitive participation. Vanina Inkx remembers her father's advice at the start of her car-racing career:

> . . . that his career as world-level car pilot had been exceptional. That my sister and myself shouldn't take it for granted trying to emulate a similar feat. That the sacrifices needed to be made were gigantic. . . . Not to stop us, but rather out of fear that we would run in head-over-heels and with our eyes shut and end up getting stuck in a cul-de-sac. (de Jonge, 1996, p. 40).

Transitions Into an Intensive Level of Training and Participation in Competitions

This transition introduces young athletes (approximately from 12 to 14 years of age) to the developmental phase in their sport careers. Youngsters have become hooked and strongly committed to their sport (Bloom, 1985), and they perceive themselves, or are perceived by their close environment, as being talented or promising "athletes" or "players," with the capabilities to achieve high-level athletic achievements. This confronts youngsters with the need to cope with, among other changes, new training loads; a higher frequency of (daily) training sessions, and a more specialized level of (technical and tactical) training; an increased need to prepare physically and psychologically for competitions; an increased equality in competitors' athletic abilities at competitions; higher expectations from significant others to show athletic proficiency; the growing demands of their athletic career and their education, other leisure interests, and psychosocial development. Young athletes will need to further their psychological skills (e.g., the development of strategies for coping with competition stress, the development of a system of psychological preparation towards high-level competitions) and pay attention to the consequences of higher training and competition loads (e.g., injury prevention, rehabilitation techniques). The importance of a supportive psychological network increases. Parents may try to support the young athlete in her or his endeavors via a more active engagement. At a task-oriented level, parents may organize transport; provide financial support for coaching, sports equipment, and use of sports infrastructure; and probably most important, organize family life as a function of the athletic demands put to the athlete (e.g., training sessions and training camps, competitions) (Carlson, 1988; Ewing & Weisner, 1996; Hill, 1993). On a socioemotional level, parents should be able to encourage and support athletes, thus providing a refuge for athletes against the growing demands of competitions (Hellstedt, 1995). This active parental involvement is exemplified by the father of Kim Hannes:

> We are at the same time taxi driver, assistant-coach, and their hardiest fans. Above all we are always expected to listen patiently, especially during those moments that aren't going as it should be ("With a Mobile Home," 1996).

Parents should also realize that their children also experience a developmental transition. More particularly, youngsters will enter a phase of life in which they will strive toward more autonomy from their parents, by way of, among other needs, developing their own individual lifestyle and identifying their own place within their psychosocial environment (Dusek, 1987). This "separation-individuation" phase, which may create an imbalance between athletes' need for more autonomy and their need for support (e.g., logistic, financial) from parents, may lead to conflicts in the athlete-parents relationships. Parents may, therefore, find themselves walking a thin line when trying to support their daughter or son in coping with this athletic career transition. Although parents may seem to become less significant to young athletes, the coach, on the other hand, may gain more importance as athletes' level of athletic proficiency rises.

In order to provide athletes efficiently and effectively with support in this transitional period, parents and coach need to develop an open and constructive relationship, based upon mutual acceptance, respect, and consultation. Consultation and cooperation are required on, among other goals, the aims and development of young athletes' sport careers, the necessity to provide athletes with the opportunity to develop a scholastic and/or academic career, the codes of behavior on playing fields, or during trips abroad. Such parents-coach consultation, based upon consensus among all involved, may provide young athletes with a more secure psychological environment to cope with the requirements put to them during this transitional period.

Transitions Into High-Level Competitive Sports

This transition brings young athletes (approximately from 17 to19 years of age) into contact with high levels of competitive sport at the national level, or even at the international level (e.g., as member of the national junior squad). It is the initial step in a career phase that requires athletes to perform at their highest level, in a consistent way, and for as long as possible. Young athletes may be confronted with the need to work toward attaining a professional status, thus focusing a period of their life almost exclusively to an all-out involvement and preparation for training and competitions. Such a professional approach may lead them to become part of a team away from home, or even abroad. This may require them to become proficient in a foreign language, to adapt to another social and cultural lifestyle. As they approach the age limit between junior and senior age-groups, young athletes will also be confronted with a world of adults who are generally experienced and proficient athletic-wise.

Notwithstanding general belief, parents do remain significant to athletes, among others, by way of regularly attending competitions at home and abroad, or via their close relationship with the athlete's coach(es). For example, Kim Hannes' father explains:

> As we wanted to keep attending competitions abroad, we needed to look for an affordable mode of transport. We eventually chose an RV. In this way, Kim could count on the home atmosphere of our family instead of being alone in a hotel room. ("With a Mobile Home," 1996).

Parents need to sustain their support by continuing to provide athletes with the possibility to take refuge from the (sometimes excessive) pressures from high-level competitions (Bakker et al., 1993), a support that is independent of their son's or daughter's athletic achievements. As Sebastien Godefroid's mother explains before the start of the final and decisive regatta at the 1996 Olympic Games:

. . . even in the worst case scenario, if everything goes wrong, Sebastien will become fifth. And this is still much better than anyone of us had dared to hope for. . . . I knew my boy has talent, but this. . . . One thing you may be sure of, whatever the result, we will be celebrating. ("Damned, I Can Win," 1996).

Although athletes will express a need to develop an independent way of life as young adult, they will remain strongly dependent upon their parents, especially in view of the financial and logistic demands put to them during this transitional period. These demands may include, among others, frequent participation in competitions and training camps, acquisition of new material or specialized clothing, and so on. As these financial demands are not always covered by the sports club or sports federation, athletes will need to look for sponsors. However, as pointed out by Kim's father, this is generally a task for parents as the athlete has already a hectic life. Financial support is generally gathered by parents within their own social networks (e.g., friends, colleagues, neighbors). Sometimes, parents are able, via these networks, to find sponsors at a community level, as was the case with Sebastien. The city council provided him with a small RV with which he traveled around Europe in order to save on travel and accommodation expenses:

And I wasn't sleeping just a couple of nights in this RV. Last year [the pre-Olympic year], I was only some 25 nights in Belgium. The rest of the year I spend in my RV. But I guess that's the price you have to pay to get to the top. ("Sebastien Godefroid," 1996).

Parental support is especially relevant as, due to their time-consuming athletic activities, athletes are not always able to develop relationships outside of the family, or outside of the sporting arena. Sebastien stated about his sailing career and his social life: "The life I lead doesn't permit me to have strong relationships. Only 25 days per year at home, and a highly insecure way of life" ("Sebastien Godefroid," 1996). Poignant is his remark on his relationships with his friends:

I'm grateful to my friends for not letting me down, although I realize that the past years I've taken a lot, and have given very little in return. I cannot keep this up after the Olympic Games. I'd like therefore to spend the next two years developing my social life. ("Sebastien Godefroid," 1996).

Parents will need to weigh the way in which they try to support their daughter or son in coping with this transition and the athlete's "growing away" from parents and family. In order not to feel let down, or disappointed by this, parents should focus on the way they have been involved throughout the athletic career. Kim Hannes' parents reflect in a similar way when responding to their past and future involvement in their daughter's squash career: "We do not feel let down or having missed out on anything. On the contrary, we've got to know many new friends abroad. . . . We've sacrificed a lot, but we've also got much in return" ("With a Mobile Home," 1996).

One of the factors that may discourage parents to remain supportive is the growing closeness of the coach-athlete relationship (Wylleman, De Knop, & Sillen, 1998). It remains, therefore, very important that parents and coach be willing to further their mutual consultative and cooperative relationship and, thus, provide the athlete with a conflict-free psychological environment. Finally, a constructive cooperation with the coach, as well as with other specialists (e.g., sports physician, sports psychologist), in which athletes are advised professionally with the opportunity for independent decision making and self-actualization, will also enhance athletes' ability to cope with this transitional period.

Transitions out of Competitive Sports

Young athletes' transition out of competitive sports has always been at the forefront of sports psychologists' attention during the past decades and has, consequently, provided a body of empirical data that is more substantial than for other transitions. Athletes may choose freely to disengage from competitive sport. As outlined by Alfermann in this volume, this voluntary choice may be related to (a combination of) personal (e.g., lack of enjoyment, change of interest) and social (e.g., deteriorating level of family support) elements (Allison & Meyer, 1988; Baillie, 1993; Seefeldt, Ewing, & Walk, 1982; Wylleman, De Knop, Menkehorst, Theeboom, & Annerel, 1993). On the other hand, young athletes may suddenly be confronted with a specific situation or with demands that inhibit them to cope with the demands of high-level competitive sport (e.g., injury). Independent of the cause for discontinuation, parents need to remain supportive and respect their child's decision to disengage from active participation in competitive sports. This may not always be easy for parents who have, throughout the athlete's sport career, invested a lot, financially, as well as emotionally, and who have, to some extent, also stood in the spotlight next to the athlete. When the end of the athletic career suddenly rises, parents will need to provide, in a speedy and concrete way, emotional support or invite expert help (e.g., sport psychologist). A need will arise for parents to help the athlete, in consultation with the coach, to change step by step the daily routine of athletic involvement into a more general lifestyle. In this way, parents may also be able to assist their child in starting out in a postathletic career (e.g., at academic level). Therefore, the transition out of high-level competitive sport does not mean that parental involvement and (emotional, financial, logistic) support will end.

Transitions Affecting Young Athletes' Involvement in Competitive Sports

During the past years, the need has been underlined to broaden sports psychologists' view on career transitions to include those nonathletic transitions that may impact, or that themselves are affected by, athletes' athletic careers (e.g., Ewing, 1998; Wylleman et al.,1998). One such transition relates to athletes' academic development. The increased importance awarded to the optimal development of talented athletes, as well as the concurrent occurrence of transitions in athletes' educational and athletic setting (Wylleman et al., 1998) has brought the specificity of the situation of student-athletes to the forefront. Causes for possible conflict between both roles are related to the need for student-athletes to excel in two domains, deemed by society as important, during one and the same period of life (Wylleman & De Knop, 1996, 1997a, 1997b). Student-athletes need to cope not only with the transitions in their athletic career, but also with the basic transitions from the secondary education to higher education level, as well as with the transitions inherent to each level of education. These transitions include at secondary level, for example, teacher-pupil relationships, choice of subject of study, academic achievements, intraclass relationships, perhaps a delayed college decision; at the higher education level, transitions relate to adjusting to campus life, selecting a subject of study or a major, making the college team, preparing for a postuniversity career. These transitions require student-athletes to adjust to, and cope with, challenges and changes occurring in the combination of academics and athletics. Concurrently, student-athletes are confronted with the duality of their situation. Possible conflict between the role of pupil/student and athlete may occur or may be imposed by the athlete's coach who forces the student-athlete to "choose" between one or the other (e.g., coaches may feel that an athlete cannot fully concentrate and be motivated for high-level sport if involved in academic study; laboratory courses, which are typically scheduled during the late afternoons, conflict with practice times and result in choosing a academic major or sport participation). However, as in Sebastien's case, going on to university seems to have been very beneficial to him:

> Combining top-level sport and university study has in fact been very good for me. My academic education at the Vrije Universiteit Brussel has prevented me becoming a maniac, obsessed by athletic achievements. Studying became in fact a type of relaxation. ("Sebastien Godefroid," 1996).

Student-athletes may be faced with time-management problems, restricted development of relationships, accruing pressure and demotivation to perform at both scholastic/academic and athletic level. In-house psychological services at school and university should provide primary prevention to student-athletes, as well as offer them support in developing their career and life. Although this may include optimizing student-athletes' study, interpersonal communication or goal-setting skills, the support provided by student-athletes' psychological network should alleviate the occurrence of problems related to, for example, their living environment, a possible identity foreclosure, injury, and overtraining (e.g., Carr & Bauman, 1996; Finch & Gould, 1996; Greenspan & Andersen, 1995; A. Petitpas et al., 1997; A. J. Petitpas, Brewer, & Van Raalte, 1996).

Parents may help young athletes to cope with the demands of combining an academic and athletic career, in the first instance, by gathering information on how a school, college or university provides guidance to its student-athletes, on the availability of support or mentoring programs for student-athletes on the priorities put on academic achievement, and on the quality of coaching provided. Secondly, parents may need to watch over their son's or daughter's daily schedule—a point illustrated by Kim's mother: "Starting point was that for Kim and Tine [her younger sister who also plays squash at international level] university and school would always prevail. This required, however, a very good planning" ("With a Mobile Home," 1996).

Such a schedule needs to provide young athletes with an opportunity to combine academic, athletic, and personal activities (e.g., leisure time) in a realistic and "livable" way, avoiding as much as possible long-term stressful situations that may lead to athletes' burnout (Wylleman & Theeboom, 1992). Consultation with the athlete and the coach should provide the opportunity to adapt (temporarily) an overloaded schedule. Parents should also be watchful for the fact that young athletes are also able to take time out to participate in activities other than academic or athletic (e.g., being together with friends). In view of the supplemental demands put on young athletes when actively combining an academic and a athletic career, it should not be surprising that student-athletes perceive their parents' influence longer and that the onset of the "separation-individuation" process may, in comparison to other talented athletes, occur at a later age (Wylleman et al., 1998).

Conclusion

Not only the way in which young athletes start out participating in competitive sport, but also the way in which their athletic careers will develop, will be influenced by their parents. This influence is generally based upon the need expressed by athletes for parental, especially emotional, support. Although the quality of the athlete-parents relationships has been shown to be of stronger influence on athletes' athletic achievements than that of the athlete-coach relationship, it is not easy to convince the sporting world of the necessity to accept that parents may play a constructive and positive role in the young athletes' sports career. This is clearly illustrated by Roger De Vlaeminck (former elite-level cyclist), who states that parents are responsible for 70% of failures among young cyclists (Heylen, 1994). Such an attitude not only is related to negative experiences in dealing with parents, but is generally also a consequence of not knowing why parents should be involved and, more specifically, not knowing how to relate to parents. However, when one takes into account parents' legal guardianship over their children, the amount of time young athletes do spend at home with their parents, and the importance young athletes themselves award to parental support, it becomes important that the sporting world (e.g., coaches, sports federations) realize that parents need to be included rather than excluded in the development of their child's athletic career. Parents (as well as coaches) need, however, to be educated on how their involvement can be beneficial to young athletes and, more particularly, on how parents may support the young athlete in coping with the transitional demands of an athletic career, as well as with those transitions affecting the development of the athletic career. It is only then that parents can be psychologically more ready to be(come) involved in the sport participation of their children (Malina, 1986) and that all support persons within the athletic, family, educational, and leisure-time settings are working in concert to provide for the athlete's needs as they traverse the sport career path.

References

Aflermann, D. (1995). Career transitions of elite athletes: Drop-out and retirement. In R. Vanfraechem-Raway & Y. Vanden Auweele (Eds.), *Proceedings of the 9th European Congress of Sport Psychology* (pp. 828–833). Brussels: European Federation of Sports Psychology.

Allison, M. T., & Meyer, C. (1988). Career problems and retirement among elite athletes: The female tennis professional. *Sociology of Sport Journal, 5,* 212–222.

American Sport Education Program (1994). *Sportparent.* Champaign, IL: Human Kinetics.

Baillie, P. H. F. (1993). Understanding retirement from sports: Therapeutic ideas for helping athletes in transition. *The Counseling Psychologist, 21,* 399–410.

Bakker, F. C., De Koning, J. J., van Ingen Schenau, G. J., & De Groot, G. (1993). Motivation of young elite speed skaters. *International Journal of Sport Psychology, 24,* 432–442.

Bloom, B. S. (Ed.). (1985). *Developing talent in young people.* New York: Ballantine.

Brustad, R. J. (1988). Affective outcomes in competitive youth sport: The influence of intrapersonal and socialization factors. *Journal of Sport & Exercise Psychology, 10,* 307–321.

Brustad, R. J. (1993). Youth in sport: Psychological considerations. In R. N. Singer, M. Murphey, & L. K. Tennant (Eds.), *Handbook of research on sport psychology* (pp. 695–717). New York: MacMillan.

Brustad, R. J. (1996). Parental and peer influence on children's psychological development through sport. In F. L. Smoll & R. E. Smith (Eds.), *Children and youth in sport. A biopsychosocial perspective* (pp. 112–124). Dubuque, IA: Brown & Benchmark.

Byrne, T. (1993). Sport: It's a family affair. In M. Lee (Ed.), *Coaching children in sport: Principles and practice* (pp. 39–47). London: E&FN Spon.

Carlson, R. (1988). The socialization of elite tennis players in Sweden: An analysis of the players' backgrounds and development, *Sociology of Sport Journal, 5,* 241–256.

Carr, C. & Bauman, N. J. (1996). Life skills for collegiate student-athletes. In E. F. Etzel, A. P. Ferrante, & J. W. Pinkney (Eds.), *Counseling college student-athletes: Issues and interventions* (pp. 281–308). Morgantown, WV: Fitness Information Technology.

Damned, I can win a medal here (1996, July 30). *Het Belang van Limburg.*

de Jonge, S. (1996, November 18). Jonge leeuwen: Vanina Ickx [Young lions: Vanina Ickx], *HUMO,* pp. 168–170, 172.

DeFrancesco, C., & Johnson, P. (1997). Athlete and parent perceptions in junior tennis. *Journal of Sport Behavior, 20,* 29–36.

Dusek, J. B. (1987). *Adolescent development and behavior.* Englewood Cliffs, NJ: Prentice-Hall.

Ewing, M. E. (1998, August). *Youth sports parents' expectations and perceptions of coaches and athletes.* Paper presented at the 28th Congress of the International Association of Applied Psychology, San Francisco, CA.

Ewing, M. E., & Weisner, A. (1996). *Parents' perceptions of the role of sport in the development of youth.* Paper presented at the annual conference of the Association for the Advancement of Applied Sport Psychology, Williamsburg, VA, USA.

Finch, L., & Gould, D. (1996). Understanding and intervening with the student-athlete to be. In E. F. Etzel, A. P. Ferrante, & J. W. Pinkney (Eds.), *Counseling college student-athletes: Issues and interventions* (pp. 223–245). Morgantown, WV: Fitness Information Technology.

Gould, D., Horn, T., & Spreeman, J. (1983). Competitive anxiety in junior elite wrestlers. *Journal of Sport Psychology, 5,* 58–71.

Gould, D., & Martens, R. (1979). Attitudes of volunteer coaches toward significant youth sport issues. *Research Quarterly, 50,* 369–379.

Greenspan, M., & Andersen, M.B. (1995). Providing psycholgical services to student athletes: A developmental psychology model. In S. Murphy (Ed.), *Sport psychology interventions* (pp. 177–191). Champaign, IL: Human Kinetics.

Hellstedt, J.C. (1987). The coach/parent/athlete relationship. *The Sport Psychologist, 1,* 151–160.

Hellstedt, J. C. (1990). Early adolescent perceptions of parental pressure in the sport environment. *Journal of Sport Behavior, 13,* 135–144.

Hellstedt, J. C. (1995). Invisible players: A family systems model. In S. M. Murphy (Ed.), *Sport psychology interventions* (pp. 117–146). Champaign, IL: Human Kinetics.

Heylen, M. (1994, April 7). Musseeuw en De Vlaeminck rijden Parijs-Roubaix [Musseeuw and De Vlaeminck will cycle Paris-Roubaix], *HUMO,* pp. 34–38.

Heylen, M. (1995, October 3). Cherchez la femme: Claudine Merckx [In search of woman behind the man: Claudine Merckx], *HUMO,* pp. 22–28.

Hill, G. M. (1993). Youth sport participation of professional baseball players, *Sociology of Sport Journal, 10,* 107–114.

Iso-Ahola, S.E. (1995). Intrapersonal and interpersonal factors in athletic performance, *Scandinavian Journal of Medicine and Science in Sports, 5,* 191–199.

Kirk, D., O'Connor, A., Carlson, T., Burke, P., Davis, K., & Glover, S. (1997). Time commitments in junior sport: Social consequences for participants and their families. *European Journal of Physical Education, 2,* 51–73.

Lee, M., & MacLean, S. (1997). Sources of parental pressure among age group swimmers. *European Journal of Physical Education, 2,* 167–177.

Malina, R.M. (1986). Competitive youth sports and biological maturation. In E. W. Brown & C. F. Branta (Eds.), *Competitive sports for children and youth* (pp. 227–246). Champaign, IL: Human Kinetics.

Malina, R.M. (1996). The young athlete: Biological growth and maturation in a biocultural context.

In F. L. Smoll & R. E. Smith (Eds.), *Children and youth in sport. A biopsychosocial perspective* (pp. 161–186). Dubuque, IA: Brown & Benchmark.

Martens, R. (1993). Psychological perspectives. In B. R. Cahill, & A. J. Pearl (Eds.), *Intensive participation in children's sports* (pp. 9–17). Champaign, IL: Human Kinetics.

Michigan joint legislative study on youth sports. (1978). Lansing, MI: State of Michigan.

Murphy, S. M. (1995). Transitions in competitive sport: Maximizing individual potential. In S. M. Murphy (Ed.), *Sport psychology interventions* (pp. 331–346). Champaign, IL: Human Kinetics.

Ommundsen, Y., & Vaglum, P. (1993). Soccer competition, anxiety and enjoyment in young boys: The influence of perceived competence and emotional involvement of significant others. In W. Duquet, P. De Knop, & L. Bollaert (Eds.), *Youth sport—A social approach* (pp. 110–117). Brussels: VUB Press.

Pearson, R. E., & Petitpas, A. J. (1990). Transitions of athletes: Developmental and preventive perspectives. *Journal of Counseling and Development, 69,* 7–10.

Petitpas, A., Champagne, D., Chartrand, J., Danish, S., & Murphy, S. (1997). *Athlete's guide to career planning. Keys to success from the playing field to professional life.* Champaign, IL: Human Kinetics.

Petitpas, A. J., Brewer, B. W., & Van Raalte, J. L. (1996). Transitions of the student-athlete: Theoretical, empirical, and practical perspectives. In E. F. Etzel, A. P. Ferrante, & J. W. Pinkney (Eds.), *Counseling college student-athletes: Issues and interventions* (pp. 137–156). Morgantown, WV: Fitness Information Technology.

Power, T. G., & Woolger, C. (1994). Parenting practices and age-group swimming: A correlational study. *Research Quarterly for Exercise and Sport, 65,* 59–66.

Régnier, G., Salmela, J., & Russell, S. J. (1993). Talent detection and development in sport. In R.N. Singer, M. Murphey, & K. Tennant (Eds.), *Handbook of research on sport psychology* (pp. 290–313). New York: MacMillan.

Reynolds, M. J. (1981). The effects of sports retirement on the job satisfaction of the former football player. In S. L. Greendorfer & A. Yiannakis (Eds.), *Sociology of sport: Diverse perspectives* (pp. 127–137). West Point, NY: Leisure Press.

Rotella, R. J., & Bunker, L. K. (1987). *Parenting your superstar.* Champaign, IL: Leisure Press.

Rowley, S. (1986). The role of the parent in youth sport. In G. R. Gleeson (Ed.), *The growing child in competitive sport* (pp. 92–99). London: Hodder & Stoughton.

Salmela, J. H. (1994). Phases and transitions across sports careers. In D. Hackfort (Ed.), *Psycho-social issues and interventions in elite sport* (pp. 11–28). Frankfurt: Lang.

Scanlan, T. K. (1988). Social evaluation and the competition process: A developmental perspective. In F. L. Smoll, R. A. Magill, & M. J. Ash (Eds.), *Children in sport* (pp. 135–148). Champaign, IL: Human Kinetics.

Scanlan, T. K., & Lewthwaite, R. (1984). Social psychological aspects of competition for male youth sport participants: I. Predictors of competitive stress. *Journal of Sport Psychology, 6,* 208–226.

Scanlan, T. K., & Lewthwaite, R. (1986). Social psychological aspects of competition for male youth sport participants: IV. Predictors of enjoyment. *Journal of Sport Psychology, 8,* 25–35.

Scanlan, T. K., Stein, D. L., & Ravizza, K. (1989). An in-depth study of former elite figure skaters: II. Sources of enjoyment. *Journal of Sport & Exercise Psychology, 11,* 65–83.

Schlossberg, N. K. (1981). A model for analyzing human adaptation to transition. *The Counseling Psychologist, 9,* 2–18.

Sebastien Godefroid wants to experience his dream in full (1996, July 16). *Gazet van Antwerpen.*

Seefeldt, V., Ewing, M. E., & Walk, S. R. (1982). *An overview of youth sports* [Paper commissioned by the Carnegie Council on Adolescents]. Washington, DC:

Sinclair, D. A., & Orlick, T. (1994). The effects of transition on high performance sport. In D. Hackfort (Ed.), *Psycho-social issues and interventions in elite sport* (pp. 29–55). Frankfurt: Lang.

Smith, R. E., Smoll, F. L., & Smith, N. J. (1989). *Parents' complete guide to youth sports.* Costa Mesa, CA: HDL.

Smoll, F. L. (1993). Enhancing coach-parent relationships in youth sport. In J. M. Williams (Ed.),

Applied sport psychology: Personal growth to peak performance (2nd ed., pp. 58–67). Mountain View, CA: Mayfield.

Stambulova, N. (1994). Developmental sports career investigations in Russia: A post-perestroika analysis. *The Sport Psychologist, 8,* 221–237.

Stambulova, N. (1998, August). Sports career transitions of Russian athletes: Summary of studies (1991–1997). In D. Alfermann (Chair), *Career transitions in sport: Determinants and consequences.* Paper presented at the 24th International Congress of Applied Psychology, San Francisco, CA.

Swain, D. A. (1991). Withdrawal from sport and Schlossberg's model of transitions. *Sociology of Sport Journal, 8,* 152–160.

Vanden Auweele, Y., & Wylleman, P. (1993). The interpersonal relationship between coaches and parents of young athletes. In S. Serpa, J. Alves, V. Fereira, & A. Paulo-Brito (Eds.), *Proceedings of the VIII World Congress of Sport Psychology* (pp. 184–187). Lisbon: International Society of Sport Psychology.

Weiss, M. R. (1993). Psychological effects of intensive sport participation on children and youth: Self-esteem and motivation. In B. R. Cahill & A. J. Pearl (Eds.), *Intensive participation in children's sports* (pp. 39–69). Champaign, IL: Human Kinetics.

Weiss, M. R. (1995). Children in sport: An educational model. In S. Murphy (Ed.), *Sport psychology interventions* (pp. 39–70). Champaign, IL: Human Kinetics.

Werthner, P., & Orlick, T. (1986). Retirement experiences of successful Olympic athletes. *International Journal of Sport Psychology, 17,* 337–363.

With a mobile home to squash tournaments. (1996, December 7–8). *Het Nieuwsblad.*

Wylleman, P., & De Knop, P. (1996, October). *Combining academic and athletic excellence: The case of elite student-athletes.* Paper presented at the International Conference of the European Council for High Ability, Vienna, Austria.

Wylleman, P., & De Knop, P. (1997a). The role and influence of the psychosocial environment on the career transistions of student-athletes. In J. Bangsbo, B. Saltin, H. Bonde, Y. Hellsten, B. Ibsen, M. Kjaer, & G. Sjogaard (Eds.), *Book of Abstracts 2nd Annual Congress of the European College of Sports Science* (pp. 90–91). Copenhagen: University of Copenhagen.

Wylleman, P., & De Knop, P. (1997b, June). *Elite student-athletes: Issues related to career development and social support.* Paper presented at the 12th Annual Conference on Counseling Athletes, Springfield, MA.

Wylleman, P., & De Knop, P. (1998, August). *Athletes' interpersonal perceptions of the "parent-coach" in competitive youth sport.* Paper presented at the 28th Congress of the International Association of Applied Psychology, San Francisco, CA.

Wylleman, P., & De Knop, P. (1999, May). *Parents' perceptions of youth sport coaches.* Paper presented at the International Conference on Youth Sports into the 21st Century, East Lansing, MI.

Wylleman, P., De Knop, P., Menkehorst, H., Theeboom, M., & Annerel, J. (1993). Career termination and social integration among elite athletes. In S. Serpa, J. Alves, V. Ferreira, & A. Paula-Brito (Eds.), *Proceedings of the VIII World Congress of Sport Psychology* (pp.902–905). Lisbon: International Society of Sport Psychology.

Wylleman, P., De Knop, P., & Sillen, D. (1998). *Former Olympic athletes' perceptions of retirement from high-level sport.* Paper presented at the 28th Congress of the International Association of Applied Psychology, San Francisco, CA.

Wylleman, P., & Theeboom, M. (1992). Stressmanagement bij jonge topatleten [Stress management for young high-level athletes]. In M. van der Meulen, H. A. B. M. Menkehorst, & F. C. Bakker (Eds.) *Jeugdig sporttalent: Psychologische aspecten van intensieve sportbeoefening* [Talented young athletes: Psychological aspects of intensive sport participation] (pp. 93–114). Amsterdam: Vereniging Sportpsychologie Nederland.

Wylleman, P., Vanden Auweele, Y., De Knop, P., Sloore, H., & De Martelaer, K. (1995). Elite young athletes, parents and coaches: Relationships in competitive sports. In F. J. Ring (Ed.), *Proceedings of the 1st Bath Sports Medicine Conference* (pp. 124–133). Bath, England: Centre for Continuing Education.

10

Sport Transitions Among Athletes With Disabilities

Jeffrey J. Martin
Wayne State University

Sport scientists have become increasingly interested in transitions out of sport. Unfortunately, little theoretically based research or applied literature is available examining transitions out of disability sport. Athletes with disabilities face challenges similar to those experienced by able-bodied athletes (Martin, 1996). The focus of this chapter, however, is to examine how leaving sport may be particularly challenging and unique for athletes with disabilities. This chapter examines the transition experience, motivation, social integration, and "quintuplet jeopardy," and discusses how these psychosocial processes influence the experience of sport withdrawal for athletes with disabilities.

Sport Transitions among Athletes with Disabilities

Sport science researchers have typically studied athletes participating "in" sport (Gill, 1997). However, the growing recognition that leaving sport has been very difficult for some athletes (Blinde & Stratta, 1992; Rosenberg, 1981) has led to an abundance of research in the last 10 years. Fortunately, it appears that most athletes successfully adjust to life without sport (Ogilvie & Taylor, 1993). In the only two published studies examining disability, most (i.e., 90%) athletes successfully left disability sport without suffering from persistent negative affect (G. Wheeler et al., 1996; G. D. Wheeler, Malone, VanVlack, Nelson, & Steadward, 1996).

The purpose of this chapter is to examine how athletes with physical disabilities (e.g., amputee, hearing impaired) withdraw from sport. It is important to examine how athletes with disabilities may experience sport withdrawal because their experiences do not mirror those of able-bodied athletes (G. Wheeler et al., 1996; G. D. Wheeler et al., 1996). Reasons for potential differences may be rooted in four broad considerations.

First, the socialization experiences of athletes with disabilities are quite different from those of able-bodied athletes (Nixon, 1988; Sherrill, Pope, & Arnhold, 1986; Sherrill & Rainbolt, 1986; Wang & DePauw, 1995; Williams, 1994; Williams & Taylor, 1994; Zoerink, 1987, 1992). For instance, contrary to able-bodied sport, more opportunities in disability sport exist for adults compared to children (Steadward, 1994).

Second, the major psychological and physical trauma that most athletes with a disability have dealt with influences the experience and quality of their athletic experience (Asken, 1991). Most athletes (i.e., 85%) have acquired disabilities (e.g., car accidents) as opposed to congenital disabilities (i.e., born with a disability).

Third, it is important to understand the pervasiveness of disability from a pragmatic perspective. Virtually all areas of life—economic, educational, social, psychological, and physiological—are affected (Chubon, 1994). Transportation difficulties (e.g., lack of appropriate transportation) and architectural barriers (e.g., curbs) are typically factors that nondisabled athletes do not have to consider. For example, at a recent world-class road race, wheelchair athletes housed on the upper floors of the hotel missed the race start as they were unable to get an empty elevator to the ground floor.

Finally, individuals with disabilities live in a world quite foreign to able-bodied people. People with disabilities are considered minorities (Kleinfield, 1979; Shapiro, 1993) and are often stigmatized (Goffman, 1963), discriminated against (Hockenberry, 1995; Yuker, 1987), and abused (Sobsey, 1994), and they feel powerless (Asch, 1986). Athletes with disabilities are not immune to the impact of the above forces.

The above factors are important considerations because they influence how athletes with disabilities experience sport and life and how they derive meaning from sport. In turn, the meaning and experience of a transition into a world without sport are shaped by these factors (Wheeler, Hutzler, et al., 1996; Wheeler, Malone, et al., 1996). In the following four sections, the transition experience, motivation, the concept of "quintuplet jeopardy," and social integration are discussed in relation to disability sport withdrawal. The objective is to provide the reader with unique information about how athletes with disabilities may experience a transition out of sport and the factors that influence sport withdrawal.

The Transition Experience

It appears that able-bodied athletes often withdraw from sport, yet remain involved in related capacities. For instance, ex-professional hockey players remained involved in sport through administration or coaching (Curtis & Ennis, 1988). Research with collegiate athletes has found that over their 4-year collegiate career, sport gradually diminished in importance (Blinde & Greendorfer, 1985), suggesting a lengthy process of "mental" disengagement. Being able to remain in sport in some capacity aids the process of leaving sport as a competitive athlete.

Unfortunately, the limited research in disability sport indicates that the opportunity for athletes with disabilities to remain in sport through administration or coaching is limited, and thus, few athletes do so (G. D. Wheeler et al., 1996). For instance, only 10% of disability sport coaches in the United States have a disability (DePauw & Gavron, 1991). The barriers and limited opportunities for sport involvement beyond the competitive realm may be exacerbated for female athletes (Olenik, Matthews, & Steadward, 1995; Sherrill, 1993b). In one report, athletes with disabilities who withdrew from sport devoted their energy towards nonsport interests (Wheeler, Malone, et al., 1996). Other retiring athletes purposely avoided sport and friends associated with sport as a coping mechanism (Wheeler, Malone, et al., 1996).

Formal programs, such as the Career Assessment Program for Athletes, which serves elite amateur athletes in the United States, and the Making the Jump program, which serves U.S. collegiate athletes (Anderson & Morris, this volume; Pearson & Petitpas, 1990), acknowledge the institutional obligations that organizations have to help able-bodied athletes successfully leave sport (Thomas & Ermler, 1988). The availability of similar programs for athletes with disabilities is lacking, or such programs are underutilized, and athletes with disabilities have indicated that they received little institutional support in the form of retirement advice in spite of their support for such programs (G. D. Wheeler et al., 1996). Evidence that many athletes with disabilities neither thought of leaving sport while participating nor prepared for retirement suggests that athletes with disabilities are unprepared for leaving sport (G. D. Wheeler et al., 1996).

However, there is reason for optimism as programs and services are available. For instance, the Athlete Career and Education program of the Australian Institute of Sport is available for elite athletes with disabilities. Of greater note is the Paralympic Employment Program (PEP) developed by the Australian

Paralympic Committee and a leading employment agency. The PEP is geared specifically to aid Paralympians in career planning, job placement, and retirement counseling (K. Smith, personal communication, April 27, 1999).

Reports that many athletes with disabilities did not think of leaving sport while participating, nor did they prepare for retirement, suggest that athletes with disabilities are unprepared for leaving sport (G. D. Wheeler et al., 1996). A variety of researchers have also suggested that athletes with no control over when they stop competing are at risk for emotional difficulties (e.g., Ogilvie & Taylor, 1993). A particularly poignant example of an athlete with no control over the end of her career has been presented by Sherrill (1993b) in an account of how a 1992 Paralympic team member was told, shortly before the start of the Games, that she would not be going because her event had been canceled. The continuing development and refinement of a controversial (Richter, Adams-Mushett, Ferrara, & McCann, 1992) classification system are still evolving and likely to continue (C. Mushett, personal communication, August 26, 1998), resulting in more elite athletes, particularly women and those with severe disabilities, experiencing abrupt endings to their careers.

In summary, athletes with disabilities may face abrupt endings to their careers, be psychologically unprepared to leave sport, receive little institutional support, and have few opportunities to truly transition out of sport by being involved in related sport capacities.

Motivation

Athletes with disabilities have motivational orientations that vary in strength similar to those of able-bodied athletes (Martin, Mushett, & Eklund, 1994; Martin, Mushett, & Smith, 1995; White & Duda, 1993). Athletes with disabilities, similar to able-bodied athletes, use sport for typical physiological (e.g., strength), psychological (e.g., competence), social (e.g., friendship), and economic (e.g., travel) reasons. Thus, by leaving sport, disabled athletes would cease to derive these sport-specific benefits. For instance, athletes examined by G. D. Wheeler and colleagues (1996) were aware of losing fitness as a result of not training or competing. Fitness and functional status are particularly important for many individuals with disabilities because they directly relate to health-related quality of life (Rejeski, Brawley, & Shumaker, 1996).

Martin (1998) speculated that athletes with disabilities have motivations that are closely related to the meaning their disability holds for them, and Asken (1991) has noted that athletes with disabilities may also hold complex motivations. Sport may be a vehicle to exhibit "ability" versus "disability" (Sherrill, 1993a) and a way for athletes to be seen as normal (G. D. Wheeler et al., 1996). In fact, athletes often reference themselves as being "beyond normal" (G. D. Wheeler et al.). Athletes may also use sport to cope with their disability (G. D.

Wheeler et al.), overcome marginalization (G. D. Wheeler et al.), develop self-determination, overcome feelings of powerlessness, and advance the disability sport movement (Martin, 1996, 1998). Clearly, leaving sport would mean that athletes could no longer meet their needs in the above areas and might present adjustment challenges not typically found among able-bodied athletes.

In summary, athletes with disabilities may hold unique and complex motivations for sport involvement. Accordingly, leaving sport means athletes are void of an activity that allowed them the opportunity to meet a variety of unique and complex needs.

Quintuplet Jeopardy

Wheeler and colleagues used the term "quintuplet jeopardy" to refer to a multitude of challenges that may accompany leaving sport (G. D. Wheeler et al., 1996). In addition to leaving sport, athletes may have to cope with their disability for the first time, deal with a chronic injury or a "secondary disability," and face fears of aging with a disability (G. Wheeler et al., 1996; G. D. Wheeler et al.). Clearly, facing simultaneous stressors taxes people's abilities to cope with any one particular issue (Schlossberg, 1984).

In some countries, athletes are introduced to competitive sport shortly (e.g., one month) after they have acquired their disability (G. Wheeler et al., 1996). Although such quick sport involvement is designed to aid adjustment, some athletes may use sport to avoid coping with their disability (G. D. Wheeler et al., 1996). Athletes have reported achieving Paralympic status and then leaving sport while still trying to adjust to their disability (G. D. Wheeler et al.).

A growing body of research examining injuries suffered by wheelchair athletes has noted chronic overuse injuries involving the shoulders and hands (Ferrara, Buckley, & McCann, 1992; Ferrara & Davis, 1990). G. D. Wheeler et al. (1996) reported that chronic injuries, combined with a lack of sport success, were associated with postsport life dissatisfaction and that athletes feared a chronic injury or a "secondary disability."

Athletes also have fears about growing old with a disability and dealing with a chronic injury at the same time. The aging and disability literature has noted that individuals with disabilities may age sooner than if they were not disabled although there is likely to be wide variation in aging across and among disability type and severity (Trieschmann, 1987). In short, people with disabilities face potential problems that are unique to aging and their disability (Ansello & Eustis, 1992).

In summary, athletes with disabilities leaving sport have to deal with athletically related concerns (e.g., loss of fitness). Additionally, they may face issues related to their initial disabling condition, contend with a chronic injury, and deal with fears about growing old with a disability condition.

Social Integration

Social support is an important factor in adjustment to sport withdrawal (Baillie & Danish, 1992). When athletes leave sport, they typically have less access to social support provided by their teammates. Elite British wheelchair athletes provided each other with support through training, racing, and traveling together to races (Williams & Taylor, 1994). By living substantial distances from each other, elite wheelchair athletes would clearly face reduced social support from teammates upon leaving sport (Williams & Taylor). G. D. Wheeler et al. (1996) noted that most retired and semiretired athletes in their investigation frequently mentioned missing friends although they had satisfying nonsport relationships.

It is important to note that many people with disabilities have less extensive social networks and opportunities for career-related social contact. For example, the United States Bureau of Census estimates that almost two thirds of individuals with severe disabilities are unemployed or underemployed (McNeil, 1993) and engage in much less social activity compared to nondisabled individuals (McNeil, 1993; Zoerink, 1992). Reduced social support (Fuhrer, Rintala, & Hart, 1992) and physical activity (Noreau & Shephard, 1995) for spinal-cord-injured individuals are related to reduced quality of life.

In summary, leaving athletics may be particularly difficult for individuals who already face reduced social integration because of limited mobility, employment opportunities, and social networks.

Summary

Athletes with disabilities likely face unique challenges when they decide to withdraw from competitive sport (G. Wheeler et al., 1996; G. D. Wheeler et al., 1996). Trauma from an acquired disability, the impact of disability on daily life, disability culture, and unique sport socialization experiences all shape the meaning sport holds for athletes with disabilities and subsequently influence their transitions out of disability sport.

Information was provided in four related areas that suggested (a) disabled athletes may be unprepared for sport withdrawal and have limited opportunities to remain connected to sport; (b) the absence of sport as a vehicle with which to meet a variety of disability-related psychosocial needs may make withdrawal particularly difficult; (c) the presence of "quintuplet jeopardy" suggests disabled athletes may have to simultaneously deal with multiple stressors or transitions; and (d) leaving sport reduces opportunities for disabled athletes to be socially integrated. Athletes with disabilities will likely face many challenges in adapting to life without sport. It is hoped that information presented in this chapter will stimulate professional discourse and continued research, ultimately benefiting the many athletes who face the challenges of sport withdrawal.

References

Asch, A. (1986). Will populism empower the disabled? *Social Policy, 16,* 12–18.

Asken, M. J. (1991). The challenge of the physically challenged: Delivering sport psychology services to physically disabled athletes. *The Sport Psychologist, 5,* 370–381.

Ansello, E. F., & Eustis, N. N. (1992). *Aging and disabilities: Seeking common ground.* Amityville, NY: Baywood.

Baillie, P. H. F., & Danish, S. J. (1992). Understanding the career transition of athletes. *The Sport Psychologist, 6,* 77–98.

Blinde, E. M., & Greendorfer, S. L. (1985). A reconceptualization of the process of leaving the role of competitive athlete. *International Review for the Sociology of Sport, 20,* 87–93.

Blinde, E. M., & Stratta, T. M. (1992). The "sport career death" of college athletes: Involuntary and unanticipated sport exits. *The Journal of Sport Behavior, 15,* 3–20.

Chubon, R. A. (1994). *Social and psychological foundations of rehabilitation.* Springfield, IL: Charles C. Thomas Publisher.

Crook, J. M., & Robertson, S. E. (1991). Transitions out of elite sport. *International Journal of Sport Psychology, 22,* 115–127.

Curtis, J., & Ennis, R. (1988). Negative consequences of leaving competitive sport? Comparative findings for former elite-level hockey players. *Sociology of Sport Journal, 5,* 87–106.

DePauw, K. P., & Gavron, S. J. (1991). Coaches of athletes with disabilities. *The Physical Educator, 48,* 33–40.

Ferrara, M. S., Buckley, W. E., & McCann, B. C. (1992). The injury experience of the competitive athlete with a disability. *Medicine & Science in Sports & Exercise, 24,* 184–188.

Ferrara, M. S., & Davis, R. W. (1990). Injuries to wheelchair athletes. *Paraplegia, 28,* 335–341.

Fuhrer, M. J., Rintala, D. H., & Hart, K. A. (1992). Relationship of life satisfaction to impairment, disability and handicap among persons with spinal cord injury living in the community. *Archives of Physical Medicine Rehabilitation, 73,* 552–557.

Gill, D. L. (1997). Sport and exercise psychology. In J. D. Massengale, & R. A. Swanson (Eds.), *The history of exercise and sport science* (pp. 293–320). Champaign, IL: Human Kinetics.

Goffman, E. (1963). *Stigma: Notes on the management of spoiled identity.* New York: Simon & Schuster.

Hockenberry, J. (1995). *Moving violations.* New York: Hyperion.

Kleinfield, S. (1979). *The hidden minority: America's handicapped.* Boston: Little, Brown and Co.

Martin, J. J. (1996). Transitions out of competitive sport for athletes with disabilities. *Therapeutic Recreation Journal, 30,* 128–136.

Martin, J. J. (1998). *Applied sport psychology considerations for athletes with disabilities.* Paper presented at the 2nd International Meeting of Psychology Applied to Sport and Exercise, Braga, Portugal.

Martin, J. J., Mushett, C., & Eklund, R. (1994). Factor structure of the Athletic Identity Measurement Scale with adolescent swimmers with disabilities. *Brazilian Journal of Adapted Physical Education Research, 1,* 87–101.

Martin, J. J., Mushett, C., & Smith, K. L. (1995). Athletic identity and sport orientation of elite athletes with disabilities. *Adapted Physical Activity Quarterly, 12,* 113–123.

McNeil, J. M., (1993). *Americans with disabilities, 1991–92: United States Bureau of the Census current population reports, P70–33.* Washington DC: United States Government Printing Office.

Nixon, H. L.(1988). Getting over the worry hurdle: Parental encouragement and the sports involvement of visually impaired children and youths. *Adapted Physical Activity Quarterly, 5,* 29–43.

Noreau, L., & Shephard, R. J. (1995). Spinal cord injury, exercise and quality of life. *Sports Medicine, 20,* 226–250.

Ogilvie, B., & Taylor, J. (1993). Career termination issues among elite athletes. In R. N. Singer, M. Murphey, & L. K. Tennant (Eds.), *Handbook of research on sport psychology* (pp. 761–775). New York: Macmillan.

Olenik, L. M., Matthews, J. M., & Steadward, R. D. (1995). Women, disability and sport. *Canadian Woman Studies, 14,* 54–57.

Pearson, R., & Petitpas, A. (1990). Transitions of athletes: Developmental and preventive perspectives. *Journal of Counseling and Development, 70,* 7–10.

Rejeski, W. J., Brawley, L. R., & Shumaker, S. A. (1996). Physical activity and health-related quality of life. *Exercise and Sport Science Reviews, 24,* 71–108.

Richter, K. R., Adams-Mushett, C., Ferrara, M. S., & McCann, B. C. (1992). Integrated swimming classification: A faulted system. *Adapted Physical Activity Quarterly, 9,* 5–13.

Rosenberg, E. (1981). Gerontological theory and athletic retirement. In S. L. Greendorfer & A. Yiannakis (Eds.), *Sociology of sport: Diverse perspectives* (pp. 119–126). Champaign, IL: Leisure Press.

Schlossberg, N. K. (1984). *Counseling adults in transitions: Linking theory to practice.* New York: Springer.

Shapiro, J. (1993). *No pity: People with disabilities forging a new civil rights movement.* New York: Random House.

Sherrill, C. (1993a). *Adapted physical activity, recreation and sport: Cross-disciplinary and lifespan.* Madison, WI: Brown & Benchmark.

Sherrill, C. (1993b). Women with disability, Paralympics, and reasoned action contact theory. *Women in Sport and Physical Activity Journal, 2,* 51–60.

Sherrill, C., Pope, C., & Arnhold, R. (1986). Sport socialization of blind athletes: An exploratory study. *Journal of Visual Impairment and Blindness, 80,* 740–744.

Sherrill, C., & Rainbolt, W. J. (1986). Sociological perspectives of cerebral palsy sports. *Palaestra, Summer,* 21–50.

Sobsey, D. (1994). *Violence and abuse in the lives of people with disabilities.* Baltimore: Brookes.

Steadward, R. D. (1994). From community participation in physical activity to Olympic integration. In H. A. Quinney, L. Gauvin, & A. E. T. Wall (Eds.), *Toward active living: Proceedings of the International Conference on Physical Activity, Fitness and Health* (pp. 171–178). Champaign, IL: Human Kinetics.

Thomas, C. E., & Ermler, K. L. (1988). Institutional obligations in the athletic retirement process. *Quest, 40,* 137–150.

Trieschmann, R. B. (1987). *Aging with a disability.* New York: Demos.

Wang, W., & DePauw, K. P. (1995). Early sport socialization of elite Chinese athletes with physical and sensory disabilities. *Palaestra, Winter,* 40–46.

Wheeler, G., Hutzler, S., Campbell, E., Malone, L., Legg, D., & Steadward, R. D. (1996). *Retirement from disability sport: A cross cultural analysis.* Paper presented at the Paralympic conference, Atlanta, USA.

Wheeler, G. D., Malone, L. A., VanVlack, S., Nelson, E. R., & Steadward, R. D. (1996). Retirement from disability sport: A pilot study. *Adapted Physical Activity Quarterly, 13,* 382–399.

White, S., & Duda, J. (1993). Dimensions of goals and beliefs among adolescent athletes with physical disabilities. *Adapted Physical Activity Quarterly, 10,* 125–136.

Williams, T. (1994). Disability sport socialization and identity construction. *Adapted Physical Activity Quarterly, 11,* 14–31.

Williams, T., & Taylor, D. (1994). Socialization, subculture, and wheelchair sport: The influence of peers in wheelchair racing. *Adapted Physical Activity Quarterly, 11,* 416–428.

Yuker, H. E. (1987). *Attitudes towards persons with disabilities.* New York: Springer.

Zoerink, D. A. (1987). Early play and recreation experiences of persons with physical disabilities: An exploration. *Adapted Physical Activity Quarterly, 4,* 293–304.

Zoerink, D. A. (1992). Exploring sport socialization environments of persons with orthopedic disabilities. *Palaestra, Spring,* 38–44.

11

Career Transitions Among Dancers

Wendy Patton and Susan Ryan
Queensland University of Technology
Australia

Abstract

This chapter is one of the few in this volume to outline the place of career transition in career theory. Following an introductory section, models of career transition are explored. Although these models have been primarily developed to explain issues in athletes' career transition, the authors believe that because of the similarity between athletes and dancers, researchers and practitioners working with each group can learn from each other in relation to career transition issues. The authors then focus on empirical work in relation to dancers' career transition and look at centers that have been developed to assist dancers in the career transition process.

Career Transitions among Dancers

Why dancers in a book about career transitions in sport? In terms of investment, commitment, and the pattern of their careers, athletes and dancers share many similarities. These include an early and enduring identification with their field, from intensive training commencing at a young age (Pickman, 1987; Saposnek, 1995). After years of dedicated training, dance students may become professional performers while teenagers (Schnitt & Schnitt, 1987), mirroring the elite level of performance required of their athletic peers who compete at national and international levels.

Saposnek (1995) emphasizes that much of this intensive commitment among dancers occurs during the stage of identity development (Erikson, 1968). Indeed some researchers have commented that intensive training in sport during adolescence contributes to a lack of exploration (i.e., identity foreclosure) and a related poor career maturity (Murphy, Petitpas, & Brewer, 1996). Thus, early athletic commitment and selective involvement in sport may restrict exploration of other career options. Hence, there may be similarities in identity development between athletes and dancers at this stage and, consequently, a parallel impact on their career development.

Commitment and endeavor, however, do not secure a career of many years' standing for dancers or athletes. Most will be faced with a professional career that will begin and end earlier than the more traditional careers that their peers will choose. Sinclair and Orlick (1993) estimate that most professional athletes retire, voluntarily or involuntarily, between 25 and 30 years of age. Similarly, few dancers continue to dance professionally after 40 years of age. Australian dancers making a career transition are generally between 25 and 30 years of age (Beall, 1989); most dancers in North America stop performing professionally by the age of 35 years (Pickman, 1987). Thus, dancers or athletes may leave their profession at a time when other professionals (e.g., doctor or lawyer) are becoming established in their careers (Paritzky, 1995).

These issues of early identification and commitment, particularly during a crucial identity development stage, and familiarity and preference for a role are identified by Baillie and Danish (1992) as likely stressors for athletes when the role is lost. Baillie and Danish discuss the importance of understanding the transition from "the role of athlete to the role of former athlete" (p. 77). We contend that because of the similarity between athletes and dancers, researchers and practitioners working with each group can learn from each other in relation to career transition issues.

In this chapter, we will outline the place of career transition in career theory and explore models of career transition. We will then focus on dancers' career transition and look at centers that have been developed to assist dancers in the transition process.

Career Theory and Transition

There is a robust body of literature outlining the many theories proffered to explain career behavior (Patton & McMahon, 1999). However, much of this theory has been directed toward career choice as opposed to career development, including career change. For example, many of the major theories, including those of Holland (1992), Dawis and Lofquist (1984), and Dawis (1996), focus on the content of career decision making, for instance, the fit between personality and environment. Other approaches in this category focus on other elements of content, for example, values (Brown, 1996) and personality (McCrae & John, 1992).

Theories that focus on content and process, for example, the work of social learning theorist Krumboltz (1979; Mitchell & Krumboltz, 1990) and sociocognitive theorists Lent, Brown, and Hackett (1994), emphasize the process of learning career behaviors. Although these theories allow for the process of career change, there is a limited focus on transition or on factors influencing this process.

The process or developmental theoretical approaches acknowledge that career choice is not a single static decision but rather a dynamic developmental process involving a number of decisions made over time, often in serial form. These approaches are referred to as life-span approaches as they view career choices as occurring throughout life. These approaches include the work of Ginzberg and his colleagues (Ginzberg, 1984; Ginzberg, Ginsburg, Axelrad, & Herma, 1951), Gottfredson (1981, 1996), and the major theorist in this category, Super (1980, 1992, 1994).

Super's theory (1980, 1992, 1994) has particular application to discussions of career transition and to the career transition of dancers. Emphasizing temporal continuity in career development across the life span through delineating a series of stages, Super describes tasks or concerns associated with each stage that may be predictable chronologically or related to situations requiring adaptive behaviors. A number of salient constructs to understanding career transition have been proposed. For example, Super describes the process of career maturity (i.e., the readiness to make educational and vocational choices) in adolescence and the related term, *career adaptability* (i.e., a sense of "planfulness" and readiness to deal with changing work and working conditions) in adulthood. In addition to describing macro life-span stages, Super acknowledges that an individual may recycle through previous stages as personal or contextual factors necessitate change. Such a theoretical proposition provides a mechanism for broader midlife career transition and, in particular, the career transition of dancers, with personal (injury) and contextual (nonrenewal of contract) factors that may contribute to the transition being identified.

Another construct delineated by Super (1980, 1992, 1994), role salience, also has particular application to understanding dancers' career transitions. *Role salience* describes the multiple life roles enacted by an individual and the importance attributed to each role. Super, Savickas, and Super (1996) assert that obsolete roles may be relinquished and new roles adopted during the process of career transition. Thus, the developmental theory of Super provides a framework for the investigation of career transition processes and issues relevant to dancers.

Career Transition Models

Most traditional theorizing about careers has envisaged fixed positions that have clear and stable boundaries and purposes. More recently, however, with rapid and dynamic changes in the world of work (detailed in Feller & Walz, 1996; Hall, 1996; Patton & McMahon, 1999), individuals can expect careers that will increasingly be discontinuous and transitional in nature, as opposed to being continuous and stable. Such a perspective on career transitions serves as a broad context in which to focus our discussion on career transition models.

It is important to distinguish here between the objective and subjective career. The objective career refers to the externally defined and visible events that define an individual' s work history. The subjective career is recognized in the attitudes, orientations, and perceptions about the career that is held by the individual. Within the changing nature of career for individuals, and in this case for dancers, an understanding of career transition needs to focus on objective and subjective careers. Louis (1980a, 1980b) proposed that a career transition occurs when an individual moves from one role to another (objective career) or changes orientation to a role already held (subjective change). Such a definition incorporates traditional job transitions, such as transfers, promotions, and redundancies, as well as subjective aspects of career, such as changes in an individual's orientation toward career. Research by Nicholson and West (1989) illustrated that an orderly step-like objective career transition process (i.e., promotions and/or lateral moves) is now the exception rather than the rule and represents only 10% of the workforce.

Louis (1980a) developed a model of career transitions that identified interrole (objective) transitions and intrarole (subjective) transitions. Interrole transitions include workforce entry or reentry, intra- and interorganizational transitions, interprofession transitions, and workforce exit. Intrarole transitions relate to the individual's adopting a new and different orientation to an existing role. These transitions can be seen to be relevant to dancers' careers, and similar examples could be cited for athletes. They include intrarole adjustment (changes to a work role as the work role changes, for example, a dancer's contributing to the choreographic process for a particular production), extra-role adjustment (adjustment to a work role as a result of change in a role outside of work, for example, career adjustment to fit with the demands of parenting), career-stage transitions (change from one career stage to another, for example, moving from performance to teaching), and life-stage transitions (a subset of extra-role adjustment, for example, modifying career activity to have children).

A number of models of career transition have been posited as relevant to an athlete's career. These include thanatology, where retirement is seen as social death, or alienation from a former group to which an individual belonged (Rosenberg, 1984). Social gerontological perspectives describe the aging of an individual and cessation of the athletic career as retirement from the workforce. Both models have been criticized as inappropriate for application to athletes' career research (e.g., Blinde & Greendorfer, 1985; Crook & Robertson, 1991), with little empirical support and limited relevance to the many athletes who leave their career in midlife, but will continue to work in alternative or related careers for another 30 years (Mason, 1993). These criticisms are equally relevant when considering the applicability of these models to dancers' career transitions.

One of a number of models of athlete career transition that may be useful for understanding issues inherent in dancers' career transitions is that of Taylor and Ogilvie (1994, 1998). As outlined in chapter 7 in this volume, they have proposed a five-step model that outlines adaptation to career transition through its developmental course. First, they suggest that causal factors that initiate the transition should be identified (e.g., internal or external factors). Second, factors related to adaptation to transition, such as developmental experiences, conceptualizations of identity, and perceptions of control, need to be specified. Third, available resources, such as coping skills, social support, and preretirement planning, need to be spelt out. Fourth, the quality of the adaptation to the transition should be described, and finally, treatment issues should be explored for problem reactions to the transition process. However, before any of these models can be used extensively in practice, empirical support for them is necessary.

Dancers' Career Transition

Taylor and Ogilvie (1994) state that the body of research devoted to athletes' career transition has evolved during the past two decades from initial writings that were based upon clinicians' and other professionals' impressions gained from assisting athletes with career transition to current, more systematic investigations examining retirement from a variety of sports. Although dancers' career transition is an even more nascent area of research, it has developed likewise in the last 10 years from anecdotal writings to include a small number of surveys and a handful of interview studies detailing the experiences of ex-professional dancers. Although limited in scope, this condensed body of work provides a pinhole view of the state of dancers' career transition research.

From survey responses of 298 ex-professional dancers in North America, Wallach (1988) identified that the average career of contemporary dancers and female ballet dancers is 10 years, with male ballet dancers performing for an average of 14 years. The median retirement age reported for female ballet dancers was 26 to 30 years of age; for the remaining groups, the median age of transition from dance was between 31 and 35 years of age. However, dancers anticipated retiring later than these ages. Male dancers expected, on average, to retire between 36 and 40 years of age; female ballet dancers, between 31 and 35 years; and female contemporary dancers, from 40 years and onward. Similarly, in a survey of 180 professional and retired dancers in Australia, Beall (1989) found that most dancers who had made a career transition were between 25 and 30 years of age, although she emphasized that many of these dancers did not expect to retire from dance until they were closer to or beyond 40 years of age. Thus, a dance student may train for a minimum of 10 years (Avery, 1994) to have a professional career that may last only the same amount of time. If the results of these two surveys are typical, then dance students and dance professionals may overestimate the age at which they will leave their performance career. Not only is this an issue relevant to dance students at the time of career choice, but it is likely also to contribute to the difficulty experienced by some dancers in adjusting to and dealing with the transition process.

According to the survey by Wallach (1988), reasons for leaving a dance career were varied and included injury (39% of female ballet dancers; 27% of female contemporary dancers; 20% of male dancers), lack of financial security (22% of female contemporary dancers), and family considerations (25% of female dancers). Wallach also identified the tendency for female dancers to be "pushed" out of performing through injury, age, frustration with the lifestyle, reduced opportunities for work, and changing technical competence. In contrast, male dancers were distinguished as generally "pulled" out of performing by a new career interest or the desire for change.

Causes for transition by the Australian dancers in the Beall (1989) report included reduced opportunities for mature dancers, injury, dissatisfaction with the disruptive lifestyle of dance, financial constraints, and family considerations. Causes for dancers' career transition have some similarity, therefore, to precursors to athletic career termination identified by Taylor and Ogilvie (1994) as clustering around four factors: chronological age, deselection, injury, and free choice.

Although the majority of dancers in Wallach's (1988) survey reported experiences of control over their decision to leave dance, 88% of respondent dancers reported emotional or physical difficulties related to retirement from their performing career. Six percent of the female dancers reported suicidal tendencies. Nearly one half of the female dancers described loss of self-esteem, loneliness, or isolation associated with the transition. Furthermore, over half of the female dancers described career confusion, with 61% of all dancers reporting an identity crisis. Nearly one half of all respondents sought assistance from counseling and other health professionals.

Consistent with Wallach's (1988) findings, Beall (1989) identified that more than one half of the Australian respondents reported difficulty with the transition experience. It is possible that dancers' experiences at the end of their performing career may emulate athletes' career transition, given that a number of studies report that athletes may experience difficulty at the end of their professional career (e.g., Werthner & Orlick, 1986; Wylleman, De Knop, Menkehorst, Theeboom, & Annerel, 1993). Not all transitions from sport are problematic, however, with some athletes reporting retirement as a positive experience (Sinclair & Orlick, 1993).

Although the described surveys provide a limited snapshot of the career transition experience for dancers, consistency of findings is evident in relation to the early age at which dancers leave their profession, the discrepancy between anticipated and actual age of retirement, the perceived distress that some dancers report during transition, and the range of precursors to retirement. These findings are supported by a clique of smaller studies of ex-professional dancers in the United States and Canada.

Mason (1993) concluded from unstructured interviews conducted with eight professional dancers who had left a dance career 2 to 10 years previously that career transition can be stressful due to a dancer's limited exposure to other career/life roles and investment in the dancer's identity. Although acknowledging limitations, such as interview bias, Mason emphasized that perceived control over the decision to leave dance and involvement in alternative activities may enhance adjustment following midlife career change.

A study of 25 former professional ballet dancers in North America concurs with these findings. Relying on current and retrospective questionnaire completion, Saposnek (1995) reported that more than three quarters of the dancers experienced identity change or loss due to transition. Minimal perceived control of transition was associated with problematic transition, with limited control related to negative emotionality including feelings of anger, alienation, fatigue, and depression. Although this is one of the few studies to employ quantitative analyses, further research needs to extend the sample size, focus on data of recent transition experiences, and use validated measures.

Following a hermeneutic approach, Paritzky (1995) extracted data from biographical questionnaire completion and a series of interviews of 15 ex-professional dancer. Although all dancers reported loss related to separation from their colleagues and the kinaesthetic element of dance, two distinct patterns of career change were identified: crisis and smooth. Crisis changers perceived the end of their dance career as a loss of their identity, had limited control over their exit from their professional dance career, and had not prepared for the transition. In contrast, smooth changers identified feelings of control regarding the decision to leave their performance career, although they cited similar reasons for career change, including age, attenuated employment opportunities, and financial insecurity. Furthermore, satisfaction with career achievements, consistent family approbation, and development of alternative identities beyond that of a performer characterized smooth changers. Paritzky concluded that smooth changers were buffered by a positive self-concept that incorporated identities beyond dance.

This research is resonant of findings from athlete transition research. As an example, strong commitment to an athletic identity was found to be inversely related to career planning prior to transition from a sporting career (Grove, Lavallee, & Gordon, 1997). During transition, athletes who perceive minimal control regarding the cause for retirement may experience greater adjustment difficulty (Lavallee, Grove, & Gordon, 1997). Athletes are more likely to make a smoother career transition, however, if they perceive that they have achieved their goals in sport, with those who feel incompetent outside of sport experiencing poorer adjustment (Sinclair & Orlick, 1993).

As a more established body of research, literature devoted to athletes' transition may inform research on dancers' transition. At this early stage in the latter's development, there appear to be some common themes between the two areas of research. This is most evident in relation to the impact that investment in the athletic or dancer identity may have on the quality of subsequent midlife career transition. Research on dancers' transition remains significantly uncharted, however, and further research findings can only provide a more accurate view of similarities and distinctions between these two subpopulations.

Career Transition Centers for Dancers

Although dancer transition research is in its infancy, increased awareness of the needs of dancers at the end of performing has led to the establishment of a number of dancer transition centers around the world. Typically, these centers provide a range of services that may include personal and career counseling, financial and/or legal advice, and mentoring relationships with ex-professional dancers who have experienced transition to a new career. Access to retraining information, training opportunities, scholarships, and other career information may be available. Financial advice, subsistence grants, and loans are provided by some centers, in addition to guidance in small business establishment and operation.

One such organization, the Dancer Transition Centre, was established in Toronto in 1985 and has regional representation in a number of other Canadian cities. Now titled the Dancer Transition Resource Centre, the organization is funded through a combination of government, corporate, private, and membership sources. By contributing to the center a small percentage of their salary, which is matched by their company, dancers can become members. Personal, academic, career, financial, and legal counseling is available through the center. A dancer-awareness program involves educational seminars designed to increase dancers' awareness of the need for preparation for midlife career transition. A public awareness program includes newspaper publication, conferences, and other activities aimed at increasing public awareness of dancer transition issues. Dancers may be eligible to receive funding through grants to improve work-relevant skills, provide retraining in a new career area (with and without subsistence support), and assist transition through special awards.

Similar centers are in operation in the United States, the United Kingdom, and the Netherlands. Less comprehensive services (some providing only financial support) are provided by dance companies in a number of other countries, including Australia, which is in the process of requesting governmental assistance to support the establishment of a dancer transition scheme.

Although these centers receive positive feedback from the dancers they assist, there appears to be little work published on the efficacy of different interventions to assist dancers with midlife career transition. A study by White and Guest (1995) attempted to detail assistance provided to a small group of dancers in Western Australia through a series of four workshops. Focusing on career change planning, communication skills, self-esteem building, and job-acquisition training, this program drew its program content from interviews conducted with 27 dancers and other personnel within the dance industry and from information from other transition schemes. Although the workshops seemed to be well received by the participants, the authors stress that further research is necessary to accurately identify the complexity of issues surrounding dancers' career transition and most appropriate methods of facilitation through this phase. Given the recent establishment of the International Organization for the Transition of Professional Dancers (see contact details at the end of the chapter), it seems likely that rigorous research into transition facilitation may be generated by its members and associates and hence identify the most efficacious forms of assistance to dancers.

Conclusion

Research examining career transitions of former professional dancers is exploratory and is not yet grounded in career development theory. From the few studies that have been conducted, a number of shared observations can be noted. These include the notion that a dancer's career is time limited; departure from a professional dance career may relate to a range of factors; some dancers will experience distress during transition; dancers may invest significantly in their identity as a dancer; and perceived control and alternative roles may facilitate transition. These studies need to be complemented, however, by further research employing larger sample sizes, valid and reliable measures, and mixed-method designs for the purposes of convergence and elaboration. Research is warranted also in program evaluation. It appears that although a number of dancer-transition centers may have internal quality assurance mechanisms, factors that may facilitate career transition in the dance population have yet to be identified using rigorous research methodology including control groups. Appropriate empirical research can only strengthen the quality of assistance provided to dancers at this critical time and ensure that they may move to the next stage of their career with greater ease.

References

Avery, C.B. (1994). Dancers' career. (Master's thesis, The American University, 1992). *Masters Abstracts International, 32,* 6.

Baillie, P. H. F., & Danish, S. J. (1992). Understanding the career transition of athletes. *The Sports Psychologist, 6,* 77–98.

Beall, C. (1989). *Dancers' transition: A report investigating the needs of professional dancers making career transitions.* Canberra: Australian Association for Dance Education.

Blinde, E. M., & Greendorfer, S. L. (1985). A reconceptualization of the process of leaving the role of competitive athlete. *International Review of Sport Sociology, 20,* 87–93.

Brown, D. (1996). Brown's values-based, holistic model of career and life role choices and satisfaction. In D. Brown & L. Brooks (Eds.), *Career choice and development* (3rd ed., pp. 337–372). San Francisco: Jossey-Bass.

Crook, J., & Robertson, S. (1991). Transitions out of elite sports. *International Journal of Sports Psychology, 22,* 115–127.

Dawis, R. V. (1996). The theory of work adjustment and person-environment-correspondence counseling. In D. Brown & L. Brooks (Eds.), *Career choice and development* (3rd ed., pp. 75–120). San Francisco: Jossey-Bass.

Dawis, R. V., & Lofquist, L. H. (1984). *A psychological theory of work adjustment.* Minneapolis: University of Minnesota Press.

Erikson, E. (1968). *Identity, youth and crisis.* New York: Norton.

Feller, R., & Walz, G. (Eds.). (1996). *Career transitions in turbulent times: Exploring work, learning and careers.* Greensboro, NC: Educational Resources Information Center.

Ginzberg, E. (1984). Career development. In D. Brown & L. Brooks (Eds.), *Career choice and development* (pp. 169–191). San Francisco: Jossey-Bass.

Ginzberg, E., Ginsburg, S. W., Axelrad, S., & Herma, J. L. (1951). *Occupational choice: An approach to a general theory.* New York: Columbia University Press.

Gottfredson, L. S. (1981). Circumscription and compromise: A developmental theory of occupational aspirations. *Journal of Counseling Psychology, 28,* 545–579.

Gottfredson, L. S. (1996). Gottfredson's theory of circumscription and compromise. In D. Brown & L. Brookes (Eds.), *Career choice and development* (3rd ed., pp.179–232). San Francisco: Jossey-Bass.

Grove, J. R., Lavallee, D., & Gordon, S. (1997). Coping with retirement from sport: The influence of athletic identity. *Journal of Applied Sport Psychology, 9,* 191–203.

Hall, D. T. (Ed.). (1996). *The career is dead—long live the career: A relational approach to careers.* San Francisco: Jossey-Bass.

Holland, J. L. (1992). *Making vocational choices: A theory of vocational personalities and work environments* (2nd ed.). Odessa, FL: Psychological Assessment Resources.

Krumboltz, J. D. (1979). A social learning theory of career decision making. In A. M. Mitchell, G. B. Jones, & J. D. Krumboltz (Eds.), *Social learning theory and career decision making* (pp. 19–49). Cranston, RI: Carroll.

Lavallee, D., Grove, J. R., & Gordon, S. (1997). The causes of career termination from sport and their relationship to post-retirement adjustment among elite-amateur athletes in Australia. *Australian Psychologist, 32,* 131–135.

Lent, R. W., Brown, S. D., & Hackett, G. (1994). Toward a unifying social cognitive theory of career and academic interest, choice, and performance. *Journal of Vocational Behavior, 45,* 79–122.

Louis, M. R. (1980a). Career transitions: Varieties and commonalities. *Academy of Management Review, 5,* 329–340.

Louis, M. R. (1980b). Surprise and sense making: What newcomers experience in entering unfamiliar organizational settings. *Administrative Science Quarterly, 25,* 226–251.

Mason, J. L. (1993). Career endings: An exploratory study of ballet dancers (Doctoral dissertation, The California School of Professional Psychology). *Dissertation Abstracts International, 54,* 2785B.

McCrae, R. R., & John, O. P. (1992). An introduction to five factor model and its applications. *Journal of Personality, 60,* 175–215.

Mitchell, L. K., & Krumboltz, J. D. (1990). Social learning approach to career decision making: Krumboltz's theory. In D. Brown & L. Brooks (Eds.), *Career choice and development: Applying contemporary theories to practice* (2nd ed., pp. 145–196). San Francisco: Jossey-Bass.

Murphy, G. M., Petitpas, A. J., & Brewer, B. W. (1996). Identity foreclosure, athletic identity, and career maturity in intercollegiate athletes. *The Sport Psychologist, 10,* 239–246.

Nicholson, N., & West, M. (1989). Transitions, work histories and careers. In M. Arthur, D. T. Hall, & B. S. Lawrence (Eds.), *Handbook of career theory* (pp. 181–201). Boston: Cambridge University Press.

Paritzky, A. B. (1995). How dancers leave dancing: A hermeneutic investigation of the psychosocial factors in career change (Doctoral dissertation, University of California, Los Angeles). *Dissertation Abstracts International, 56,* 829A.

Patton, W. & McMahon, M. (1999). *Career development and systems theory: A new relationship.* Pacific Grove, CA: Brooks/Cole.

Pickman, A. (1987). Career transitions for dancers: A counselor's perspective. *Journal of Counseling and Development, 66,* 200–201.

Rosenberg, E. (1984). Athletic retirement as social death: Concepts and perspectives. In N. Theberge & P. Donnelly (Eds.), *Sport and the sociological imagination* (pp. 245–258). Fort Worth: Texas Christian University Press.

Saposnek, S. A. (1995). *After the ballet: The effects of career transition on sense of identity, self-concept and body image.* Unpublished manuscript, Reed College, Portland, OR.

Schnitt, J. M., & Schnitt, D. (1987). Psychological issues in a dancer's career. In A. J. Ryan & R. E. Stephens (Eds.), *Dance medicine: A comprehensive guide* (pp. 334–349). Chicago: Pluribus Press.

Sinclair, D. A., & Orlick, T. (1993). Positive transitions from high-performance sport. *The Sport Psychologist, 7,* 138–150.

Super, D. E. (1980). A life-span, life-space approach to career development. *Journal of Vocational Behavior, 13,* 282–298.

Super, D. E. (1992). Toward a comprehensive theory of career development. In D. Montross & C. Shinkman (Eds.), *Career development: Theory and practice* (pp. 35–64). Springfield, IL: Thomas.

Super, D. E. (1994). A life-span, life-space perspective on convergence. In M. L. Savickas & R. W. Lent (Eds.), *Convergence in career development theories* (pp. 63–76). Palo Alto, CA: Consulting Psychologists Press.

Super, D. E., Savickas, M. L., & Super, C. M. (1996). The life-span, life-space approach to careers. In

D. Brown & L. Brooks (Eds.), *Career choice and development* (3rd ed., pp. 121–178). San Francisco: Jossey-Bass.

Taylor, J., & Ogilvie, B. C. (1994). A conceptual model of adaptation to retirement among athletes. *Journal of Applied Sport Psychology, 6,* 1–20.

Taylor, J., & Ogilvie, B. C. (1998). Career transition among elite athletes: Is there life after sports? In J. M. Williams (Ed.), *Applied sport psychology: Personal growth to peak performance* (3rd ed., pp. 429–444). Mountain View, CA: Mayfield.

Wallach, E. (1988, February). Life after performing: Career transition for dancers. *Dance/USA,* 5–11.

Werthner, P., & Orlick, T. (1986). Retirement experiences of successful Olympic athletes. *International Journal of Sport Psychology, 17,* 337–363.

White, B., & Guest, G. (1995). *Career options for dancers.* Perth: Arts Training Australia.

Wylleman, P., De Knop, P., Menkehorst, H., Theeboom, M., & Annerel, J. (1993). Career termination and social integration among elite athletes. In S. Serpa, J. Alves, V. Ferreira, & A. Paula-Brito (Eds.), *Proceedings of the VIII World Congress of Sport Psychology* (pp. 902–906). Lisbon: International Society of Sport Psychology.

Contact Details for the International Organization for the Transition of Dancers

President
Philippe Braunschweig
IOTDP
Av. Bergieres 6 CH-1004
Lausanne
Tel: 41 21 643 24 05
Fax: 41 21 643 24 09
Email: braunsph@fastnet.ch

Paul Bronkhorst
Theater Instituut Nederland
Heerengracht 168
PO Box 19304
1000 GH Amsterdam Holland
Tel: 31 20 623 51 04
Fax: 31 20 623 70 39
Fax: 31 20 620 00 51
Email: tinresearch@gn.apc.org

Garry Neil, Joysanne Sidimus
Dancer Transition Resource Centre
66 Charles Street East, Suite 202
Toronto Ontario M5B 1G3 Canada
Tel: 1 416 595 56 55
Fax: 1 416 595 00 09
Email: gtneil@mail.interlog.com

Linda Yates
Dance Companies Resettlement Fund
Dancers Trust
Rooms 222-226 Africa House
64-78 Kingsway
London WC2 B6BG
Tel: 44 171 404 6141
Fax: 44 171 242 33 31

Ann Bary
Career Transition for Dancers Inc.
1727 Broadway
New York 100019
Tel: 1 212 581 70 43
Fax: 1 212 262 90 88

12

Within-Career Transitions of the Athlete-Coach-Parent Triad

John H. Salmela, Bradley W. Young, and Jamie Kallio
University of Ottawa
Canada

Abstract

The within-career transitions of athletes as they evolve from novices to experts are traced in a somewhat predictable fashion along with concurrent changes in the lives of both their parents and coaches. Using the developmental framework of B. S. Bloom (1985) and the expertise research methodology of Ericsson and colleagues (Ericsson, Krampe, & Tesch-Römer, 1993; Ericsson & Lehmann, 1996), insights into the career transitions of the microstructure of practice are presented for selected sports. The transitions in parental roles are documented across the duration of the athletes' careers in terms of the initial nurturing process, as well as their social and financial support. The importance of various skilled coaches who must also evolve within their careers to meet the various demands of developing athletes is also highlighted.

Within-Career Transitions
of the Athlete-Coach-Parent Triad

There are a number of career initiation and termination transitions that have been reported in the literature from both psychological and sociological perspectives. The various antecedents of entering sport, remaining committed to its practice, dropping out during this initial period, and being deselected from the talent pool and the later retirement process have all undergone the scrutiny of researchers (Taylor & Ogilvie, 1994).

However, there have been a number of research initiatives that have addressed both the overall within career patterns of exceptional performers, as well as those of their parents and coaches in sport and other domains of accomplishment (B. S. Bloom, 1985). Attention has also been directed to the microstructure of athletes' careers (i.e., the means by which these sport performers have evolved from one stage of athletic progress to the next) (Ericsson, Krampe, & Tesch-Römer, 1993; Helsen, Starkes, & Hodges, 1998; Salmela, 1994). The intent of this chapter is to document some of the critical conditions for athletic development by illuminating significant within-career events related to the physical reality of training and competing within a specific sport (e.g., starting age, cultural constraints, access to facilities, demands of the sport). Further, this chapter will highlight certain benchmarks and transitional episodes that appear common in the evolution of sporting careers. The discussion will be framed within the context of the athlete-coach-parent triad.

Transitions for Athletes

One of the most significant large-scale studies that focused upon the within-career evolution of exceptional performers in sport, as well as within the arts and sciences, was carried out by B. S. Bloom (1985). What was remarkable in these retrospective accountings of the evolution of the career paths of Olympic swimmers, world-class tennis players, concert pianists, sculptors, research mathematicians, and research neurologists was the robust similarities of their overall career profiles, once normalized for starting ages.

B. S. Bloom (1985) was interested in the process of talent development in young people, beginning with their early years and ending with their rise to international prominence. Via in-depth, structured interviews with 120 talented individuals from a wide breadth of fields, Bloom identified three consistent developmental phases of expert performers across their careers: the early, middle, and late years.

The first phase began when individuals were casually introduced to activities within their domain. This often involved instruction from a local coach/teacher who was caring, thoughtful, and well respected in the community. The coach/teacher provided the performer with significant positive feedback that was garnered for effort rather than for achievement and was rarely critical of the child's performance. B. S. Bloom (1985) also found that parents played a significant role by providing necessary encouragement and motivation needed to maintain their child's interest, also with a lesser emphasis on performance outcome.

During the middle years, individuals began to set performance goals and were committed to them. For the tennis players, the sport became more than a "game"; it became "real business." As one player described it: "I was now eating, sleeping and breathing tennis" (B. S. Bloom, 1985, p. 236). During this period, players began to receive acclaim, rewards, and recognition by significant others within their sport. Bloom also reported that most athletes began to feel the necessity of more advanced forms of coaching.

During the early years, the initial coaches excelled at nurturing a stimulating outlook towards tennis. The same players later felt that they required a more skilled coach to refine both technique and strategy and to tailor their game to maximize personal strengths and compensate for any weaknesses.

The teacher/coach during the middle years was typically more skilled or a reputable leader within a larger geographical area. Skill development now became a top priority for the performer and coaches demanded more arduous practices, and greater commitment and discipline were directed towards competitive outcomes. One player reported:

> [My coach] would watch me play this boy . . . and then say if I lost, he would point out why I lost. If it were a stroke deficiency, we'd work on that stroke. If it were tactics, he would show me and explain what I should have done. (B. S. Bloom, 1985, p. 242).

During the later stage, exceptional athletes often sought out a still more accomplished coach, an individual widely recognized as a master teacher or expert in their sport. Individuals who were capable of reaching the third stage effectively adopted an urge to mastery in their performance domain; they were totally obsessed by their chosen activity and did whatever it took to progress to the top echelon. In concurrence, their families decidedly made a full-time commitment and, in doing so, incurred new burdens and sacrifices, such as increased financial demands or their family's relocation in search of better coaching.

Transitions for Coaches

As might be expected, it has also been shown that expert coaches also pass through a number of identifiable phases in the development of their own coaching careers. Schinke, Bloom, and Salmela (1995) identified career steps in the development of coaching expertise. Top Canadian basketball coaches traced their career evolution, beginning with their athletic interests and moving to the path that took them from apprentice, to developing, to expert levels of coaching. It was reported that coaches progressed through seven stages, both as athletes and coaches, that were labeled as early, elite, and international sport participation, and novice, developmental, national, and international coaching.

The first three stages pertained to the coaches' athletic careers, beginning with their initiation to, and early involvement within, the sporting domain. The final four stages centered on the evolution of their coaching careers. During the novice coaching stage, the coaches obtained initial, often volunteer, coaching appointments, either at community centers or public schools, or as player-coaches. During the developmental stage, the coaches earned their first paid positions working with aspiring competitors. After a number of years and a significant accumulation of both winning and losing experiences, they evolved to the national stage and had their first opportunity to work with university or provincial teams with their principal goal being the personal development of their athletes. Later at the international level, the coaches readjusted their priorities so that performance results were placed above all other concerns. This change in orientation was partly attributed to the fact that coaches were now accountable to more people, including national sport-governing bodies, the media, and the public.

Within-career transitions have also been shown to reflect culturally driven motives. Foreign-born expert judo coaches have demonstrated an obligation to alter their Japanese-based or European-based belief system to conform to the Canadian sport reality (Moraes & Salmela, 1998). For both micro (seasonal) and macro (across-career) durations, expert coaches have been shown to evolve along with their athletes through dynamic transitions in both communication skills (G. A. Bloom, Schinke, & Salmela, 1998) and team building (Schinke, Draper, & Salmela, 1997). Those interactions that were fostered over a longer temporal period tended to be repeated with increasing efficacy across their careers. Finally, G. A. Bloom, Durand-Bush, Schinke, and Salmela (1998) have shown how the mentoring of coaches at various stages in their careers has resulted in maximum personal development.

Transitions for Parents

B. S. Bloom (1985) alluded to different roles in each of the three career stages for the parents of athletes who would eventually attain exceptional levels of performance. During the early stage, they were supportive of the nurturing atmosphere created by the entry-level coach and did not attempt to undermine the process-oriented training, for example, by pushing their children to achieve competitive results before they were "hooked" with the love of the activity itself. During the middle years, the parents were again supportive of the more intense and demanding outcome-oriented training environment. They accepted the prerequisite sacrifices and adjustments required of them (e.g., heightened financial support and rescheduling of their lives around the achievements of their child). During the late years, when the athletes' lives were completely dedicated towards their practice of sport, the parents played a less immediate role in the training environment, but often still provided social and financial support for these more autonomous athletes.

More recently, Côté and Hay (in press) studied the roles of parents in their child's early developmental years in the sport of rowing. These same children would eventually achieve exceptional rowing careers. The advantage of actually gathering data during this developmental training period was that the participants' recollections of past and current events were temporally linked, easier to recall, and therefore, more accurate. Côté and Hay were able to break down B. S. Bloom's (1985) early years into three distinct periods: the sampling, specializing, and investment years.

The sampling years predated B. S. Bloom's (1985) period of working with a coach and was an interval during which the parents encouraged their children to experiment with different enjoyable activities for their pure pleasure. The children were not pressured to chose one sport discipline in preference over another, but rather they were encouraged to sample the benefits of various sport and musical activities. Once a bond was created with one sport discipline, the specializing period began, and more focused attention was directed towards this single discipline although still maintaining a playful environment, possibly with a coach. During the investment years, parents began to redirect time, energy, and finances towards the pursuit of an appropriate training environment for their young children. It is important to note that these three stages all occurred within Bloom's characterization of the early years, or shortly thereafter.

Côté and Hay (in press) believe that although the portrayal of these developing athletes' behaviors in the early years could be construed as goal-directed, serious training, or what Ericsson et al. (1993) called "deliberate practice," they were actually playful activities. In that these children were totally and joyfully immersed in the moment and process of training, rather than being goal driven, Ericsson et al. termed these activities "deliberate play."

The Evolving Microstructure of Practice

Ericsson and associates (Ericsson et al., 1993; Ericsson & Lehmann, 1996) studied the developmental microstructure of exceptional performance in music from the viewpoint that the achievement of expertise in any domain was the result of maximal adaptations to the constraints of goal-oriented, structured practice. These maximal adaptations to practice were exhibited not only in athletes' landmark performances, but also in training transitions. Ericsson et al. argued that reaching a high level of expertise was not principally due to innate abilities, but was the result of cumulative, sustained, and effortful training activities designed to optimize improvement, a process that was labeled "deliberate practice." The fundamental view of the deliberate practice perspective is best summarized as follows:

> In contrast to play, deliberate practice is a highly structured activity, the explicit goal of which is to improve performance. Specific tasks are invented to overcome weaknesses, and performance is carefully monitored to provide cues for ways to improve it further . . . the amount of time an individual is engaged in deliberate practice is monotonically related to that individual's acquired performance. (Ericsson et al., 1993, p. 368).

Resources, including time, energy, and access to competent teachers and training facilities, as well as sustaining high levels of effort and motivation, were identified as constraints inhibiting the process of deliberate practice.

Ericsson and associates (Ericsson et al., 1993; Ericsson & Lehmann, 1996) provided a time frame for the development of expertise. A 10-year rule of necessary preparation was invoked as a necessary, but not sufficient, condition for the acquisition of exceptional performance in a domain. This time frame was derived from Simon and Chase's (1973) research in chess in which they found that international chess masters required, on average, 11.7 years from the first time they learned the rules until they achieved the grandmaster level. Ericsson et al.'s research also extended B. S. Bloom's (1985) framework to include a fourth developmental phase for eminence: "The criteria for eminent performance goes beyond expert mastery of available knowledge and skills and requires an important and innovative contribution to the domain" (Ericcson et al., p. 370).

Ericsson and colleagues (Ericsson et al., 1993; Ericsson & Lehmann, 1996) introduced two significant methodological breakthroughs for the understanding of the development of exceptional performance that are highly useful when considering within-career transitions in sport. The first was the documentation of daily life activities, both practice and nonpractice, of the studied musicians over the course of their careers by means of retrospective recall. This enabled the detailing of quantity of practice activities over the developmental span of their careers in music. Second, they advanced a methodology for studying performers' perceptions of their own training that would be instrumental for discriminating between play and deliberate practice. A list of practice activities was elaborated, and the musicians were subsequently asked to judge their own experiences in each category of practice according to measures of relevance (of the practice to improving their performance), effort (required to perform the practice activity), and pleasure (how enjoyable they perceived the actual process of practice). The combination of these two methodologies permitted the functional documentation of the microstructure of practice across the careers of these musicians. These findings have since been replicated within the sport domain in soccer (Helsen et al., 1998), wrestling (Starkes, Deakin, Allard, Hodges, & Hayes, 1996), middle-distance running (Young, 1998; Young & Salmela, 1998) and biathlon (Kallio & Salmela, 1998). Attention will be now directed towards within-career transitions and the microstructure of practice within these two latter sport disciplines.

Middle-Distance Running

Young and Salmela (1998) recently studied 81 national, provincial, and club-level Canadian middle-distance runners and have illuminated several trends regarding career initiation and transitions. Aided by their own training diaries, rather than retrospective recall, the runners longitudinally reconstructed their own practice patterns for the initial 9 years of their careers. The researchers performed analyses that indicated benchmarks for athletes' initiation into the sport of running, and the formative role of the coach in the early years of systematic training, and suggested a significant transitional period after 9 years of practice.

Biographical data revealed comparable entry moments into middle-distance running for all performance levels. In general, the runners began running at 12.3 years of age, started systematic training with a coach at 14.4 years, and commenced full-time, year-round practice for running at 15.9 years. Although not statistically significant, it was interestingly noted that the club runners typically exhibited earlier starting ages than those of their more elite counterparts. This finding intimated that starting age was not a robust determinant of eventual performance level, but rather the subsequent process of skill acquisition was of far more importance.

Further analyses contrasted the three eventual performance groups for accumulated kilometers run, as well as for accumulated amounts of practice in the most relevant activities for improving performance. The two more elite groups consistently compiled greater amounts of training than the club runners. Across the initial 7 years of systematic practice, the national and provincial athletes exhibited relatively the same patterns for accumulated amounts of practice. However, from 7 years to 9 years of training, there appeared to be a transition; the national runners demonstrated a marked increase in amounts of practice relative to their provincial peers. The athletes who eventually achieved national status, increased their total amounts of training, ran more kilometers, and perhaps most important, invested more training in the most relevant activities for improving performance, including the amount of time working with a coach.

Ericsson and colleagues (Ericsson et al., 1993; Ericsson & Lehmann, 1996) alluded to the importance of the coach or teacher in facilitating the process of deliberate practice. For example, in the absence of coaches or teachers, they found that subjects usually played rather than practiced. Second, feedback was crucial, and expert performers needed to be taught and corrected when errors occurred.

To assume effective learning, athletes ideally should be given explicit instructions about the best method and be supervised by a teacher to allow individualized diagnosis of errors, informative feedback, and remedial training. The instructor has to organize the sequence of appropriate training tasks and monitor improvement to decide when transitions to more complex and challenging tasks are appropriate (Ericsson et al., 1993).

In sum, although the role of the coach was deemed important by Ericsson and colleagues (Ericsson et al., 1993; Ericsson & Lehmann, 1996), their comments were limited to the instructional process, which, in reality, is but one of many roles of expert coaches. Other important dimensions also include training both the physical and mental systems, organizing team and individual procedures, and building a cohesive team (Côté, Salmela, Trudel, Baria, & Russell, 1995).

Young and Salmela (1998) compared the three eventual performance groups for accumulated amounts of work with a coach. One striking feature was the significant differences between the two elite groups and the less skilled club runners, particularly during the early years of their careers. After 3 years of training, the national and provincial runners had accumulated 210 hours and 139 hours of work with a coach, respectively, compared to a paltry total of 22 hours for the club runners. These findings pointed towards the formative role of a coach in the development of middle-distance runners, particularly early in the their careers. Although not quite as dramatic, work with a coach still distinguished between eventual performance groups after 9 years; the national group had accumulated on average 217 hours of more work with a coach than the provincial group had.

These findings underscore the fundamental importance of establishing initial athlete-coach interactions because the developing athlete benefits from an optimal training environment and increases the efficiency of skill acquisition. This is vital during the early years when the athlete's skill acquisition is greatest and the symbiotic relationship between amounts of practice and performance gains is strongest (Young & Salmela, 1998). The role of the running coach is to enable an athlete to overcome each of the three constraints of skill acquisition—the resource, effort, and motivational constraints (Ericsson et al., 1993). An effective coach is a resource of knowledge and training material and can effectively streamline the process of skill acquisition by imparting sound strategies for performance enhancement. The coach also coordinates aspects of organization, training, and competition in order to balance maximal bouts of effort with sufficient recovery (Côté et al., 1995). Finally, coaches provide external motivation and encouragement within the training environment.

The notion of a transitional period after 9 years of training is not a novel one; rather, it seemingly corroborates other results in sport. Based on accumulated practice trends, 9 years into a career has been identified as a watershed period for skill acquisition for soccer and field hockey players (Helsen et al., 1998). In those sports, there were ever widening discrepancies between skill groups for accumulated amounts of practice beyond 9 years. The fact that discrepancies between provincial and national middle-distance runners were not apparent until after 9 years of systematic training reaffirms the long process of specialized running practice required to eventually achieve national-level status. Additionally, this trend lends further credibility to the notion that a 10-year period of domain-specific preparation is a necessary, although insufficient, prerequisite of exceptional performance (Ericsson et al., 1993; Simon & Chase, 1973). At the very least, the 9-year "gap" demarcates another transition on a lengthy road to middle-distance running excellence.

Young and Salmela (1998) also employed the methodology of Ericsson and colleagues (Ericsson et al., 1993; Ericsson & Lehmann, 1996) for rating the nature of practice activities by asking the runners to rate a current list of training activities according to their perceptions of four dimensions: relevance, effort, enjoyment, and concentration. Results indicated no significant differences between the performance groups for the activity ratings; the national, provincial, and club runners all perceived the same set of training activities as most relevant for athletic improvement. Yet, as the analyses for the quantity of accumulated practice previously indicated, differences did exist with regard to how much training the groups actually did accumulate. These trends suggest that the less skilled runners' shortcoming is not "knowing what to practice," but rather actually "doing the practice." It is quite possible that the national-level athletes are far more able than their provincial and club counterparts to sustain the high levels of motivation required to perform the most relevant activities.

Biathlon

Using a similar methodology, Kallio and Salmela (1998) also expanded research into the developmental aspects of expertise to the sport of biathlon. Biathlon is an interesting sport in that it requires high intensity, strength and endurance in skiing at one moment, then steadiness and fine motor control during the shooting phase. The sample included a provincial-level group and an expert group consisting of world- and Olympic-level biathletes, and an Olympic gold medalist.

Analyses of biographical data indicated that entry into the sport was later for biathletes than for middle-distance runners (Young & Salmela, 1998); on average, the biathletes began their sport at 17 years of age. Reconstructive analyses of career practice patterns demonstrated three trends: First, the expert-level performers accumulated significantly more training hours than their provincial counterparts did across their careers; second, the expert biathletes consistently increased their training volumes across their careers; and third, the provincial biathletes demonstrated inconsistencies and greater fluctuations in their activity patterns. The provincial group's inconsistent training patterns across their careers suggest that many of these athletes adopt a "recreational path to training" in which they oscillate between treating biathlon as a sport and a recreational activity. In terms of individual training activities, the expert biathletes spent significantly more time doing biathlon-specific activities of high intensity (e.g., combination skiing and shooting) and simulation-type activities related to shooting (e.g., dry firing without bullets, precision firing without fall-down targets).

Kallio and Salmela (1998) found discrepancies between the performance groups with regard to how they perceived their own training activities. The expert biathletes were more likely to report the need to incorporate substantial levels of physical effort and concentration within biathlon-specific training activities than were their provincial counterparts. Thus, the experts rated long-interval skiing, short-interval skiing, and hard combination training (shooting and skiing) as far more relevant for improving their performance than the provincial group did. These results can potentially be attributed to differential career learning processes, dissimilar entry ages into the sport, and unequal access to adequate coaching for the two groups of biathletes. As such, the provincial biathletes failed to gain a true understanding of the processes and conditions necessary to attain the exceptional levels of performance in the sport. Alternatively, international biathletes had received the necessary instruction and experiential bases to realize the relevance of these activities.

A second pattern that emerged centered upon the biathletes' perceptions of enjoyment and effort. For example, the provincial group rated cross-training and particularly distance skiing as highly relevant and as forms of training that demanded relatively low physical effort and little concentration and were highly enjoyable in which to participate. The expert group, on the other hand, although recognizing the same effort, enjoyment, and concentration attributes, did not judge cross-training or distance skiing to be very relevant for improving their performance. Provincial biathletes also exhibited an aversion for activities requiring high levels of physical effort or concentration; in those cases, they rated the activities as unenjoyable. The expert biathletes judged the same activities to be relatively enjoyable. These results indicated that biathletes of different performance levels did not share similar perceptions of relevance, effort, or enjoyment. In addition, the provincial biathletes' extremely high enjoyment rating for activities that required low concentration and low physical effort appears to reinforce the aforementioned notion of a "recreational path to training."

There were also differences between the performance groups in terms of the relevance they accorded to working with a coach. Provincial skiers did not rate working with a coach as relevant, thereby indicating their failure to appreciate the benefits of working with an instructor. Asked to comment, a Canadian national coach responded:

> Athletes taking the recreational path like to be alone. They do not like to receive daily advice from somebody who requires effort from them. They don't like someone on a daily basis to tell them that you must go and do this 100 times.

This may also explain the provincial group's tendency to rate distance skiing as highly relevant: "They like long distance training because no one, e.g., a coach, requires anything from them," reported the same national coach. Kallio and Salmela's (1998) findings suggest that the provincial biathletes are not willing to engage in structured, deliberate training with a coach. It seems that the provincial biathletes have not undergone the transition from B. S. Bloom's (1985) early years to the middle years of systematic training. In fact, the national coach reinforced this notion by claiming: "In comparison to European athletes who spend 7 to 9 years, many North American biathletes spend almost 15 years in the investment years of their career." The extensive time spent in playing, rather than practicing deliberately, during the investment years is in part a reflection on the lack of experienced coaching in an unstructured, unregulated system. This effectively results in the dropout of aspiring biathletes or their forced change to another sporting career.

Conclusion

The various within-career transitions that athletes experience are inextricably linked to the concurrent changes in the lives of both their parents and coaches. The complex interactions in the athlete-coach-parent triad explain, in part, the difficulty in charting or predicting athletic outcomes for a given individual in sport. For all three actors, however, there appears to be a growing body of evidence that suggests that the parameters for the development of exceptional performance in sport do follow a number of fairly well-delineated transitional steps.

The athlete must first be incubated within an environment created by parents and coaches who are willing to support the child's love for the activity and foster a bond between the activity and the child. The youth in sport must then acclimate to a more goal-directed mode in which both the athlete and the parents begin to rigorously commit more training and resources to the "mission." If commitment to progress to the later stages is desirable, an obsession to master the performance domain demands the reduction of competing life activities. Parental roles begin to change, lives revolve around a child's athletic accomplishment, and expert coaching is successively sought.

Practice activities during this period are directed towards improving performance, and what was formerly play or casual practice now takes on a work-like personality. In that this period can span more than 10 years, the importance of a skilled coach is central to keeping practice activities on track, while also planning for the recuperation of energy resources. The transition to the phase of perfection again demands an escalation of commitment and resources as well as novel outlooks towards training, coaching, and parenting.

References

Bloom, B. S. (Ed.). (1985). *Developing talent in young people.* New York: Ballantine.

Bloom, G. A., Durand-Bush, N., Schinke, R. J., & Salmela, J. H. (1998). The importance of mentoring in the development of coaches and athletes. *International Journal of Sport Psychology, 29,* 267–281.

Bloom, G. A., Schinke, R. J., & Salmela, J. H. (1998). The development of communication skills by elite basketball coaches. *Coaching and Sport Science Journal, 2 (3),* 3–10.

Bloom, G. A., Salmela, J. H., & Schinke, R. J. (1995). Expert coaches' views on the training of developing coaches. In R. Vanfraechem-Raway & Y. Vanden Auweele (Eds.), *Proceedings of the 9th European Congress of Sport Psychology* (pp. 401–408). Brussels: European Federation of Sports Psychology.

Côté, J., & Hay, J. (in press). Family influences on youth sport performance and participation. In J. M. Silva & D. Stevens (Eds.)., *Psychological foundations of sport* (2nd ed.). Champaign, IL: Human Kinetics.

Côté, J., Salmela, J. H., Trudel, P., Baria, A., & Russell, S. J. (1995). The coaching model: A grounded assessment of expert gymnastics coaches' knowledge. *Journal of Sport & Exercise Psychology, 17,* 1–17.

Ericsson, K. A., Krampe, R. T., & Tesch-Römer, C. (1993). The role of deliberate practice in the acquisition of expert performance. *Psychological Review, 100,* 363–406.

Ericsson, K.A., & Lehmann, A. C. (1996). Expert and exceptional performance: Evidence of maximal adaptation to task constraints. *Annual Review of Psychology, 47,* 273–305.

Helsen, W. F., Starkes, J. L., & Hodges, N. J. (1998). Team sports and the theory of deliberate practice. *Journal of Sport & Exercise Psychology, 20,* 12–34.

Kallio, J., & Salmela, J. H. (1998). Development of expert performance in biathlon [Abstract]. *Journal of Applied Sport Psychology, 10* (Suppl.), S90.

Moraes, L. C., & Salmela, J. H. (1998). Development of characteristics of expert Canadian, Japanese, and European expert judo coaches [Abstract]. *Journal of Applied Sport Psychology, 10* (Suppl.), S89.

Salmela, J. H. (1994). Phases and transitions across sport careers. In D. Hackfort (Ed.), *Psycho-social issues and interventions in elite sports* (pp. 11–29). Frankfurt: Lang.

Schinke, R. J., Bloom, G. A., & Salmela, J. H. (1995). The career stages of elite Canadian basketball coaches. *Avante, 1,* 48–62.

Schinke, R. J., Draper, S. P., & Salmela, J. H. (1997). A conceptualization of team building in high performance sport as a season-long process. *Avante, 3,* 57–72.

Simon, H. A., & Chase, W. G. (1973). Skill in chess. *American Scientist, 61,* 394–403.

Starkes, J. L, Deakin, J. M., Allard, F., Hodges, N. J., & Hayes, A. (1996). Deliberate practice in sports: What is it anyway? In K. A. Ericsson (Ed.), *The road to excellence: The acquisition of expert performance in the arts and sciences, sports and games* (pp. 81–106). Mahwah, NJ: Erlbaum.

Taylor, J., & Ogilvie, B. C. (1994). A conceptual model of adaptation to retirement among athletes. *Journal of Applied Sport Psychology, 6,* 1–20.

Young, B. W., & Salmela, J. H. (1998). Athletes' perceptions of deliberate practice in Canadian middle distance running [Abstract]. *Journal of Applied Sport Psychology, 10* (Suppl.), S89–90.

Young, B. W. (1998). *Deliberate practice and skill acquisition in Canadian middle distance running.* Unpublished master's thesis, University of Ottawa.

Author Note

This research was funded in part by grant 410-97–0241 of the Social Sciences and Humanities Research Council of Canada.

13

The End of An Era: The Case of Forced Transition Involving Boston University Football

Leonard Zaichkowsky, Elizabeth King, and John McCarthy
Boston University

Abstract

The termination of the Boston University football program in 1997 provided a unique opportunity to look into an unusual aspect of career transition of the athlete: forced career transition. This chapter presented the results of studies conducted by Duffy, Nascimento, Schwager, and Zaichkowsky (1998) on the role identity of team members after the event and by McCarthy (1998) on the effect of the event on players one year later. Further research findings are also presented on how the events affected the coaching and support staff of the program. This case study hopes to give insight into the emotional impact forced termination of a group may have on those individuals and on organizational morale.

The End of an Era: The Case of Forced Transition Involving Boston University Football

Focusing primarily on the process of the athlete's experiences as she or he moves from an intensive involvement in sport into life in the absence of sport, the subject of athletic career transition has become a prolific area of interest for researchers over the past few decades. For an experience to be classified as transitional, there should be personal awareness of a discontinuity in one's life space and required new behaviors arising from the newness of the situation, the novelty of the required behaviors, or both." (Crook & Robertson, 1991, p. 122). As an athlete retires from their exclusive involvement in sport, making a transition to everyday life, the process of adjustment can be emotionally difficult. In the absence of sport, athletes may struggle to locate/identify themselves outside of the context of sport, resulting in confusion, low self-esteem and self-confidence.

Zaichkowsky, Lipton, and Tucci (1997) in their study of the transition of collegiate student-athletes out of sport found that 20% of the young men and women who participated in the study reported experiencing emotional difficulty involved in the process of leaving their sport. Indeed, "every transition has the potential to be a crisis, a relief or a combination of both, depending on the individual's perception of the situation"(Sinclair & Orlick, 1993, p. 138). Crook and Robertson (1991) conclude in their review of athletic retirement literature that many athletes experience a sense of loss as they move through the adjustment period.

The factors that contribute to the reasons for career transition and termination have been linked to the quality of the adjustment process (Gordon, 1995; Taylor & Ogilvie, 1994). Extant research also suggests that adjustment problems can occur when retirement from sport is involuntary, due to external circumstances, or beyond the control of the athlete him- or herself. In addition to the confusion already felt with regard to self-definition in the absence of sport, athletes are also subject to feelings of having no control or input in their decision to retire, compounding the already emotionally volatile situation. As a fundamental piece of the psychological aspects of career transition, identity has a strong influence on the quality of an athlete's adjustment process to life beyond sport. "Regardless of the events that precipitate involuntary retirement, athletes who are forced to retire tend to be more resistant to and less well prepared for retirement than those who retire voluntarily" (Crook & Robertson, 1991, p.120).

A Case of Forced Transition

In October 1997, the Boston University men's football program, steeped in over a century of tradition, was unexpectedly terminated. As one of the few schools in the history of collegiate football to eliminate its football program, Boston University created a situation that left many of the individuals associated with the former team displaced and facing major transitional changes, including the termination of numerous athletic careers. Under this unique circumstance, researchers took the opportunity to study the impact and the effects of this administrative decision on the football players, coaches, and support staff who were left to deal with the consequences.

In their first study performed at Boston University, Nacimento, Duffy, Schwager, and Zaichkowsky (1998) evaluated the initial impact of involuntary career transition and termination on the identities of the members of the football team after the football program was suddenly eliminated by the university administration. A second study looked at the retrospective impressions of eight players, four of whom transferred to other universities whereas four remained at Boston University (McCarthy, 1998). The third and fourth studies involved the impact the decision had on coaches and support staff, and the feelings of players who remained at Boston University almost one year after the news was broken to them about the termination of the football program.

Study I: The Players

Thirty players on full scholarship to Boston University for Division I-AA football were selected, all of whom were on the Boston University team roster at the time the program was terminated in October 1997. The sample of players consisted of freshmen, sophomores, juniors, and seniors, ranging in age from 18 to 22. Twenty-two of the players were redshirted (i.e., not scheduled to participate in athletic competition) during their freshman year.

A variation on the Athletic Identity Measurement Scale (AIMS; Brewer, Van Raalte, & Linder, 1993) was implemented to assess each student-athlete's athletic identity. Questionnaires, created by the research team, were also given to the athletes to complete. The student-athletes participating in the study were asked to comment on their personal football experience. They were also asked to identify themselves in order of importance on a numerical scale of 1 to 8 by using a designation (if applicable) such as brother, athlete, son, student, football player, friend, boyfriend, or father.

As described by Brewer, Van Raalte, and Petitpas in this volume, athletes with a strong athletic identity may experience premature identity foreclosure and emotional confusion following the termination of their athletic career, particularly in the case of forced retirement. Thus, an exclusive athletic identity would be a potential risk factor for emotional disturbance upon the termination of the athletic career (Brewer et al., 1993). Additionally, athletic identity has been positively associated with identity foreclosure (Good, Brewer,

Petitpas, Van Raalte, & Mahar, 1993; Marcia, 1996; Petitpas, 1978). In light of this information, Nacimento et al. (1998) hypothesized that individuals with strong and exclusive commitment to the athletic role would be less prepared for postsport careers than would individuals less interested in the athletic role.

Nacimento et al. (1998) also noted the importance of considering the individual differences in transitional experience due to environment, social, and family situations. Adaptations of the Kübler-Ross (1969) stage model of grief have been utilized by some sport psychologists to help explain the processes endured by athletes as they face transition out of sport. It has been assumed that an athlete, like others suffering from loss, would pass through similar stages of shock, denial, anger, depression, and acceptance.

The results of this study were consistent with the findings of earlier studies (e.g., Murphy, Petitpas, & Brewer, 1996), which suggested that the younger players held stronger athletic identities than did those older players who had already begun to move toward the transition they would have to make from sport into other areas of their lives at the commencement of their collegiate athletic career. Similarly, Pearson and Petitpas (1990) found that the most challenging transition for many college student athletes was from the status of player to the status of nonplayer. This study also examined the effect of the elimination of a football program on the player's sense of identity and the factors involved in coping with the transition, and the findings support the expectations of Pearson and Petitpas, which were that the older players would already have entered into their transition out of sport whereas the younger players would be faced with a less diversified choice, not having considered life beyond sport, questioning their identity and self-worth. Of the players who participated in this study, 16 transferred to other universities to continue to play football. The remaining 14 players stayed at Boston University, in the absence of their sport, to "ensure a future" for themselves.

Study II: The Players' Perceptions

Approximately 6 months after the termination of the Boston University football program, eight team members who had participated in Study I were selected to take part in a qualitative study. Two student-athletes were randomly selected from each collegiate year (i.e., freshman, sophomore, junior, and senior). Four of the selected players continued their enrollment at Boston University whereas the other four players had transferred to other universities in the United States. All eight players were active, noninjured members of the 1997 Boston University football team. The purposes of Study II involved eliciting opinions held about the support services offered by Boston University to former members of the football team, feelings of satisfaction from former team members toward Boston University from a holistic perspective, and identification of specific forced-transition issues brought to the surface as a result of the termination of the program.

The results of this study included the shared reaction of the eight individuals to the termination of the football program as simply "shock." The qualitative responses of the players, regardless of age or collegiate year, consisted of similar reactions to the elimination of the football program. The decision to end the program was neither expected nor welcomed. Additionally, there was widespread disappointment in the inadequacies in and lack of support offered to the players following the termination of the program. Each of the players felt strong degrees of animosity toward the way in which the administration made its decision to eliminate the football program as well as for the rationale behind the decision. Emotions ranged from betrayal to abandonment, and no player was able to state that he knew the clear and exact reason as to why the program had been eliminated. Each of the eight players also acknowledged having some degree of transition to deal with. In this unique case, these issues had to be considered with a certain degree of immediacy due to the importance of the life decisions that had to be made by the players regarding their academic and athletic careers.

In the discussion of Studies I and II, Nacimento et al. (1998) identified the need for the development of programs to assist athletes in the career transition process. They suggested that athletes might need assistance in adapting their lives to encompass other, more diverse, areas of interest. Career development programs such as the NCAA CHAMPS/Life Skills Program are effective and well-received by participants (Ferrante, Etzel, & Lantz, 1996). Findings made throughout these studies support the fact that athletes transitioning out of sport would benefit from both intervention and support services. Currently, at Boston University, the CHAMPS/Life Skills Program is not available to student-athletes as a resource for specific issues such as transition from sport to life and career.

Study III: The Coaches

A qualitative study was performed to gain insight into the perspectives of the 10 member coaching staff almost one year after the termination of the football program. As one coach stated, "You are not a coach until you've been fired," meaning it was not inconceivable that the individuals on the staff were unaware of the sometimes volatile nature of job security on the Division I-AA level. Because the head coach had been hired only one and a half years before the elimination of the program and had been assured by the administration at that time that the program was in a secure position, other staff members may have developed a false sense of security with regard to their own job status. This sense of ease may have intensified feelings of shock and dismay when the announcement to cut the program was made because of the unexpected nature of the situation. The Boston University football program had enjoyed a 93-year history that included many moments of athletic excellence. In 1993, Boston University boasted an undefeated season, a feat unprecedented in the Yankee Conference, which led to consecutive play-off seasons from 1993 through 1994. The coaches may have imagined losing their jobs after a 1–10 losing season in 1996, but none could have predicted the abandonment of the football program in its entirety by the fall of 1997.

The seven full-time staff members were continued for 6 months after the end of the season, which enabled them to take an ample amount of time to seek employment elsewhere. Conversely, the three part-time staff members were forced to look for employment immediately. Rather than in a more typical situation in which a head coach might take some of his or her staff with them to their new appointment, this group of coaches was forced to scatter, professionally, in very separate directions. Two coaches moved up to the professional level through becoming involved with the Canadian and World leagues. Two coaches remained at the same level (Division I-AA), situations in which the head coach became an assistant and a part-time coach was able to maintain his part-time status. One coach moved on to the Division II level, and three other coaches are now teachers and coaching assistants at the high school level. Only 2 of the 10 coaches have left coaching altogether; one obtained a sales position, and the other is now a part-time graduate student while working part-time for an investment firm.

The interviews for Study III were conducted over the phone. The participants were informed of the intended uses for their responses to the questions and of their being privy to the findings. Because the interviewer had a close relationship with the coaches, the questions were asked in a casual, conversational manner.

The questions posed to the coaches focused on three different periods of time beginning with their reaction to the initial decision to eliminate the football program, moving to their view of the termination one year later, and finally gathering their thoughts on future ramifications of the experience. The coaches responded in various ways to the questions in that each coach had an immediate reaction to the situation, followed by a secondary response through which implications regarding the way the decision affected them becomes clear. Immediate responses included emotions of shock, denial, anger, and ultimately, acceptance. These reactions are similar to those held by the players themselves, which tended to follow the Kübler-Ross (1969) stage model of grief. The involuntary nature of the situation created an atmosphere of confusion for everyone involved in the end of the Boston University football legacy. "It was crazy, because it did not have to happen that way," stated one coach whose sentiments imply that there may have been a less invasive method that could have been employed to approach the situation more carefully. Another colleague had this to say about the loss suffered when one's intrinsic involvement in professional life is suddenly eliminated: "I was furious. It was a shame for so many of us who invest so much of ourselves into something which the school did not ultimately value." After their first reactions, the coaches were then able to consider how they were affected on an individual basis. The secondary response was characterized by a sense of confusion as well as the pressure to somehow find a new job in the midst of a difficult situation. "I was confused. I asked myself, 'Where do I go from here?' because it [this job] had been a good opportunity for me." Another coach responded, "Suddenly I felt a tremendous sense of pressure both personally and professionally." A third coach indicated the mental anguish he associated such a large degree of change: "It made me think that I did not want to coach at that level [Division I-AA] any more and go through that job insecurity thing again." The feelings of pain and mistrust of those in the decision-making roles were felt by players and coaches alike.

The second segment of the interview asked the coaches to talk about their retrospective views of the situation one year later. The sentiment here indicated that, at this juncture, a strong feeling of loss had replaced the initial shock and disbelief over the course of a year. Coaches said: "I feel like I lost something fun, working with those guys and the coaches" and "We tried to build something [the football program] the right way, and we will never get to see what could have been." The sense that their work and commitment had been taken from them with no forewarning contributed to the emptiness that accompanied such feelings of loss: "Where I work now doesn't have the same sense of camaraderie that we had." The fact that they realized that they could never retrieve what had been taken from them indicated that their emotional position was somewhere beyond denial, yet not at the level of acceptance.

The third and final part of the interview asked the coaches to consider any of the long-term effects the elimination of the football program might have on them, if any. Some of the coaches felt positive about the experience at this point: "It was a blessing in disguise—I now have more time to myself"; "It helped me to consider things outside of football that I may not have"; and "It could not have worked out better for me personally, I love where I am now." Others felt more negatively affected: "I am a more skeptical person now, especially of administrators," "I miss college football because it is something special—not many have the feeling of working together to accomplish something" and "I may not have a career opportunity like that again; it was two steps backward for me." Still others maintained a more accepting attitude

CHAPTER 13

towards the situation: "Things happen for a reason" or "It worked out the way it was supposed to." These responses illustrated the individuality of the transition process for coaches. Because of the emphasis on individual perceptions of the situation, they may have had a very different experience from that of someone else in a similar position (Sinclair & Orlick, 1993).

The pattern of responses to the termination of the football program can be compared to the Kübler-Ross (1969) stages of grief and bereavement as these responses showed a progression through the initial shock and denial of the situation to anger and then on to acceptance, though not all of the coaches have necessarily reached this point in their transition. The coaches not only lost their employment, but also lost their shared sense of purpose that comes from such intense and exclusive involvement in a team sport such as football. Though all of the coaches have moved on to various new endeavors, there is some question as to whether they would have been able to navigate through the situation more easily had there been a network of support and assistance created by Boston University in anticipation of this transition period. Those who had to endure the transition process in the absence of assistance suggested that counseling, aptitude and interest testing, as well as basic career search skills would have helped them through such a difficult experience.

Study IV: The System

The sports medicine department, academic advisement staff, strength and conditioning staff, facilities manager, and football secretary were also given the opportunity to indicate the affects of the elimination of the football program on their personal and professional lives.

For the sports medicine department, the loss of the football program was crushing:

> I was devastated. I worked so closely with those guys, and to see what they had to go through, I was so disappointed. . . . It [the loss of the program] ruined my program. Football was the key part of how our athletic trainers could get hands on experience. . . . It [the loss of the program] may have messed up my career. I feel I have been training for 18 years to get to the skill level to run a program well, and just when I get to that place they pull the rug out from underneath us. . . . It hurts my chances of other jobs in the field that include football.

Many other organizations within the athletic department, aside from the football players and coaches, were also significantly affected by the termination of the football program.

The academic advisement staff had the following comments:

Emotionally I was very sad. I enjoy working with all our athletes, and contrary to popular belief, football players are no more difficult than any other sport. There are so many of them that I will miss. . . . A year later, I feel disoriented, waiting for football to start. I find I have more time to myself, but my responsibilities have shifted toward other athletes. . . . In the long term, if I wanted to apply for a job in a big program, I would have to start over at another school. If I wanted to do that, it [the loss of the program] would be a stumbling block.

Again, concerns about career progression and future professional opportunities were addressed.

The strength and conditioning staff did not experience the same level of personal disruption as some of the other departments. However, their professional lives were equally affected: "It affected me professionally because if I still wanted to do strength and conditioning for a school that had football I would have to get a job elsewhere and be an assistant again." The facilities manager and the football secretary had this to say, respectively, "I am still devastated, and that won't change; it eroded my trust in this administration" and "I felt like I was losing whole part of my family; it is not the same; I feel like I don't belong here anymore." The effects of the termination of the Boston University football program were far-reaching. The surprising decision left many individuals apprehensive of administration and incredulous at the lack of open communication and support from the administration to the athletic department.

Even those who were indirectly linked to the termination of the Boston University football program could relate to the processes the remaining players would have to endure as a part of the transition they would have to make from player to nonplayer. As quoted in an October 28, 1997 article in the *Boston Herald*, the head coach of the Northeastern University football team, Barry Gallup, had the following reaction to the situation: "I feel bad for the student athletes. Now they have to go through a transition and it will work out for some, and for some it won't." Those involved intrinsically in sport are aware of the difficulties that potentially lie within the transition process.

Conclusion

Organizations around the world have a common thread: They are composed of people. Groups within organizations also have varying degrees of interdependence. Loss of a group or even a highly valued member of an organization can affect the total organizational system. Often times it is difficult for organizational leadership to calculate what the overall culture may lose by a decision to cut a certain program. What is more, because such decisions are often unpopular and difficult, decision makers may want to spare themselves the anguish of knowing too much about those who might be affected. This scenario is replayed all too often in organizations everywhere.

The termination of the Boston University football program had profound effect upon the lives of those involved with the program. Unfortunately, the players were forced to cope with the disbanding of an organization into which they had personally invested much. Many of the coaches involved with the team were also facing their own difficult transition process and were not available to assist the players as they faced the loss of their status as athletes within the university. Moreover, it appeared that the support staff seemed even more affected in the long term than the investigators initially expected because, as compared to the coaches who were forced to move on to new situations, they remained. As the University moved beyond the decision to terminate a football program by transforming the locker rooms, offices, and the playing field, evidence supports the notion that the transition was not as elementary for the former players. It is clear that the University miscalculated the traumatic effect this action had upon the entire morale of the athletic department, and perhaps the entire University and its alumni.

What can be learned from this case study? In today's rapidly changing society, programs, divisions of companies, and entire departments can become obsolete or worse cost-ineffective and thus be subject to termination. Decision makers need to consider many different human aspects of the situation if they are to act responsibly. Administrators, management, and leadership of organizations of schools, businesses and politicians need to consider seriously what the ramifications of a decision are and how best to mitigate its negative impact. The termination of the Boston University program can serve as a case study for those interested in understanding the emotional costs of such action.

References

Brewer, B. W., Van Raalte, J. L., & Linder, D. E. (1993). Athletic identity: Hercules' muscles or Achilles' heel? *International Journal of Sport Psychology, 24,* 237–254.

Crook, J. M., & Robertson, S. E. (1991). Transitions out of elite sport. *International Journal of Sport Psychology, 22,* 115–127.

Ferrante, A. P., Etzel, E. F., & Lantz, C. (1996). Counseling college student-athletes: The problem, the need 1996. In E. F. Etzel, A. P. Ferrante, & J. W., Pinkney (Eds.), *Counseling college student-athletes: Issues and interventions* (2nd ed., pp. 3–26). Morgantown, WV: Fitness Information Technology.

Good, A. J., Brewer, B. W., Petitpas, A. J., Van Raalte, J. L., & Mahar, M. T. (1993). Athletic identity, identity foreclosure, and college sport participation. *Academic Athletic Journal, 8,* 1–12.

Gordon, S. (1995). Career transitions in competitive sport. In T. Morris & J. Summers (Eds.), *Sport psychology: Theory, applications and issues* (pp. 474–501). Brisbane: Jacaranda Wiley.

Kübler-Ross, E. (1969). *On death and dying.* New York: Macmillan.

Marcia, J. E. (1996). Development and validation of ego-identity status. *Journal of Personality and Social Psychology, 3,* 551–558.

Murphy, G. M., Petitpas, A. J., & Brewer, B. W. (1996). Identity foreclosure, athletic identity, and career maturity in intercollegiate athletes. *The Sport Psychologist, 10,* 239–246.

Nascimento, A., Duffy, D., Schwager, E., & Zaichkowsky, L. (1998) The end of an era: An investigation on forced transition of Boston University football players. *Journal of Applied Sport Psychology, 10,* (Suppl.), S109.

Pearson, R. E., & Petitpas, A. J. (1990). Transitions of athletes: Developmental and preventive perspectives. *Journal of Counseling and Development, 69,* 7–10.

Petitpas, A. (1978). Identity foreclosure: A unique challenge. *Personnel and Guidance Journal, 56,* 558–561.

Sinclair, D. A., & Orlick, T. (1993). Positive transitions from high-performance sport. *The Sport Psychologist, 7,* 138–150.

Taylor, J., & Ogilvie, B. C. (1994). A conceptual model of adaptation to retirement among athletes. *Journal of Applied Sport Psychology, 6,* 1–20.

Zaichkowsky, L., Lipton, G., & Tucci, G. (1997). Factors affecting transition from intercollegiate sport. In R. Lidor & M. Bar-Eli (Eds.), *Proceedings of the IX World Congress of Sport Psychology* (pp. 782–784). Netanya, Israel: International Society of Sport Psychology.

Appendix A

Career Transitions in Sport: An Annotated Bibliography

David Lavallee
University of Teesside
England

Paul Wylleman
Vrije Universiet Brussel
Belgium

Dana Sinclair
Human Performance International
Canada

Career Transitions in Sport: An Annotated Bibliography[1]

The purpose of this bibliography is to provide researchers, practitioners, and others interested in career transitions in sport with an annotated reference list on the topic. Pertinent references (viz., references focusing on career transitions in sport, athletic career termination, or retirement from sport) were initially identified by conducting a literature search using SPORTdiscus and PsycLIT. A number of journals considered likely to publish relevant citations were also reviewed, including *Dissertation Abstracts International, International Journal of Sport Psychology, International Review for the Sociology of*

---

1. A total of 270 references were generated on the topic of career transitions in sport. However, 44 references were not available to be annotated. These additional citations are provided in the reference list at the end of the bibliography (D. Anderson, 1996; D. K. Anderson, 1998; Asselin, 1992; Brandmeyer & Alexander, 1989; Brock & Kleiber, 1994; Butlin, 1980; Deiters, 1996; Denison, 1994, 1996; Figler & Figler, 1984; Fish, Grove, & Eklund, 1997; Fortunato, 1996; Fortunato & Marchant, in press; Gordon, 1988; Grandisson & Vezina, 1997; Hinitz, 1988; Hurley & Mills, 1993; Lantz, 1995; Lewis, 1993; Loppnow, 1990; Mayocchi, 1998; Mayocchi & Hanrahan, 1997; McCann, 1995; Missler, 1996; Murphy et al., 1989; Neyer, 1996; Owens, 1994; Posthuma, 1992; Reece, Wilder, & Mahanes, 1996; Riesterer & Etzel, 1992; Sowa, Yusuf, & Mass, 1996; Sparkes, 1998; Stambulova, 1998; Tate & Joshua, 1996; Tian, Li, & Zhan, 1993; Ungerleider, 1994; Urofsky, 1997; Weimer, 1987; Weiss, 1992; Wendel & Shefsky, 1994; G. Wheeler et al., 1996; G. D. Wheeler et al., 1994).

Sport, Journal of Applied Sport Psychology, Journal of Sport Behavior, Journal of Sport and Social Issues, Quest, Sociology of Sport Journal, and *The Sport Psychologist.* Last, an extensive manual search was conducted using the reference lists from the citations identified in the computer and journal searches.

As indicated in Table 1, a total of 226 references (94 theoretical/applied references; 132 empirical references) on career transitions in sport are reported in this bibliography,[2] including 80 conference presentations (e.g., papers, posters, proceedings), 64 journal articles (sociology, 19; psychology, 19; other, 25), 27 book chapters/books, 11 monographs/reports, 29 dissertations/theses, and 15 other citations (e.g., magazine articles). The total distribution of research also included 80 separate studies. The breakdown of these investigations is as follows: competition level (professional, 27; Olympic/elite-amateur, 29; collegiate, 15; amateur, 5; across competition levels, 4); country of origin (Australia, 16; Canada, 11; Europe, 13; United States, 37; multinational, 3); gender (female, 9; male, 31; both females and males, 40); and methodology (qualitative, 23; quantitative, 47; both qualitative and quantitative, 10).

Table 1
Summary of References on Career Transitions in Sport

Type of Reference	1950–69	1970–79	1980–89	1990–98	Total
Conference Presentation	1	2	30	47	80
Journal Article	2	4	26	32	64
Book Chapter/Book	1	2	11	13	27
Monograph/Report	0	0	6	5	11
Dissertation/Thesis	0	3	8	18	29
Other	0	0	11	4	15
Total	4	11	92	119	226

2. An earlier version of this annotated bibliography was published by the Australian Council for Education Research in the *Australian Journal of Career Develpment.*

Career Transition Bibliography

Abraham, A. (1986). *Problems of identity with rhythmical gymnastics: A study on effects of sport specific constitutions of identity on finding the identity after the termination of a career in top-class athletics.* Schorndorf: Karl Hofmann.

• The results of a study conducted on the personality development of female gymnasts both during and after their retirement from sport are presented in this book. The issue of identification with the athlete role during the competitive career is discussed, along with the psychophysical difficulties that accompany a strong athletic identity upon career termination. Suggestions for athletes, coaches, and officials are presented.

Adelman, C. (1990). *Light and shadows on college athletes: College transcripts and labor market history.* Washington DC: United States Government Printing Office.

• This study examines the long-term educational and labor market careers of college varsity athletes in the *National Longitudinal Study of the High School Class of 1972.* After comparing athletes who attended 4-year colleges with their nonathlete counterparts, it was found that varsity football and basketball players enter college with relatively lower high school academic records, yet graduate from college at only a slightly lower rate. In addition, at age 32, ex-varsity football and basketball players had a higher rate of home ownership, lower rate of unemployment, and higher degree of economic mobility. Finally, former athletes were less likely to claim that their higher education was relevant to their current occupation.

Aflermann, D. (1995). Career transitions of elite athletes: Drop-out and retirement. In R. Vanfraechem-Raway & Y. Vanden Auweele (Eds.), *Proceedings of the 9th European Congress of Sport Psychology* (pp. 828–833). Brussels: European Federation of Sports Psychology.

• This paper presents the results of two studies focusing on elite athletes' perceptions with causes and consequences related to their retiring and/or dropping out from high-level sport in West Germany. The first study, which asked 50 female track and field athletes to complete a questionnaire at two ages (16–18 and 20–24), revealed that the major causes for dropping out were related to motivational problems and lack of social support. In a second study, 96 former athletes completed a questionnaire that focused on coping with the end of their sporting career. These athlete reported that physical challenge, self-esteem, and the desire to win were important reasons to continue their sports career, whereas involvement in professional (nonsport) activities, health problems, and age were reasons for retirement. A majority of former athletes also reported few negative consequences related to ending their careers in sport, with the exception to health problems and an imbalanced lifestyle.

Aflermann, D., & Gross, A. (1997). Coping with career termination: It all depends on freedom of choice. In R. Lidor & M. Bar-Eli (Eds.), *Proceedings of the IX World Congress on Sport Psychology* (pp. 65–67). Netanya, Israel: International Society of Sport Psychology.

Aflermann, D., & Gross, A. (1998). Erleben und bewaeltigen des karriereendes im hochleistungssport [How elite athletes perceive and cope with career termination]. *Leistungssport, 28 (2),* 45–48.

• This paper investigates differences in the career termination adjustment process among a sample of 90 former elite-level athletes (34 female; 56 male) representing 20 different sports in Germany. Participants in the study who voluntarily retired were compared with those who were forced to end their careers in terms of the quality of adjustment, as well as coping strategies. Results suggested that individuals who retired for voluntary reasons experienced significantly more positive reactions to their adjustment. Moreover, the former athletes who ended their careers involuntarily employed more coping strategies during the career transition process. In particular, these individuals reported using more emotion-focused coping strategies, whereas those who ended their careers by choice preferred more problem-related coping styles.

Ahlgren, R. (1995, October). *Perspectives of former high school football players on the process of sport career termination and transition from sport.* Paper presented at the annual conference of the Association for the Advancement of Applied Sport Psychology, New Orleans, USA.

• Eleven former high school football players participated in this interview study. Results indicated that participation in competitive sport was a central experience in the former athletes' lives and that the transition process had a negative impact at four specific points during the 18 months immediately following career termination.

Allison, M. T., & Meyer, C. (1984, July). *Career problems and retirement among elite athletes: The female tennis professional.* Paper presented at the annual meeting of the Olympic Scientific Congress, Eugene, OR, USA.

Allison, M. T., & Meyer, C. (1988). Career problems and retirement among elite athletes: The female tennis professional. *Sociology of Sport Journal, 5,* 212–222.

• Qualitative techniques (i.e., networking and snowball sampling) were used to describe the competitive and retirement experiences of elite female tennis professionals. Twenty athletes completed an extensive semistructured questionnaire focusing on childhood and adolescent socialization experiences, career experiences and aspirations, and retirement experiences. Results suggested that athletes perceived retirement to be an opportunity to reestablish more traditional societal roles and lifestyles, rather than a traumatic process.

Anderson, D. (1993). *Research tour: Elite athlete education programs.* Melbourne: Victorian Institute of Sport.

• This research report outlines the career transition and education programs for elite athletes in Australia, Canada, United Kingdom, and the United States. The services offered in each program are delineated, and names of the program directors are provided where available. A summary of contemporary issues concludes this report.

Andrews, D. S. (1981). Socialization agents and career contingencies affecting the elite hockey player during his active and post-active occupational role. *Arena Review, 5,* 54–63.

• This article reviews the pertinent literature on the socialization process of hockey players into, during, and after a career in elite-level sport. This process is compared to that of nonathletes, and it is suggested that socialization problems need to be addressed by the management of sporting associations at the elite level.

Arviko, I. (1976). *Factors influencing the job and life satisfaction of retired baseball players.* Unpublished master's thesis, University of Waterloo, Canada.

• Drawing on gerontological theory, this study analyzed the postplaying adjustments of professional baseball players. Results suggested that most respondents experienced relatively high levels of adjustment difficulties.

Baillie, P. H. F. (1987). *Career transition in elite and professional athletes: A model of adjustment to retirement with implications for counselling.* Unpublished master's thesis, The University of Toronto, Canada.

• This thesis presents a five-factor model of adjustment to athletic career termination. Mental preparation for retirement, specific plans for retirement, and unfinished business in sports are the predictor factors in the model, whereas emotional adjustment and functional adjustment to retirement serve as outcome factors. This theoretical conception forms the foundation of later studies (see Baillie, 1990, 1992).

Baillie, P. H. F. (1990). *Career transition in elite and professional athletes: Three case studies of preparation and adjustment to retirement from competitive sport.* Unpublished master's thesis, Virginia Commonwealth University, Richmond, USA.

• Three case studies are presented in this thesis as illustrations of the career transition process experienced by elite-level athletes. Semistructured interviews were conducted in order to assess the participant's personal histories, extent of preretirement career planning, and postretirement adjustment. Comparisons between the three former athletes are made, with a focus on the factors predicting the degree of adjustment to retirement from competitive sport.

Baillie, P. H. F. (1992a). *Career transition in elite and professional athletes: A study of individuals in their preparation for adjustment to retirement from competitive sports.* Unpublished doctoral dissertation, Virginia Commonwealth University, USA.

Baillie, P. H. F. (1992b, October/November). *Career transition in elite and professional athletes: A study of individuals in their preparation for and adjustment to retirement from competitive sports.* Colloquium presented at the annual conference of the Association for the Advancement of Applied Sport Psychology, Colorado Springs, USA.

• In this research project, 260 former athletes were surveyed in terms of their mental preparation for retirement, specific plans for retirement, achievement of sport-related goals prior to career termination, and emotional and functional adjustment to retirement. The participants in this sample were drawn from distinct populations in order to compare the career transition experiences of former professional, Olympic, and collegiate athletes. Suggestions are provided for the improvement of pre- and postretirement programs for elite athletes.

Baillie, P. H. F. (1993). Understanding retirement from sports: Therapeutic ideas for helping athletes in transition. *The Counseling Psychologist, 21,* 399–410.

• This article discusses therapeutic strategies for assisting athletes in transition. The meaning of being an athlete is described by drawing on empirical and theoretical research, and various career counseling issues are presented. Suggestions are outlined on interventions that can assist athletes prior to, during, and following their retirement from sport.

Baillie, P. H. F., & Danish, S. J. (1992). Understanding the career transition of athletes. *The Sport Psychologist, 6,* 77–98.

• Beginning with the early identification of the athlete role and continuing on through to the retirement from active participation in sport, this paper provides an overview of the various aspects related to the career transition process. Research on the influence of participation in high-level sport in the development of athletes' self-perception is discussed, as are the mechanisms related to coping with career termination. The applicability of various theories on the retirement is also reviewed. The article concludes with a discussion of specific therapeutic and counseling interventions, which can be applied with athletes in transition.

Baillie, P. H. F., & Lampron, A. (1992). Retirement from sport: Studies show wide range of experiences and expectations, *Olympinfo, 8,* 4.

• This article describes two surveys conducted in Canada on the experience of preparing for and adjusting to athletic career termination. Whereas the first study examines the preparation for retirement among a sample of former athletes (see Baillie, 1992), the second survey assesses the career transition expectations among a sample of active athletes. Respondents in both studies expressed strongly the need to have access to career transition programs.

Bardaxoglou, N., & Vanfraechem-Raway, R. (1993). Systemic approach of the social reinsertion of top level athletes. In S. Serpa, J. Alves, V. Ferreira, & A. Paula-Brito (Eds.), *Proceedings of the VIII World Congress of Sport Psychology* (pp. 810–813). Lisbon: International Society of Sport Psychology.

Bardaxoglou, N., & Vanfraechem-Raway, R. (1995). The life line inventory: A new tool for interviewing the athlete in transition career. In R. Vanfraechem-Raway & Y. Vanden Auweele (Eds.), *Proceedings of the 9th European Congress of Sport Psychology* (pp. 834–840). Brussels: European Federation of Sports Psychology.

Bardaxoglou, N., & Vanfraechem-Raway, R. (1997). Mental strategies used after the life line inventory. In R. Lidor & M. Bar-Eli (Eds.), *Proceedings of the IX World Congress of Sport Psychology* (pp. 97–99). Netanya, Israel: International Society of Sport Psychology.

• Employing a neurolinguistic programming model, these papers introduce the life line inventory as a counseling tool that can be employed when working with athletes in transition. The methodology for employing this systemic approach is provided, and the development of various mental strategies for successfully changing behavior during a career transition is discussed.

Blann, F. W. (1985a). *The relationship of level of intercollegiate athletic competition and student's educational and career plans.* Paper presented at the annual meeting of the American Alliance of Health, Physical Education, Recreation, and Dance.

Blann, F. W. (1985b). Intercollegiate athletic competition and students' educational and career plans. *Journal of College Student Personnel, 26,* 115–119.
 • Athletes from two National Collegiate Athletic Association (NCAA) Division 1 and two NCAA Division III member institutions (265 female; 303 male) participated in a study examining the relationships of students' sex, class, and competitive level of participation in intercollegiate athletics and their ability to formulate mature educational and career plans. Results utilizing Task 2 of the Revised Student Development Task Inventory (SDTI-2; Winston, Miller, & Prince, 1979) and a demographic questionnaire suggested that participation in intercollegiate athletics at a high level of competition may detrimentally affect students' ability to formulate mature educational and career plans.

Blann, F. W. (1992). Coaches' role in player development. *Journal of Applied Research in Coaching and Athletics, 7,* 62–76.
 • This article examines the coaches' role in the career transition process for elite athletes. The Professional Athletes' Career Transition Program (PACTP) developed from a series of studies conducted by Blann and Zaichkowsky (1989) is outlined. The nine modules of the PACTP are summarized, as well as the benefits to athletes, coaches, management, and players' associations.

Blann, F. W., & Zaichkowsky, L. (1986). *Career/life transition needs of National Hockey League players.* Final report prepared for the National Hockey League Players' Association, USA.

Blann, F. W., & Zaichkowsky, L. (1987a). *Career/life transition needs of a National Hockey League players' spouses perspective.* Report prepared for the National Hockey League Players' Association, USA.

Blann, F. W., & Zaichkowsky, L. (1987b). *An assessment of National Hockey League players' career transition needs.* Paper presented at the annual meeting of the American Alliance of Health, Physical Education, Recreation, and Dance.

Blann, F. W., & Zaichkowsky, L. (1988). *Major League Baseball players' post-sport career transition needs.* Preliminary report prepared for the Major League Baseball Players' Association, USA.

Blann, F. W., & Zaichkowsky, L. (1989). *National Hockey League and Major League Baseball players' post-sport career transition surveys.* Final report prepared for the National Hockey League Players' Association, USA.
 • These reports present the results of two in-depth surveys conducted on the

career transition needs of active professional baseball and ice hockey players. The Professional Athletes' Career Transition Inventory (PACTI) was developed and employed to assess career awareness, postathletic career plans, life satisfaction, and the most and least helpful aspects of career planning programs among 117 male National Hockey League players (and their spouses) and 214 male Major League Baseball players. Conclusions are based on athletes' needs, and implications are provided for athletes, coaches, and sport managers.

Blinde, E. M., & Greendorfer, S. L. (1985). A reconceptualization of the process of leaving the role of competitive athlete. *International Review for the Sociology of Sport, 20,* 87–93.
• This article examines the appropriateness of social gerontology and thanatology as theoretical frameworks for studying sport retirement. As such, alternative notions derived from a database of former female and male intercollegiate athletes (see Greendorfer & Blinde, 1985) are discussed. The concepts of long-term development, role aptitude, and anticipatory socialization are also suggested for future research in the area of athletic transition.

Blinde, E. M., & Stratta, T. M. (1992). The "sport career death" of college athletes: Involuntary and unanticipated sports exits. *Journal of Sport Behavior, 15,* 3–20.
• In-depth interviews were conducted with 20 college athletes (18 female; 2 male) who experienced an involuntary and unanticipated career termination. The social psychological processes associated with this type of transition were examined, and it was found that this sample experienced considerable adjustment difficulties. It was concluded that involuntary retirement from intercollegiate sport may require special attention in the literature.

Bookbinder, H. (1955). Work histories of men leaving a short life span occupation. *Personnel and Guidance Journal, 34,* 164–167.
• This early article reports the findings of a study conducted with 121 retired professional baseball players. The various types of postathletic careers were examined, and it was found that the most frequently held jobs were in the professional and managerial classification. The majority of participants reported that they were satisfied with their jobs.

Botterill, C. (1982). What "endings" tell us about beginnings. In T. Orlick, T. Partington, & J. H. Salmela (Eds.), *Proceedings of the 5th World Congress of Sport Psychology* (pp. 164–166). Ottawa: Coaching Association of Canada.
• This article provides an overview of the various phases that athletes may experience when terminating their sports career. Using anecdotal accounts of

former Canadian athletes, the author suggests that there is a need for counseling and preparing athletes to cope with the career end. The specific issues emphasized are the athlete-coach relationship, financial support, and detraining opportunities.

Botterill, C. (1988). Preventing burnout and retirement problems. *Canadian Academy of Sport Medicine, 8,* 28–29.

• This article proposes that a high percentage of former athletes experience serious trauma upon retirement from competition and suggests that narrow identities and lack of self management skills contribute to their adjustment difficulties. Recommendations for the prevention of adaptation problems are outlined.

Boydell, C., & Lothian, S. F. (1993). *Adjustment to involuntary disengagement from organized athletics.* Report prepared for the Ministry of Tourism and Recreation, Ontario, Canada.

• This report describes a research project on involuntary withdrawal from elite-level sport. A series of investigations focusing on the perceptions and reactions associated with retirement from different levels of sport is outlined. It is suggested that the information gained is of use to coaches, sports administrators, and counselors.

Brandmeyer, G., & Alexander, L. (1981, May/June). Cognitive interpretations in light of contractual change: A sociology of knowledge analysis from the perspective of former ballplayers. In A. Ingham & E. Broom (Eds.), *Proceedings of the 1st Regional Symposium for the International Committee for the Sociology of Sport* (pp. 454–461). Vancouver: University of British Columbia.

• This paper qualitatively analyzed the transitions made by 18 professional baseball players to nonsporting careers by focusing on the adjustment to life after sport and attitudes toward organized baseball as a social enterprise. The paper was presented as part of a conference on career patterns and career contingencies in sport, a symposium that brought together theoretical, sociohistorical, and contemporary analytical approaches to understand the structure of professional and amateur sport and the structural constraints and opportunities that affect athletic careers.

Broom, E. F. (1982). Detraining and retirement from high level competition: A reaction to "Retirement from high level competition" and "Career crisis in sport." In T. Orlick, J. T. Partington, & J. H. Salmela (Eds.), *Proceedings of the 5th World Congress of Sport Psychology* (pp. 183–187). Ottawa: Coaching Association of Canada.

• This paper comments on the retirement-related articles by Svoboda and Vanek (1982) and Ogilvie and Howe (1982). Case studies are presented, and the need for retirement counseling is emphasized.

Chamalidis, P. (1995). Career transitions of male champions. In R. Vanfraechem-Raway & Y. Vanden Auweele (Eds.), *Proceedings of the 9th European Congress of Sport Psychology* (pp. 841–848). Brussels: European Federation of Sports Psychology.

Chamalidis, P. (1997). Identity conflicts during and after retirement from top-level sports. In R. Lidor & M. Bar-Eli (Eds.), *Proceedings of the IX World Congress of Sport Psychology* (pp. 191–193) Netanya, Israel: International Society of Sport Psychology.

Chamalidis, P. (1998). *Masculine identity in high-level sport: The glory and grief of the champion.* Unpublished doctoral dissertation, University of Rene Descartes, Paris, France.

• In-depth interviews and projective tests were used in these studies to assess 25 Greek and 15 French former elite athletes' self-concept, motivation to participate and to terminate participation in competitive sport, and experiences with losing the active role as an athlete. Most participants in this study had already accepted the end of their sporting careers and had gone on to develop successful postathletic careers. However, several athletes who had their careers ended abruptly stated that they experienced an unanticipated sense of loss. The masculine identity construction is highlighted in this research.

Coakley, J. J. (1983). Leaving competitive sport: Retirement or rebirth? *Quest, 35,* 1–11.

• This article, which is one of the most cited in the career transition literature, critically examines the available research on retirement from interscholastic, amateur, and professional sport. By employing a developmental perspective, the widespread assumption that athletic career termination is always a traumatic event is challenged. This point of departure in the literature suggests that various factors influence the quality of adjustment, and therefore, retirement itself is not inherently stressful.

Cramer-Hamman, B. (1994). *Predicting successful adjustment to disengagement from collegiate athletics.* Unpublished doctoral dissertation, University of North Carolina, Chapel Hill, USA.

• This study surveyed 23 male and female collegiate athletes in terms of their preretirement planning and decision making, athletic identity, social support, and nature of career termination. Results revealed that the best model for predicting successful adjustment among athletes who disengage from collegiate sports includes social support and career planning.

Crook, J. (1986). *Retirement from elite sport: Implications for counselling.* Unpublished master's thesis, University of Alberta, Canada.

Crook, J. M., & Robertson, S. E. (1991). Transitions out of elite sport. *International Journal of Sport Psychology, 22,* 115–127.

* A critique of two analytical models (viz., social gerontology and thanatology) referred to in the literature on retirement from high-level sport is provided, along with a review of the relevant literature on identity factors related to the process of coping with the career transition. A counseling-based approach is discussed as an alternative model.

Curtis, J., & Ennis, R. (1988). Negative consequences of leaving competitive sport? Comparison findings for former elite-level hockey players. *Sociology of Sport Journal, 5,* 87–106.

* Former Canadian junior hockey players and a representative sample of males in the general population were compared on measures of life satisfaction, employment status, and marital status. Survey results revealed no evidence of negative consequences of disengagement from high-performancesport even when the comparisons were controlled for time since retirement. However, feelings of loss reported by the former players at the time of disengagement suggested the perception of adjustment difficulties.

Danish, S. J., Owens, S. S., Green, S. L., & Brunelle, J. P. (1997). Building bridges for disengagement: The transition process for individuals and teams. *Journal of Applied Sport Psychology, 9,* 154–167.

* This article provides an overview of the reasons why disengagement occurs. Schlossberg's (1981) model of transition, Danish and D'Augelli's (1980) life-span development framework, and Tuckman's (1965) model of group development are examined in order to explain the potential impact the disengagement process has on both individuals and teams. Relevant interventions are discussed.

Doms, J. R., & Dixon, D. N. (1992, August). *Career development difficulties of athletes: Implications for counseling.* Paper presented at the annual meeting of the American Psychological Association, Washington DC.

* This paper focuses on the academic and career development difficulties experienced by intercollegiate athletes. The role of the counselor in working

with this population is described, and a psychoeducational intervention model is outlined.

Edwards, J., & Meier, K. (1984, July). *Social breakdown/reconstruction and athletic retirement: An investigation of retirement and retirement adjustment in National Hockey League players.* Paper presented at the annual meeting of the Olympic Scientific Congress, Eugene, OR, USA.
 • This study investigated the transition experiences of 83 former professional ice hockey players. The participants retired, voluntarily or involuntarily, between 1972 and 1979. Data were collected on a number of variables including preretirement planning, socioeconomic status, social support, sporting achievements, health status, reasons for career termination, and initial feelings following retirement. Statistically significant support for a social breakdown/reconstruction paradigm of retirement adjustment was obtained.

Farrell, C. S. (1992). Professional counseling needs to assist college athletes in transition. *Black Issues in Higher Education, 8,* 22–23.
 • This informational article emphasizes the risks facing athletes in the transition to a nonsports life, particularly at the collegiate level. Adjustment programs are supported and the need for such programs to assist athletes as they enter the sporting system, and not just as they prepare to leave it, is discussed.

Fish, M. B. (1994). *Non-selection as a factor contributing to retirement from Australian sport.* Unpublished honours thesis, Edith Cowan University, Perth, Western Australia.
 • This study assesses the career transition experiences of 15 Australian athletes (7 female; 8 male) who were deselected from the sports of cricket, field hockey, or water polo. Results from in-depth interviews suggested that participants perceived their sporting associations, officials, teammates, and family members as lacking in understanding of the issues of nonselection. The short- and long-term effects of this specific reason for retirement are discussed. Recommendations, including the need for greater professionalism in areas such as player relations, selection procedures, and athlete support, are provided.

Fortunato, V., Anderson, D., Morris, T, & Seedsman, T. (1995). Career transition research at Victoria University of Technology. In R. Vanfraechem-Raway & Y. Vanden Auweele (Eds.), *Proceedings of the 9th European Congress of Sport Psychology* (pp. 533–543). Brussels: European Federation of Sports Psychology.

• This article outlines a research program in the area of career education and transition at Victoria University of Technology. The content of the Australian Athlete Career and Education program is described as well as an empirical study outlining its effectiveness (see Morris & Anderson, 1994a, 1994b). Research conducted with 52 Australian League Football players is also outlined. In this study, it was found that those athletes who had terminated their career on a voluntary basis and/or remained actively involved in their sport (e.g., as a coach) experienced more positive transitions than did those who ended their careers due to injury or deselection.

Gorbett, F. J. (1985). Psycho-social adjustment of athletes to retirement. In L. K. Bunker, R. J. Rotella, & A. S. Reilly (Eds.), *Psychological considerations in maximizing sport performance* (pp. 288–294). Ithaca, NY: Mouvement.

• The purpose of this paper is to discuss the sociopsychological adjustment process of transitional athletes. The transition theories of Schlossberg (1981) and Hopson (1981) are outlined, and a preretirement counseling program for athletes is proposed.

Gordon, S. (1995). Career transitions in competitive sport. In T. Morris & J. Summers (Eds.), *Sport psychology: Theory, applications and issues* (pp. 474–501). Brisbane: Jacaranda Wiley.

• This book chapter provides an overview of career transitions in sport, with a specific emphasis on research conducted in Australia. The content includes references to both the theoretical and applied literature, and a conceptual model of the career transition process for athletes. An overview of career assistance programs for athletes in Australia, Canada, United Kingdom, and the United States is also described, as well as recommendations for prevention and treatment interventions.

Gordon, S., & Lavallee, D. (1995). *Career assistance programming for cricket.* Unpublished manuscript, Department of Human Movement, The University of Western Australia, Nedlands.

• In this survey, nine former first-class male cricket players in Australia were asked to describe their reasons for athletic retirement and provide suggestions regarding career assistance programming for elite-level cricket players. The need to assist individuals with financial adjustment was cited as a priority, whereas the opportunity to develop vocational skills during their playing careers was unanimously suggested by the sample. Recommendations for national and state cricket associations are provided.

Greendorfer, S. L. (1983, October). *Letting the data speak: The reality of sport retirement.* Paper presented at the annual meeting of the North American Society for the Sociology of Sport, St. Louis, USA.

Greendorfer, S. L. (1985, April). *Implication of sport retirement research for the practitioner.* Paper presented at the annual meeting of the American Alliance for Health, Physical Education, Recreation, and Dance, Atlanta, GA.

Greendorfer, S. L (1986, June). *Life after athletics.* Paper presented at the 10th Session of the United States Olympic Academy, Colorado Springs.

Greendorfer, S. L, & Blinde, E. M. (1985). "Retirement" from intercollegiate sport: Theoretical and empirical considerations. *Sociology of Sport Journal, 2,* 101–110.

Greendorfer, S. L. & Blinde, E. M. (1987). Female sport retirement: Descriptive patterns and research application. In L. Vander Velden & H. Humphrey (Eds.), *Psychology and sociology of sport* (pp. 167–176). New York: AMS Press.

Greendorfer, S. L., Blinde, E., & Kleiber, D. A. (1984, July). *Theoretical and empirical considerations of intercollegiate sport "retirement".* Paper presented at the annual meeting of the Olympic Scientific Congress, Eugene, OR, USA.

Greendorfer, S. L., & Kleiber, D. A. (1982, November). *Sport retirement as social death: The college athlete.* Paper presented at the annual meeting of the North American Society for the Sociology of Sport, Toronto, Canada.

• Former intercollegiate athletes (697 female; 427 male) were surveyed in this comprehensive series of studies relative to their commitment to a sport role, educational and occupational preparation, postcareer sport participation, social interests, and adjustment to sport retirement. Results indicated that participants did not experience great adjustment difficulties and that gender differences were minimal. An alternative conceptualization of the transition process is offered, and the relevance of research to coaches and athletes is demonstrated. For further details of this program of research, refer to Kleiber and Brock (1992) and Kleiber, Greendorfer, Blinde, and Sandall (1987).

Griffiths, A. (1983). Retiring stars: Gone and soon forgotten. *Champion, 7 (2),* 16–17.

• In this article, individual stories and personal accounts highlight the crises that many Canadian high-performanceathletes have experienced as a result of retirement. The question of who should prepare athletes for transitions is addressed, and differing views are presented.

Griffiths, L. L. (1982). Life after sports. *Women's Sport, 9,* 10.

• This brief educational report on retirement from sport views transition from a crisis perspective. Practical strategies for avoiding or minimizing the possible problems associated with the adjustment process are outlined for both current and transitional athletes.

Gross, S. (1987, October). *The retirement of professional hockey players: Approaching the problem from a career perspective.* Paper presented at the annual meeting of the Canadian Society for Psychomotor Learning and Sport Psychology, Alberta.
* This study is based on data collected from surveys with 115 active and 514 retired professional ice hockey players, as well as qualitative interviews with a subsample of 30 participants. It is reported that the degree of identification with sport is negatively correlated with a successful shift in career identity and positively correlated with the degree of emotional adjustment following career termination. A suggestion is made that career change and developmental issues should be the focus of intervention strategies.

Grove, J. R., Lavallee, D., & Gordon, S. (1997). Coping with retirement from sport: The influence of athletic identity. *Journal of Applied Sport Psychology, 9,* 191–203.
* In this study, 48 former elite-level Australian athletes (28 female; 20 male) supplied information about their financial, occupational, emotional, and social adjustment to retirement from sport. Athletic identity at the time of retirement was also assessed, along with self-reported use of various coping strategies. Results indicated that acceptance, positive reinterpretation, planning, and active coping were the most frequently used coping strategies during the career transition process. At the same time, athletic identity at the time of retirement exhibited significant relationships to coping processes, emotional and social adjustment, preretirement planning, and anxiety about career decision making. Suggestions for future research and implications for career transition programs are discussed.

Grove, J. R., Lavallee, D., Gordon, S., & Harvey, J. H. (1998). Account-making: A model for understanding and resolving distressful reactions to retirement from sport. *The Sport Psychologist, 12,* 52–67.
* This paper examines the account-making model of Harvey, Weber, and Orbuch (1990) as a framework for understanding negative emotional reactions to retirement from competitive sport. Theoretical aspects of the model are summarized, and a case study is presented to illustrate the central role of account-making in the adjustment process. The article concludes with suggestions for

ways in which practitioners can facilitate account-making and thereby assist athletes to cope with distressful reactions to retirement from sport.

Haerle, R. K. (1975). Career patterns and career contingencies of professional baseball players: An occupational analysis. In D. W. Ball & J. W. Loy (Eds.), *Sport and social order* (pp. 461–519). Reading, MA: Addison-Wesley.

• This chapter describes and evaluates the organizational constraints that operate in the occupational environment of professional baseball. The results of a study conducted with 335 retired male baseball players are presented, with a specific focus on the background of the athletes before their playing careers, the structural and interpersonal characteristics during their sporting careers, and the transition into a postbaseball occupation.

Hallden, O. (1965). The adjustment of athletes after retiring from sport. In F. Antonelli (Ed.), *Proceedings of the 1st International Congress of Sport Psychology* (pp. 730–733). Rome.

• In one of the first empirical examinations of retirement from sport, a sample of 61 amateur Swedish athletes were surveyed in terms of their adaptation to career termination. Utilizing both quantitative and qualitative methodologies, 45 athletes reported experiencing emotional adjustment difficulties. No specific conclusions are presented in this study.

Hallinan, C. (1986, October/November). *Forced disengagement and the student-athlete.* Paper presented at the annual meeting of the North American Society for the Sociology of Sport, Las Vegas, USA.
Hallinan, C., & Snyder, E. (1988). Forced disengagement and the college athlete. *Arena Review, 11,* 28–34.

• This study investigated the nature and psychosocial consequences of forced disengagement from sport. Four female athletes who were deselected from their college teams were interviewed in regards to their backgrounds, personal characteristics, athletic involvement, and reaction to the disengagement process. The findings are presented using the model of Kubler-Ross (1969).

Hanion, T. (1988, September/October). Life after the Olympics: Helping athletes cope when it's all over. *American Coach,* p. 5.

• This article describes the development of Career Assistance Program for Athletes (CAPA), a program developed by the United States Olympic Committee. An interview with the pilot project coordinator is reported in which the reasons for the initiation of program are outlined.

Hare, N. (1971). A study of the black fighter. *The Black Scholar, 3 (3),* 2–9.
• In this study of the postretirement careers of boxers, it was concluded that many athletes experience adjustment difficulties. More specifically, family socioeconomic background and minority status were significant variables in the adjustment process in that poor financial resources of low-income families and job discrimination further exacerbated transition adjustments.

Hawkins, K., & Blann, F. W. (1993). *Athlete/coach career development and transition.* Canberra: Australian Sports Commission.

Hawkins, K., & Blann, W. (1994, June). *Coping with the end of an athletic career.* Paper presented at the annual meeting of the International Association for Physical Education in Higher Education, Berlin.

Hawkins, K., Blann, F. W., & Zaichkowsky, L. (1994, August). *International perspectives on athlete/coach career development and transition.* Paper presented at the 10th Commonwealth and Scientific Congress, University of Victoria, Canada.

Hawkins, K., Blann, F. W., Zaichkowsky, L., & Kane, M. A. (1994). *Athlete/coach career development and transition: Coaches' report.* Canberra: Australian Sports Commission.
• These papers and reports provide a review of an extensive research project that surveyed the career transition needs of elite athletes and coaches in Australia. Quantitative data were collected from 124 athletes (55 female; 69 males) and 29 coaches (7 female; 22 male), and interviews were conducted with 11 athletes (6 female; 5 male) and 21 coaches (6 female; 15 male). The piloting of the questionnaires used in the study is provided in Hawkins and Blann (1993), along with copies of instruments developed for the project (see Hoskin & Hawkins, 1992). Overall, the results suggested that athletes had a higher awareness of the need for career development than did the coaches who were surveyed, although there were gender differences in this awareness. Conclusions, recommendations, and further avenues of research are provided for both athletes and coaches.

Hewett, K. R. (1994). *The career orientation of elite athletes in the Australian context: A qualitative analysis.* Unpublished honours thesis, The University of Western Australia, Nedlands.
• A case study approach was employed in this thesis to examine the similarities and differences in career orientation among five elite Australian athletes. The central research question was why elite-level athletes do or do not pursue a vocational career in cooperation with their sport. Results suggested

that a number of factors played a vital role in the athletes' vocational choices, including the elite sport coach, the age of entering sport, wider life experiences outside of sport, and academic achievement. Motivation towards a postathletic career also changed as a result of impeding retirement from sport, prolonged injury, unexpected omissions from team selection, and/or the experiences of peers. A discussion of these triggers highlights the importance of the timing of interventions in career transition programs for elite athletes.

Hill, P., & Lowe, B. (1974). *The inevitable metathesis of the retiring athlete.* Paper presented at the annual meeting of the Eastern District Association of the American Alliance on Health, Physical Education, Recreation, and Dance, New York.

Hill, P., & Lowe, B. (1974). The inevitable metathesis of the retiring athlete. *International Review of Sport Sociology, 4,* 5–29.

• The primary purpose of this paper, which is one of the earlier works published in the area, was to develop a clearer understanding of the sport transition process by examining perspectives from gerontology. The relevance of Sussman's (1972) model for the sociological study of retirement in general to the study of retirement from sport is presented.

Hoskin, D., & Hawkins, K. (1992). *Career awareness and transition for Australian athletes and coaches: The design and validation of a measuring instrument.* Paper presented at the annual meeting of the International Association for Physical Education in Higher Education, VIC, Australia.

• The *Australian Athletes Career Transition Inventory* (AACTI) and *Australian Coaches Career Transition Inventory* (ACCTI) were designed and validated with 56 athletes (48 female; 8 male) and seven coaches (2 female; 5 male) in order to collect data on the career transition needs of elite-level athletes and coaches in Australia. This project served as a pilot study for further studies conducted by Hawkins, Blann, and colleagues (see Hawkins & Blann, 1993; Hawkins, Blann, Zaichkowsky, & Kane, 1994).

Huck, B. (1982). When the bubble bursts: What happens to the amateur athletes when it's all over? *Canadian Skater, 9,* 5–7.

• This journalistic account of athletic retirement quotes former high-performance athletes and highlights the issue of organizational responsibility in the establishment of career counseling and detraining programs for athletes.

Jackson, S. A., Dover, J. D., & Mayocchi, L. M. (1998). Life after gold: I. Experiences of Australian Olympic gold-medallists. *The Sport Psychologist, 12,* 119–136.

Jackson, S., Mayocchi, L., & Dover, J. (1998). Life after winning gold: II. Coping with change as an Olympic gold medallist. *The Sport Psychologist, 12*, 137–155.
  • In these qualitative investigations, the experiences encountered by 18 Australian athletes who won Olympic gold medals between the years 1984–1992 were assessed. Interviews were conducted with each athlete, as well as 10 coaches of Olympic gold-medallists. The findings focus on the following components: experience at the Olympics, experience in the year following the Olympics, athlete's performance and career after the Olympic win, experience as a gold-medallist in general, and recommendations provided for future athletes and coaches at the Olympic level.

Jegathesan, M. (1993, June). *Staying in the race.* Paper presented at the International Sports Science Conference, Singapore.
Jegathesan, M. (1994). Staying in the race. *New Studies in Athletics, 9 (4),* 7–8.
  • This paper examines the potential physical and psychological adjustment problems associated with the end of a career in sport. The responsibilities of sporting organizations are discussed.

Johns, D. P. (1985, November). *The short career of the female gymnast.* Paper presented at the annual meeting of the North American Society for the Sociology of Sport, Boston, USA.
  • Thirty female gymnasts who had recently retired from competitive sport were assessed in terms of their participation in gymnastics and reasons for career termination. Results found the major reasons for retiring to be social evaluation, desire to be part of the teenage subculture, and injury. Skill acquisition was also identified as the most enjoyable aspect of participation in sport.

Johns, D. P. (1995). Transitions: Problems in the convergence of athletic, educational and vocational careers. In R. Vanfraechem-Raway & Y. Vanden Auweele (Eds.), *Proceedings of the 9th European Congress of Sport Psychology* (pp. 517–523). Brussels: European Federation of Sports Psychology.
  • This paper comments on the transitional demands experienced by former elite wrestlers. Drawing on the available literature regarding athletes' reactions to the career end, the ongoing transitions that wrestlers encounter are discussed. The aim of the author is to encourage sport organizations to facilitate transition interventions for athletes.

Jollimore, M. (1986). Athletes for hire: Career centre helps athletes discover life after sport. *Champion, 10,* 42–45.

• This journalistic article focuses on the establishment of Canada's *Olympic Athlete Career Centre* (OACC) in 1985. The article briefly outlines the rationale for developing the OACC and its initial concept as a job placement agency.

Kane, M. A. (1991). *The metagonic transition: A study of career transition, marital stress, and identity transformation in former professional athletes.* Unpublished doctoral dissertation, Boston University, MA, USA.

Kane, M. A. (1995). The transition out of sport: A paradigm from the United States. In R. Vanfraechem-Raway & Y. Vanden Auweele (Eds.), *Proceedings of the 9th European Congress of Sport Psychology* (pp. 849–856). Brussels: European Federation of Sports Psychology.

• This research provides a holistic perspective on retirement from sport by examining transition as a life event rather than as a career change. Data collected from 19 former professional athletes in the United States and their spouses revealed that the *metagonic* transition, where *meta* refers to change and *agon* indicates a challenge, often lasts several years. Discussions focus on the separate stages that athletes in transition face upon retirement.

Kearl, M. C. (1982). Holy exits: Symbolic portrayals of good career conclusions in professional sports. *Gerontologist, 22,* 121.

Kearl, M. C. (1982, November). *Holy exits: A theory of finite time, social endings, and good retirements.* Paper presented at the annual meeting of the Gerontological Society of America, Boston.

Kearl, M. C. (1986). How to quit: On the finitudes of everyday life. *Sociological Inquiry, 56,* 283–303.

• These papers elaborate on the psychology of social endings (e.g., retirement, divorce, death). It is argued that some ending are recognized as being better than others and that culminating behaviors associated with role conclusions can contribute to both social and personal order. Retirement from professional sport is considered in terms of how the quality of an athlete's career conclusion influences the way in which she or he is remembered after retirement.

Kirby, S. L. (1986a). *High performance female athletes retirement.* Unpublished doctoral dissertation, University of Alberta, Canada.

Kirby, S. L. (1986b). *Ageism in sport: A condition of high performance female athlete retirement.* Paper presented at the 5th Canadian Congress on Leisure Research, Halifax, Nova Scotia.

• The purpose of this research was to discover how and under what conditions female athletes leave high-performance sport. Survey data and selected interviews generated results under the following headings: decisions to leave, injury and/or ill health, barriers to continued participation, and the retirement path. Findings indicated that retiring from high-performance sport with pride, honor, and dignity was the norm.

Kleiber, D. A., & Brock, S. C. (1992). The effect of career-ending injuries on the subsequent well-being of elite college athletes. *Sociology of Sport Journal, 9,* 70–75.

• In a previous study investigating transition outcomes in the context of college sport, Kleiber, Greendorfer, Blinde, and Sandall (1987) found that a career-ending injury was the only predictor of later life satisfaction. Using the same cohort, this study examined the athletes subsequent depression of well-being (as measured by life satisfaction and self-esteem). Results indicated that of those athletes who had been injured, only those who had an investment in playing professional sport were likely to show lower self-esteem and life satisfaction 5 to 10 years later.

Kleiber, D. A., & Greendorfer, S. L. (1983). *Social reintegration of former college athletes: Male football and basketball players from 1970–1980.* Unpublished manuscript, Champaign, IL, USA.

Kleiber, D., Greendorfer, S., Blinde, E., & Sandall, D. (1987). Quality of exit from university sports and subsequent life satisfaction. *Journal of Sport Sociology, 4,* 28–36.

• As part of a larger study of the postparticipation experience of former university athletes (see Greendorfer & Blinde, 1985), this investigation examined the effect of role performance in intercollegiate basketball and football on life satisfaction. Using Kearl's (1986) analysis of exits and social endings in everyday life as a theoretical departure point, survey results for 427 male athletes revealed that although good career endings may not affect subsequent life satisfaction, bad career endings may. It is noted that findings from this study may not be applicable to all intercollegiate athletes.

Koukouris, K. (1989). *Disengagement of advanced and elite Greek male athletes from organized competitive sport.* Unpublished doctoral dissertation, Victoria University.

Koukouris, K. (1991a). Quantitative aspects of the disengagement process of advanced and elite Greek male athletes from organized competitive sport. *Journal of Sport Behavior, 14,* 227–246.

Koukouris, K. (1991b). Disengagement of advanced and elite Greek male athletes from organized competitive sport. *International Review for the Sociology of Sport, 26,* 289–306.

Koukouris, K. (1994). Constructed case studies: Athletes' perspectives on disengaging from organized competitive sport. *Sociology of Sport Journal, 11,* 114–139.

Koukouris, K. (1996, November). Greek athletes' perspectives of disengaging from organized competitive gymnastics. In Y. Theodorakis & A. Papaionnan (Eds.), *Proceedings of the International Congress on Sport Psychology* (pp. 116–121). Komotinis, Greece.
• This line of research examined the disengagement process among 113 former Greek athletes from the sports of athletics, rowing, and volleyball. Initial findings revealed that the majority of athletes reacted in a positive way to their career end and remained involved in sport on a recreational level. Follow-up individual interviews with 34 athletes from the original sample also suggested that a combination of internal and external factors from the sporting environment influence the adjustment process to athletic career termination.

Lavallee, D., Gordon, S., & Grove, J. R. (1995, June). *Athletic identity as a predictor of zeteophobia among retired athletes.* Paper presented at the 12th Annual Conference on Counseling Athletes, Springfield, MA, USA.
• Athletic identity, adjustment to retirement, and anxiety associated with career decision making and exploration (i.e., zeteophobia) were assessed among a sample of former Australian athletes (see Grove, Lavallee, & Gordon, 1997). Results indicated that athletic identity correlated positively with psychosocial adjustment to retirement and zeteophobia, and negatively correlated with the amount of preretirement career planning. Discussion focuses on the relationship between athletic identity and the quality of adaptation to athletic retirement.

Lavallee, D., Gordon, S., & Grove, J. R. (1996). A profile of career beliefs among retired Australian athletes. *Australian Journal of Career Development, 5 (2),* 35–38.
• In this study, current career beliefs and perceptions of life skills learned in sport that are transferable to postathletic career occupations were examined. Results revealed several areas of career development that have particular relevance to elite athletes. Further analyses also demonstrated that the type of sport athletes participate in can have a significant impact on career development. Future research directions in the area are elaborated, and implications for professional practitioners are discussed.

Lavallee, D., Gordon, S., & Grove, J. R. (1997). Retirement from sport and the loss of athletic identity. *Journal of Personal and Interpersonal Loss, 2,* 129–147.

• This study examines how a sample of Australian athletes coped with severe emotional adjustment to career termination. After identifying 15 former elite athletes (11 female; 4 male) who experienced a distressful reaction to athletic retirement, the coping strategies used during the career transition process were examined qualitatively. Athletic identity at the time of retirement and each individual's present athletic identity were also assessed quantitatively. Results suggested that the process of confiding is a significant moderator of distress following career termination, along with changes in athletic identity. Suggestions are presented for future research on treatment strategies for distressful reactions to retirement from sport.

Lavallee, D., Grove, J. R., & Gordon, S. (1995). Account-making as a treatment model for distressful reactions to athletic retirement. In R. Vanfraechem-Raway & Y. Vanden Auweele (Eds.), *Proceedings of the 9th European Congress of Sport Psychology* (pp. 857–864). Brussels: European Federation of Sports Psychology.

• This paper presents a brief outline of a treatment model proposed by Grove, Lavallee, Gordon, and Harvey (1998) for athletes who have experienced severe emotional adjustment to career termination. A review of the empirical studies that have specifically examined distressful reactions to athletic retirement is provided, followed by a three-phase treatment program. This proposed intervention consists of identifying athletes who have experienced an unhealthy career transition, assessing whether or not these individuals have worked through their adjustment difficulties in a follow-up survey, and implementing a counseling-based intervention with the identified athletes who have yet to reach closure.

Lavallee, D., Grove, J. R., & Gordon, S. (1995, September). Coping with retirement from sport: The influence of athletic identity. In S. Hanrahan (Chair), *Coping processes in sport.* Symposium conducted at the annual meeting of the Australian Psychological Society, Perth.

• Self-reported use of coping strategies, athletic identity, and the perceived quality of adjustment to retirement were assessed in this study with retired Australian athletes (see Grove, Lavallee, & Gordon, 1997). Results indicated that acceptance, positive interpretation, planning, and active coping were the most frequently used coping strategies during the career transition process. Athletic identity at the time of retirement also exhibited significant relationships to coping processes and adjustment to career termination.

Lavallee, D., Grove, J. R., & Gordon, S. (1997). The causes of career termination from sport and their relationship to postretirement adjustment among

elite-amateur athletes in Australia. *The Australian Psychologist, 32,* 131–135.
• In this study, 48 former elite-amateur athletes in Australia supplied information about the primary reason for their retirement from sport and the degree of adjustment required. Comparisons between athletes who retired for voluntary and involuntary reasons indicated that involuntary career termination was associated with significantly greater emotional and social adjustment upon career termination. The individuals who experienced the greatest adjustment difficulty also perceived the least personal control over the reasons for retirement. Implications for professional and applied work are discussed.

Lavallee, D., Grove, J. R., Gordon, S., & Ford, I. W. (1998). The experience of loss in sport. In J. H. Harvey (Ed.), *Perspectives on loss: A sourcebook* (pp. 241–252) Philadelphia: Bruner/Mazel.
• The concept of loss as it applies to elite-level athletes in examined in this chapter, with a specific focus on symbolic losses experienced in competitive sport. Empirical and theoretical research that has been directed at exploring the losses associated with athletic injuries, performance slumps, and retirement from sport is reviewed. In the concluding section, it is proposed that athletic identity plays a central role in the experience of loss in sport.

Lerch, S. H. (1979). *Adjustment to early retirement: The case of professional baseball players.* Unpublished doctoral dissertation, Purdue University, IN, USA.
Lerch, S. H. (1981). The adjustment to retirement of professional baseball players. In S. L. Greendorfer & A. Yiannakis (Eds.), *Sociology of sport: Diverse perspectives* (pp. 138–148). West Point, NY: Leisure Press.
Lerch, S. H. (1982a). The life satisfaction of retired ballplayers. *Baseball Research Journal, 11,* 39–43.
• Survey data from 511 retired baseball players were examined for the purpose of developing a theoretical model explaining the variation in life satisfaction among retired athletes. Results suggested that life satisfaction was related to high levels of present income, positive preretirement attitudes, good health, and education. Moreover, the vast majority of respondents experienced little or no difficulty in the transition from sport. Policy implications for retiring baseball players and the baseball establishment are discussed.

Lerch, S. H. (1982b). *Athletic retirement as social death: An overview.* Paper presented at the annual meeting of the North American Society for the Sociology of Sport, Toronto, Canada.
Lerch, S. H. (1984a). Athlete retirement as social death: An overview. In

N. Theberge & P. Donnelly (Eds.), *Sport and the sociological imagination* (pp. 259–272). Fort Worth: Texas Christian University Press.
• The analogy of retirement from sport to death is developed using two perspectives prominent in the study of death and dying. The thanatological models of Glaser and Strauss (1965) and Kübler-Ross (1969) provide parallels between the social death of the athlete and the physically dying hospital patient. Shortcomings of this analogy are noted.

Lerch, S. H. (1984b). The adjustment of athletes to career ending injuries. *Arena Review, 8 (1),* 54–67.
• This discussion paper speculates on the adjustment outcomes of athletes forced to retire due to injuries producing severe disabilities. Four categories of disability are outlined: partial and temporary, complete and temporary, partial and permanent, and complete and permanent. The author hypothesizes that problems for severely disabled former athletes are particularly acute, but that these individuals may possess certain personal characteristics that may make their adjustment easier than that of their non-athletic counterparts.

Levy, M. A., & Burke, K. (1986a, October). *The life after sport center: A program proposal.* Paper presented at the annual meeting of the Association for the Advancement of Applied Sport Psychology, Jekyll Island, GA, USA.
Levy, M. A., & Burke, K. (1986b). The life after sport clinic: A program proposal. *Journal of Applied Research in Coaching and Athletics, 1,* 212–225.
• The goals and objectives of the Life After Sports Clinic (LASC) program for retired athletes are outlined. The manner in which interventions are assessed and analyzed is also discussed, including a means of evaluating the LASC. As described, the focus of the program is on assisting athletes in making informed career decisions.

Lide, W. E. (1981). Forced retirement among former professional football players with short-term careers. (Doctoral dissertation, The Ohio State University, 1994). *Dissertation Abstracts International, 42,* 600A.
Lide, W. E. (1986, October/November). *Forced retirement among former professional football players with short-term careers.* Paper presented at the annual meeting of the North American Society for the Sociology of Sport, Boston, USA.
Lide, W. E. (1987, October/November). *The successful former professional athlete vs. the less successful professional athlete.* Paper presented at the annual meeting of the North American Society for the Sociology of Sport, Las Vegas, USA.

• Career patterns, education level, and adjustment to retirement were qualitatively examined among 28 male former football players who were forced to retire after competing at the professional level from 1 to 4 years. Results revealed that successful former players had fewer adjustment problems than did less successful former players. Moreover, the majority of participants perceived that their present degree of success hinged on their present economic state, family situation, and status.

Martin, J. J. (1996). Transitions out of competitive sport for athletes with disabilities. *Therapeutic Recreation Journal, 30,* 128–136.

• This article discusses the career transition experience for athletes with disabilities who compete in competitive sport. The related research is discussed, and suggestions are provided for how therapeutic recreation specialists can assist athletes with disabilities with the career transition process. Research directions in the area are outlined.

Mayocchi, L., & Hanrahan, S. (1994, May). *Transferable skills and high-performance athletes: Research in progress.* Poster presented at the Australian Behaviour Modification Association Update, Sunshine Coast, QLD.

Mayocchi, L., & Hanrahan, S. (1995, July). *Transferable skills for career change: What do we really know?* Poster presented at the Australian Industrial and Organisational Psychology Conference, Sydney.

Mayocchi, L., & Hanrahan, S. J. (1997). *Adaptation to a post-athletic career: The role of transferable skills.* Belconnen, ACT: Australian Sports Commission.

• These papers outline which skills are potentially transferable from one occupation to another and examine which factors influence this process. The current research and practice in the area are reviewed, with an emphasis on the application of transferable skills in career assistance programs for athletes. Suggestions and populations for future research in this area are provided.

Mayocchi, L., & Hanrahan, S. (1996, September). *The effects of individual and work-environment factors on elite athletes' use of transferable skills in a nonsporting career.* Poster presented at the annual meeting of the Australian Psychological Society, Sydney.

• This study assesses the influence of several individual and work-related factors on the use of transferable skills in non-athletic careers among 242 elite-level athletes. A significant positive effect was found between job enthusiasm and the use of transferable skills. Moderating effects between the use of skills in sport and encouragement from supervisors, coworker support, quality of management, and self-efficacy were also identified. Implications for athletic career transition programs are discussed.

McLaughlin, P. (1981a). Retirement: Athlete's transition ignored by system. *Champion, 5 (2)*, 15–16.
McLaughlin, P. (1981b). Retirement: Experts suggest a new approach to quandary. *Champion, 5 (3)*, 14–15.
• This two-part series on retirement from high-performance sport reports anecdotal information obtained from informal interviews with elite athletes, as well as individuals working within the Canadian sport structure. Several individual experiences of adjustment difficulties occurring as a result of retirement are detailed. The need for sport retirement services from an organizational perspective is also discussed.

McInally, L., Cavin-Stice, J., & Knoth, R. L. (1991, August). *Life after football: Retirement adjustment for the professional players.* Paper presented at the annual meeting of the Western Psychological Association, San Francisco, USA.
McInally, L., Cavin-Stice, J., & Knoth, R. L. (1992, August). *Adjustment following retirement from professional football.* Paper presented at the annual meeting of the American Psychological Association, Washington DC.
• These papers present the results of a study conducted with 367 retired professional male football players randomly selected from the *National Football League Alumni Directory.* The survey focused on educational and career aspiration, sources of stress prior to and during the sporting career, circumstances surrounding career termination, and adjustment to athletic retirement. Results indicated that the majority of respondents required some adjustment during their career transition, but those who had strong familial support and engaged in preretirement preparation for a subsequent occupation experienced the least adjustment difficulties.

McKnight, J. N. (1995, October). *The transition experience of an ex-professional football player.* Paper presented at the annual conference of the Association for the Advancement of Applied Sport Psychology, New Orleans, USA.
• This case study examines the career transition experience of a retired professional football player. Results of three in-depth interviews revealed the predominant reasons for career termination, initial reactions to retirement, and several factors related to the quality of adjustment.

McPherson, B. D. (1977, May). *The occupational and psychological adjust-*

ment of former professional athletes. Paper presented at the annual meeting of the American College of Sports Medicine, Chicago.

McPherson, B. D. (1978). Former professional athletes' adjustment to retirement. *Physician and Sports Medicine, 6,* 52–59.

McPherson, B. D. (1980). Retirement from professional sport: The process and problems of occupational and psychological adjustment. *Sociological Symposium, 30,* 126–143.

• These articles examine the following four processes that may account for the social situation of former athletes: socialization into the career, career patterns and contingencies, the decision-making process concerning retirement, and adjustment to retirement as well as the transition to a second career.

Menkehorst, G. A. B. M., & van den Berg, F. J. (1997). Retirement from high-level competition: A new start. In R. Lidor & M. Bar-Eli (Eds.), *Proceedings of the IX World Congress on Sport Psychology* (pp. 487–489). Netanya, Israel: International Society of Sport Psychology.

• The findings reported in this paper are based on a large-scale study examining the career transition experiences of Dutch elite athletes. Questionnaires focusing on adjustment to retirement and coping with stress were administered to 77 former athletes from a variety of sports, and results suggested a number of specific areas that required adjustment (e.g., psychological, financial, occupational, and social adjustment). Further analyses revealed that problem-oriented, cognition-changing, and emotion-regulating coping strategies were employed throughout the career transition process and that problem-oriented coping had the most positive effect on reducing psychological adjustment.

Messner, M. (1985). The changing meaning of male identity in the lifecourse of the athlete. *Arena Review, 9 (2),* 31–60.

Messner, M. A, (1992). *Power at play: Sport and the problem of masculinity* (pp. 108–128). Boston: Beacon Press.

• This article and book (chapters 6 and 7) discuss disengagement from the athletic career and life after sport. Issues of class differences, public success, and social support are examined in terms of an athlete's identity during the career transition process.

Mihovilovic, M. (1968). The status of former sportsmen. *International Review of Sport Sociology, 3,* 73–93.

Mihovilovic, M. O. (1974). *Vrhunski sportasi: Bioloski, phiholoski, socioloski, ekonomski i sportski element iz zivota I rada vrhunskih sportasa jugoslavije.* [Top sportsmen: Biological, psychological, social, economic, and sports elements from the life and work of Yugoslav top sportsmen]. Zagreb, Yugoslavia: Institute of Social Research.

• In one of the first empirical attempts to analyze retirement from sport, a descriptive survey was conducted with 44 former male Yugoslavian soccer players. Results focus on some of the factors involved in the career termination experience, including the reasons for retirement, social support networks, and mechanisms for staying involved in sport. Conclusion discusses methods to facilitate the career transition process.

Morgan, W. P. (1986, September). *Athletes and nonathletes in later life.* Paper presented at the 23rd World Congress of Sports Medicine, Brisbane, Australia.

• In this study, former athletes and nonathletes were administered the Minnesota Multiphasic Personality Inventory (MMPI; Hathaway & McKinley, 1967) at the ages of 18 and 38. Whereas the focus of this paper is on the comparison of the two groups, the results suggest that the retired athletes possessed more desirable mental health patterns in later years. Thus, this study may be of interest to researchers conducting longitudinal assessments of former elite-level athletes.

Morris, T., & Anderson, D. (1994a, September). *Career education, perceived performance and mood state in elite athletes.* Paper presented at the annual meeting of the Australian Psychological Society, Wollongong.

Morris, T., & Anderson, D. (1994b, October). *Career education, perceived performance and mood state in elite athletes.* Paper presented at the annual conference of the Association for the Advancement of Applied Sport Psychology, Lake Tahoe, NV, USA.

• These papers present the results of a study conducted with a sample of elite athletes in Australia. A single-case design was employed to examine the impact of the Australian Athlete Career and Education (ACE) Program on athletic performance and rating on the Profile of Mood States (POMS; McNair, Lorr, & Droppleman, 1971) over the course of one year. Results suggested that there was evidence of stability in perceived performance and a positive impact on mood states.

Munroe, K. J., & Albinson, J. G. (1996). *Athletes' reactions immediately after and four months following involuntary disengagement at the varsity level.* Paper presented at the Joint Conference of the North American Society for the Psychology of Sport and Physical Activity and the Canadian Society for Psychomotor Learning and Sport Psychology, Ontario, Canada.

• The experiences of 12 female athletes following deselection from varsity teams were examined in this paper. Interviews were conducted with each participant within one week of involuntary disengagement, as well as 4 months later. Psychological affect, emotions, and coping strategies were assessed in terms of the conceptual model of career termination proposed by Taylor and Ogilvie (1994).

Murphy, S. M. (1995). Transition in competitive sport: Maximizing individual potential. In S. M. Murphy (Ed.), *Sport psychology interventions* (pp. 331–346). Champaign, IL: Human Kinetics.

• This chapter focuses on how helping professionals can assist athletes in making optimal transitions out of competitive sport. The motivation of elite athletes, nature of career transitions, and factors related to the transition process are reviewed prior to outlining specific strategies for assisting athletes. Career planning assistance and individual counseling are suggested as the most effective interventions.

Ogilvie, B. C. (1983). When a dream dies. *Women's Sport, 5 (12),* 68.

Ogilvie, B. C. (1987). Counseling for sports career termination. In J. R. May & M. J. Asken (Eds.), *Sport psychology: The psychological health of the athlete* (pp. 213–230). New York: PMA.

Ogilvie, B. C. (1989, April). *Traumatic effects of sports career termination.* Paper presented at the Western Psychological Association/Rocky Mountain Psychological Association Joint Annual Convention, Reno, NV, USA.

• The psychosocial processes associated with retirement from sport are outlined with a focus on the common characteristics of athletic retirement and the consequences of forced career termination. Illustrative case studies are utilized to describe the special concerns of elite athletes.

Ogilvie, B. C., & Howe, M. (1982a). Career crisis in sport. In T. Orlick, J. Y. Partington, & J. H. Salmela (Eds.), *Proceedings of the 5th World Congress of Sport Psychology* (pp. 176–183). Ottawa: Coaching Association of Canada.

Ogilvie, B. C., & Howe, M. (1982b). Career crisis in sport. *Sports Science Periodical on Research and Technology in Sport, November,* 1–6.

Ogilvie, B. C., & Howe, M. (1986). The trauma of termination from athletics. In J. M. Williams (Ed.), *Applied sport psychology* (pp. 365–382). Palo Alto, CA: Mayfield.

• These articles and book chapter discuss the factors that are related to termination from elite-level sport. In particular, the authors describe in detail how the causes of retirement, identity issues, social support, and socioeconomic status postretirement have an impact on the quality of adjustment to career termination. Specific recommendations for sport psychological guidance are provided, as are illustrative case studies.

Ogilvie, B. C., & Taylor, J. (1993a). Career termination issues among elite athletes. In R. N. Singer, M. Murphey, & L. K. Tennant (Eds.), *Handbook of research on sport psychology* (pp. 761–775). New York: Macmillan.

Ogilvie, B. C., & Taylor, J. (1993b). Career termination in sports: When the dream dies. In J. M. Williams (Ed.), *Applied sport psychology: Personal growth to peak performance* (2nd ed., pp. 356–365). Mountain View, CA: Mayfield.

• These highly recommended chapters provide a comprehensive overview of the ending of athletes' sporting careers by reviewing historical, conceptual, and theoretical perspectives. The authors outline the causes for career termination and factors contributing to the quality of adjustment to the career end. Recommendations for prevention and guidance are provided, as well as suggestions for further research.

Orlick, T., & Werthner, P. (1987). *Athletes in transition*. Toronto: Olympic Athlete Career Centre.

• The information presented in this booklet is designed to educate current and transitional athletes about the experience of retirement. Material focuses on what feelings and thoughts to expect at the time of retirement, as well as on recommendations for athletes (competing and transitional) on making a career transition.

Orlick, T., & Werthner, P. (1992). *New beginnings: Transitions from high performance sport workbook*. Toronto: Olympic Athlete Career Centre.

• This workbook was developed in conjunction with a transition seminar provided to national teams by the Canadian Olympic Association. The objective of this resource booklet is to assist current and transitional athletes in the identification of strengths, skills, and interests for the purpose of defining new directions and options for a second career.

Parker, K. B. (1994). "Has-beens" and "wanna-bes": Transition experiences of former major college football players. *The Sport Psychologist, 8,* 287–304.

• The aim of this study was to gain insight into seven former college football players' experiences with career transition. Utilizing phenomenological interview techniques, each participant was asked to discuss what life has been like since playing in his last collegiate football game. Results showed that players' level of enjoyment with the game decreased when transferring from high school to the collegiate level.

Parker, K. B., DeSensi, J., & Beitel, P. A. (1992, October/November). *Transitions from intercollegiate sport: A qualitative approach.* Paper presented at the annual conference of the Association for the Advancement of Applied Sport Psychology, Colorado Springs, USA.
• Four former collegiate athletes (one female, team sport; one female, individual sport; one male, team sport; one male, individual sport) participated in this assessment of the perceptions and experiences of individuals as they leave competitive sport. Qualitative interviews described sport career termination as a process, identified the importance of preretirement planning, and outlined the pressures associated with athletic retirement.

Pearson, R. E., & Petitpas, A. J. (1990). Transitions of athletes: Developmental and preventive perspectives. *Journal of Counseling and Development, 69,* 7–10.
• This article describes the developmental patterns and transitions commonly experienced by athletes. The reasons for cessation from active participation in sport are outlined, including not making the team, athletic injuries, and athletic retirement. The factors that contribute to transition-related stress, as well as barriers to successful transitions, are also delineated. The article concludes with a description of prevention-oriented interventions for athlete.

Perna, F. M. (1991). Life satisfaction, psychological development and perceived mentoring at career termination of collegiate male athletes (Doctoral dissertation, Boston University). *Dissertation Abstracts International, 52,* 1694A.

Perna, F. (1992, October/November). *An examination of injury and post-athletic career adjustment.* Paper presented at the annual conference of the Association for the Advancement of Applied Sport Psychology, Colorado Springs, USA.

Perna, F. M., Zaichkowsky, L., & Bockner, G. (1996). The association of mentoring with psychosocial development among male athletes at termination of college career. *Journal of Applied Sport Psychology, 8,* 76–88.
• In this comparative study, perceptions of the incidence and impact of mentoring upon life satisfaction and psychosocial development were assessed among 43 male collegiate athletes and 33 nonathletes 2 weeks prior to graduation. Results indicated that mentoring occurs with similar frequency among athletes and nonathletes, and that no significant between-group differences existed with regard to occupational plan. In addition, an analysis of athletes who were injured suggested that perhaps an optimal level of adversity (e.g., slight injuries as compared to no injuries and severe injuries) may be growth promoting in terms of post athletic career transitions. Finally, mentoring was found to be a useful model from which to assess the coach-athlete relationship.

Petitpas, A. J., Brewer, B. W., & Van Raalte, J. L. (1996). Transitions of the student-athlete: Theoretical, empirical, and practical perspectives. In E. F. Etzel, A. P. Ferrante, & Pinkney, J. W. (Eds.), *Counseling college student-athletes: Issues and interventions* (2nd ed., pp. 137–156). Morgantown, WV: Fitness Information Technology.

• This chapter examines the major transitions experienced by student-athletes from both theoretical and empirical perspectives. Developmental models (e.g., Danish, Petitpas, & Hale, 1993; Schlossberg, 1981) are suggested as useful frameworks for understanding the transitions of this population, and the extant research on intercollegiate athlete adjustment to transition is reviewed. A conceptual framework for planning transition-specific counseling services for athletes is also presented by reviewing three existing intervention programs.

Petitpas, A., Champagne, D., Chartrand, J., Danish, S., & Murphy, S. (1997). *Athlete's guide to career planning: Keys to success from the playing field to professional life*. Champaign, IL: Human Kinetics.

• This self-help book provides athletes with a guide to planning their careers both during and after their participation in sport. Transitions that high school, collegiate, and professional athletes often face are discussed, with a focus on coping skills, social support, and career development. The exploration, planning, and acquisition of a career is also reviewed in depth and includes several job search strategies (e.g., résumé writing, interviewing techniques) and exploratory exercises. A comprehensive list of sport-related careers and career resources is provided.

Petitpas, A., Danish, S., McKelvain, R., & Murphy, S. (1990a). *A career assistance program for elite athletes*. Paper presented at the annual conference of the Association for the Advancement of Applied Sport Psychology, San Antonio, TX, USA.

Petitpas, A., Danish, S., McKelvain, R., & Murphy, S. (1990b). A career assistance program for elite athletes. *Journal of Counseling and Development, 70*, 383–386.

• This article outlines the development of the Career Assistance Program for Athletes (CAPA), an initiative of the United States Olympic Committee to assist Olympic-level athletes in coping with the transition out of active participation in competitive sport. A model of lifespan development is employed to describe the formulation of the program, followed by an evaluation of a CAPA workshop conducted with 142 athletes. Implications for counselors working with athletes are discussed.

Redmond, J. (1994). *Retirement experiences of former elite female netball players.* Unpublished master's thesis, Edith Cowan University, Perth, Western Australia.
• This study examined the career termination experiences among a sample of female netball players in Australia. Results of a three-stage interview process revealed that retirement was an individual experience, a transition that included a phase of assimilation, and a situation where athletic identity remained upon career termination. Schlossberg's (1984) model of transition is discussed, and recommendations from the participants are provided.

Reynolds, M. J. (1981). The effects of sports retirement on the job satisfaction of the former football player. In S. L. Greendorfer & A. Yiannakis (Eds.), *Sociology of sport: Diverse perspectives* (pp. 127–137). West Point, NY: Leisure Press.
• The purpose of this paper was to present some of the preliminary analyses of a research project on the development of a theoretical model of athletic retirement. Questionnaires measuring the variables of self-esteem, job congruency and job satisfaction were returned by a sample of 596 former professional football players and provided only partial confirmation of the research model.

Rosenberg, E. (1978). *Measures, correlates, and models of major league baseball playing careers.* Unpublished doctoral dissertation, University of Southern California, USA.
• This study discusses baseball as an occupation by evaluating past work in the area and examining new modes of description, explanation, and prediction of length of playing career professional sport. Hypotheses tested include patterns of playing attrition and differences in length of playing career distribution by cohort, race, position, and player competence. Findings revealed that major league playing career attrition rates resemble natural mortality rates and that controlling for player competence nullifies the relationship between race and career length. The analysis includes consideration of alternative postplaying career opportunity structures.

Rosenberg, E. (1980). Social disorganizational aspects of professional sports careers. *Journal of Sport and Social Issues, 4,* 14–25.
• The career of the professional team athlete is discussed in the context of social disorganization (i.e., defined as either structure or process, personal or institutional). Conditions leading to social disorganization are delineated, as

are the locations and type of social disorganization likely to be encountered by the athlete. Issues such as institutionalized racial discrimination, violence, stigma of failure, and athletic retirement are examined as potential sources of disorganization. Careers in sport are compared to nonsport careers, and four disorganizational elements unique to sport careers are elaborated (viz., superfluity of formal education, accelerated social mobility, inevitability of a second career, and nature of athletic retirement).

Rosenberg, E. (1981a). Gerontological theory and athletic retirement. In S. L. Greendorfer & A. Yiannakis (Eds.), *Sociology of sport: Diverse perspective* (pp. 119–126). West Point, NY: Leisure Press.

• The appropriateness of social gerontology theory as an explanatory framework for examining the antecedents and consequences of athletic retirement is discussed. A review of the major theoretical approaches in social gerontology reveals that activity, subculture, continuity, social breakdown/reconstruction, and exchange theories have relevance for athletic retirement. Social breakdown/reconstruction and exchange theories are proposed to be the most salient.

Rosenberg, E. (1981b). *Professional athletic retirement: Bringing theory and research together.* Paper presented at the 1st Regional Symposium of the International Committee for the Sociology of Sport, Vancouver, Canada.

Rosenberg, E. (1981c). *Professional athletic retirement.* Paper presented at the annual meeting of the Pacific Sociological Association, Portland, Oregon.

Rosenberg, E. (1981d). Professional athletic retirement. *Arena Review, 5,* 1–11.

• In an early examination of athletic transition, these papers assess the immediate postcedent of retirement (i.e., the first postplaying job), as it was hypothesized that any adjustment problems experienced by an athlete will be most severe at the precise moment of transition. Data provided by 21 of 24 professional baseball teams in North America on former players' first jobs after leaving professional sport (each member of the cohort first entered the major league between 1950 and 1954) revealed that nearly two thirds (65.7%) of the sample remained in baseball in some capacity. These results are limited, however, because the teams had information for only 102 of the 400 cohort members, a finding that is suggested to be the most meaningful in the study.

Rosenberg, E. (1982, November). *Athletic retirement as social death: Concepts and perspectives.* Paper presented at the annual meeting of the North American Society for the Sociology of Sport, Toronto, Canada.

Rosenberg, E. (1984). Athletic retirement as social death: Concepts and perspectives. In N. Theberge & P. Donnelly (Eds.), *Sport and the sociological imagination* (pp. 245–258). Fort Worth: Texas Christian University Press.

• These papers provide a discussion of the relevance of the concept of social death as a model for understanding retirement from sport. The analytical perspective taken is that the application of concepts and conceptual frameworks from thanatology may be beneficially applied to an understanding of the psychodynamics of athletic transition.

Salazar, M. J. (1992). Retirement adjustment of professional athletes (Doctoral dissertation, Widener University, 1991). *Dissertation Abstracts International, 53,* 1076B.

• Employing Erikson's (1963) theory of psychosocial development, this study outlines the risks associated with athletes who base their identity on their participation and performance in sport. An analysis of Schlossberg's (1981) model of human adaptation to transition is presented. Recommendations are also made for changes at youth, collegiate, and professional levels of sport.

Salmela, J. H. (1994). Phases and transitions across sport careers. In D. Hackfort (Ed.), *Psycho-social issues and interventions in elite sport* (pp. 11–28). Frankfort: Lang.

• In this chapter, the construct of transition is presented from a developmental perspective. The nature of how elite athletes make the transitions across their sport careers and evolve through its various phases, from their beginnings in play through to the retirement process is addressed. The transitions that occur within an individual's career as the athlete progresses from novice to master are defined, as are the relative and changing roles of their coaches and families.

Schaefer, U. (1992). *Retirement and adjustment process of top level athletes.* Unpublished doctoral dissertation, Hungarian University for Physical Education and Sport.

• This study surveyed 296 elite Hungarian athletes (who had ended their careers between 1952 and 1989) in terms of their adjustment to athletic career termination. The retirement period was examined in terms of the relationship between casual attribution factors and selected adjustment processes. Gerontological theories of aging are employed to explain the results.

Schilling, G. (1995). Career transitions of athletes: What has to be done? In R. Vanfraechem-Raway & Y. Vanden Auweele (Eds.), *Proceedings of the 9th*

European Congress of Sport Psychology (pp. 865–866). Brussels: European Federation of Sports Psychology.

• This paper presents three recommendations for what has to be done in the area of career transition in sport. First, due to the fact that career termination is an inevitability, it is suggested that athletes prepare for a professional career outside of sport. Second, it is recommended that further research be conducted with athletes in the midst of a transition. Last, it is suggested that elite athletes work with their governing organizations in planning for their retirement.

Schmid, J., & Schilling, G. (1997). Self-identity and adjustment to the transition out of sports. In R. Lidor & M. Bar-Eli (Eds.), *Proceedings of the IX World Congress on Sport Psychology* (pp. 608–610). Netanya, Israel: International Society of Sport Psychology.

• In this study, 135 physical education students from Switzerland were assessed in terms of their athletic identity, commitment to sports, social support, extent to which they engaged in career exploration, potential manifestations associated with a career transition out of sport, and self-reported level of athletic performance. Results suggested that individuals experience greater adjustment difficulties to the extent that they identify with and commit to their sport. In addition, highly significant correlations were found among athletic performance, athletic identity, and commitment to sports. Discussion focuses on possible prevention of psychosocial adjustment difficulties associated with athletic career termination.

Schwendener-Holt, M. J. (1995). The process of sport retirement: A longitudinal study of college athletes (Doctoral dissertation, Southern Illinois University, 1994). *Dissertation Abstracts International, 56,* 4037B.

• This longitudinal study examined the process of athletic retirement among 22 collegiate swimmer and divers. Each participant was interviewed at the middle and end of their final sport season, as well as 3 months after the season. The results, which are discussed in relation to gerontological retirement theories, suggest that athletic career termination is a gradual and anticipated process.

Shaffer, K. A. (1992). Identity, self-esteem, and self-concept upon retirement from elite level sport (Master's thesis, University of Alberta, 1990). *Masters Abstracts, 30,* 246.

• Comparisons were made between samples of competitive and retired athletes in this study. Results showed that former athletes scored higher on measures of identity and self-esteem, but that these concepts were not dependent on whether the retired athletes remained involved in sport (e.g., as a coach) after career termination. Self-reports also indicated that the retired athletes, on average, were happier at the time of the interview than when they were competing in sport.

Shahnasarian, M. (1992). Career development after professional football. *Journal of Career Development, 18,* 299–304.

• The primary purpose of this paper is to outline career development issues encountered by former professional football players in order to better facilitate individual transitions. The mission statement of the Sports, Careers, Options, Research, and Education (SCORE) Foundation is also discussed.

Sheedy, J. (1990). Retirement from sport. *Sport Health, 8,* 35–36.

• This article outlines a number of career termination issues among amateur and professional athletes, including the predominant reasons for retirement and changes that an athlete can expect to encounter upon career termination. Suggestions for professionals who may be in a position to assist athletes in transition are also presented.

Silverstone, A., & Frederick, C. M. (1993). *Transitions: Making the move from high school to college athletics.* Paper presented at the annual conference of the Association of the Advancement of Applied Sport Psychology, Montreal, Canada.

• Twenty first-year college athletes were surveyed in terms of their transition from high school to collegiate sport. Results of in-depth interviews suggested that college athletes are subject to several stressors that their nonathlete counterparts do not experience. Suggestions for interventions are provided.

Sinclair, D. A. (1990a). *The dynamics of transition from high performance sport.* Unpublished doctoral dissertation, University of Ottawa, Canada.

• The purpose of this study was to examine and explore the transition experiences of Canada's high-performance athletes within Charner and Schlossberg's (1986) theoretical framework to determine the predisposing factors and effects of the transition process. Questionnaire data from 199 retired high-performance athletes (100 female; 99 male) suggested that adjustment to retirement may not be as distressing or problematic for as many national team athletes as previously thought. Charner and Schlossberg's transitional framework received support in terms of overall fit.

Sinclair, D. A. (1990b). Retirement from sport. *National coaching certification program.* Ottawa: Coaching Association of Canada.

• This section of the coaching theory manual discusses the potential difficulties encountered by transitional athletes, outlines the factors associated with a successful transition, and provides coaches with strategies for assisting athletes with the retirement process while the athletes are still competing as well as when they retire.

Sinclair, D. A., & Orlick, T. (1993). Positive transitions from high-performance sport. *The Sport Psychologist, 7,* 138–150.
• Retired high-performance athletes completed the Athlete Retirement Questionnaire developed for this study (see Sinclair, 1990a). Analysis showed that those athletes who adjusted smoothly tended to retire after they achieved their sport-related goals. In addition, athletes who had a more difficult transition tended to feel incompetent outside of sport and to feel that keeping busy was not an effective coping strategy. Practical implications are presented.

Sinclair, D. A., & Orlick, T. (1994). The effects of transition on high performance sport. In D. Hackfort (Ed.), *Psycho-social issues and interventions in elite sports* (pp. 29–55). Frankfurt: Lang.
• This overview article reviews much of the sport transition literature, presents contemporary research findings related to the transitional athlete including recommendations for athletes in transition, and offers strategies for structural and organizational change within the elite sport system that may improve the transition experience of the individual.

Stambulova, N. B. (1993). Two ways of sport career psychological description. In S. Serpa, J. Alves, V. Ferreira, & A. Paula-Brito (Eds.), *Proceedings of the VIII World Congress of Sport Psychology.* Lisbon: International Society of Sport Psychology.
• This paper discusses two theoretical models to describe the development of the sports career. The synthetic model is a based upon the framework that consists of four concepts (viz., space, time, information, and energy) and an integrative component (viz., the sport career). The objective characteristics of the sport career, which are to be complemented with athletes' subjective perceptions of their sport career, include the following: level of satisfaction and success, length and age limits, level of generalization-specialization, level of athletic performances, and costs of the sport career (e.g., time, energy, money, health). The analytic model is based upon the evolution of a sport career in different (predictable) transition phases (each of which may lead to the occurrence of a crisis). The seven following transitions can be identified with this model: start of the sport specialization, transition toward a level of intensive

training, transition from mass sport to amateur sport, transition from junior to adult sport, transition from amateur to professional sport, transition from actively performing toward the end of the sport career, and end of the sport career.

Stambulova, N. B. (1994). Developmental sports career investigations in Russia: A post-perestroika analysis. *The Sport Psychologist, 8,* 221–237.
• This article presents an overview of psychological aspects related to the sports career of Russian athletes before and during the perestroika. The closed nature of the country, lack of information available to sport psychologists, and influence of the centralized communistic government on the development of the sports sciences were identified to be of significant influence on athletes' sports career. However, during and after the perestroika, Russian sport psychologists were able to exchange more freely information with other colleagues, which gave a new impulse to the development of sport psychology in Russia. Theoretical models, including a synthetic and analytic model of the development of the sports career, which came forth from this new impulse, are presented (see Stambulova, 1993).

Stambulova, N. B. (1995a). Sports career satisfaction of Russian athletes. In R. Vanfraechem-Raway & Y. Vanden Auweele (Eds.), *Proceedings of the 9th European Congress of Sport Psychology* (pp. 526–532). Brussels: European Federation of Sports Psychology.
• This paper presents the results of a study using the synthetic model to describe the development of the sports career (see Stambulova, 1993) in which 206 Russian athletes (121 female; 85 male) from different sports were asked to assess their level of satisfaction with the development of their sport career. Results revealed that three groups could be identified, namely, those who were very satisfied (34%), who were not very satisfied (49%), and those who were not satisfied (17%) with the way in which their sport career had developed. The level of satisfaction with the sport career was found to depend upon the following factors: level of correspondence between goals and results, costs of the sport career, level of social recognition, level of generalization-specialization, premature ending of the sport career, and gender.

Stambulova, N. B. (1995b). Career transitions of Russian athletes. In R. Vanfraechem-Raway & Y. Vanden Auweele (Eds.), *Proceedings of the 9th European Congress of Sport Psychology* (pp. 867–873). Brussels: European Federation of Sports Psychology.

Stambulova, N. B. (1997a). Sports career psychological models and its applications. In R. Lidor & M. Bar-Eli (Eds.), *Proceedings of the IX World Congress of Sport Psychology* (pp. 655–657). Netanya, Israel: International Society of Sport Psychology.

Stambulova, N. B. (1997b). Transitional period of Russian athletes following sports career termination. In R. Lidor & M. Bar-Eli (Eds.), *Proceedings of the IX World Congress of Sport Psychology* (pp. 658–660). Netanya, Israel: International Society of Sport Psychology.

• These papers present the results of a three-stage study using the analytic model to describe the sport career (see Stambulova, 1993). Initially, a total of seven transitions occurring during the sport career were identified from written essays by 402 student-athletes from Russia. In the second stage, 90 Russian athletes (47 female; 43 male) were invited to agree or disagree as to whether they had experienced these seven transitions during their careers in sport. Finally, 95 former elite-level athletes (63 females; 32 males) from Russia completed a questionnaire related specifically to their retirement from sport.

Stark, E. (1986). Life after sports. *Psychology Today, 19 (1),* 57.

• This article describes the Professional Athletes Career Enterprises (PACE), an organization founded by Steve Garvey, the former professional baseball player. As outlined, the PACE center for career development provides career counseling for active athletes and a vocational placement service for retired athletes.

Stronach, A. (1993). Life after sport: Retirement from elite level sport. *The New Zealand Coach, 2,* 10–11.

• This article describes retirement from elite-level sport in terms of the coach's role in the career transition process. The issues an athlete in transition may face are outlined, and the responsibilities for both the retiring athlete and coach are discussed. An emphasis is placed on a balanced life during the competitive years.

Svoboda, B., & Vanek, M. (1982). Retirement from high level competition. In T. Orlick, J. T. Partington, & J. H. Salmela (Eds.), *Proceedings of the 5th World Congress of Sport Psychology* (pp. 166–175). Ottawa: Coaching Association of Canada.

• This paper reports the findings from a study conducted with 163 former Czechoslovakian Olympic athletes (30 female; 133 male). A number of factors contributing to the overall quality of adjustment to retirement were assessed, including the reasons for retirement and coping strategies. Coaches' views on the career transition process of athletes are also provided.

Swain, D. A. (1990). *The experience of withdrawing from professional sport.* Unpublished doctoral dissertation, University of British Columbia, Canada.

Swain, D. A. (1991). Withdrawal from sport and Schlossberg's model of transitions. *Sociology of Sport Journal, 8,* 152–160.

• In-depth interviews were used to describe the career experiences of 10 athletes who had voluntarily withdrawn from the sports of hockey, horse racing, football, and racquetball. The findings indicated that withdrawal from sport was a process rather than an event. The study supports and extends a model proposed by Schlossberg (1984) that considers the individual's subjective perception of the transition experience.

Tate, G. F. (1993). *The effects of the transformation in the Olympic Games on the athletic retirement transition process: American Olympians and retired National Football League athletes.* Unpublished doctoral dissertation, Temple University, Philadelphia, USA.

• This study assesses 599 retired athletes who competed in the Olympics between 1948 and 1988 in terms of their participation in sport, career termination, and long-term, postathletic retirement. Results indicated significant differences in family relationship, job satisfaction, financial satisfaction, and overall life satisfaction. In addition, the 1980–1988 Olympians recorded statistically higher levels of postathletic career uncertainty when compared to the 1948–1956 Olympians. Finally, when these athletes were compared to a sample of retired professional football players, there were no significant differences found in the quality of family relations, health, and life satisfaction.

Taylor, J., & Ogilvie, B. C. (1994). A conceptual model of adaptation to retirement among athletes. *Journal of Applied Sport Psychology, 6,* 1–20.

Taylor, J., & Ogilvie, B. C. (1998). Career transition among elite athletes: Is there life after sports? In J. M. Williams (Ed.), *Applied sport psychology: Personal growth to peak performance* (3rd ed., pp. 429–444). Mountain View, CA: Mayfield.

• This article and book chapter provide a comprehensive overview of the career termination literature by presenting a conceptual framework for the athletic retirement process. By emphasizing the career end as a transition, this domain-specific model focuses on the causal factors that initiate the retirement process, developmental factors related to retirement adaptation, coping resources that affect the responses to retirement, quality of adjustment to retirement, and intervention issues.

Thomas, C. E., & Ermler, K. L. (1986, June). *Life after competition: Moral obligations of the athletic establishment.* Paper presented at the 10th Session of the United States Olympic Academy, Colorado Springs.

Thomas, C. E., & Ermler, K. L. (1988). Institutional obligations in the athletic retirement process. *Quest, 40,* 137–150.

• The focus of this philosophical paper is on the responsibility of sport organizations to assist amateur athletes during the career transition process. A rationale is outlined by discussing the issues of autonomy, beneficence, and nonmaleficence as they relate to athletes in transition. Methods for meeting the moral obligations of the athletic establishment are described.

United States Olympic Committee (1988). *Career assessment program for athletes: 1988–1989 seminar workbook.* Colorado Springs: Author.

• The Career Assistance Program for Athletes (CAPA) developed this workbook to assist athletes in the career transition process. Agendas are provided for both young and older athletes, with group seminar exercises focusing on self-exploration, career exploration, and career implementation.

United States Olympic Committee (1993). *Positioning yourself for success: An employment counseling handbook for athletes.* Colorado Springs: Author.

• This handbook was developed by the United States Olympic Committee to assist athletes in preparing for postathletic careers. Information and exercises are provided on personal values, transferable skills, and occupational interests. Job search strategies and tools and a resource list are also included.

Vamplew, W. (1984). Close of play: Career termination in English professional sport. *Canadian Journal of History of Sport, 15,* 64–79.

• The causes of career termination, career length, and postretirement adjustment issues were assessed among English professional athletes in the sports of horse racing, football, soccer, and cricket for the years of 1870 to 1914. Analysis of archival data revealed that the main causes of career cessation were injury, misbehavior, breaking club rules, and criticism of superiors. Results also suggested that only a few athletes remained in sport as coaches.

Van-Oosten, M. (1985). After the thrill is gone. *Champion, 9,* 16–21.

• This anecdotal article highlights the potential stress associated with the transition from high-performance sport, especially for unprepared athletes. The rationale for establishing Canada's Olympic Athlete Career Centre as a program to assist retiring athletes is briefly discussed.

Washington, A. M. (1981). *Adjustment to retirement among women professional golfers with respect to two selected social theories of aging.* Unpublished master's thesis, University of North Carolina, Greensboro, USA.

Washington, A. M. (1984). *Consideration of selected social theories of aging as evidenced by patterns of adjustment to retirement among professional football players.* Unpublished doctoral dissertation, University of North Carolina, Greensboro, USA.
 • Three social theories of aging (viz., disengagement theory, identity crisis theory, and activity theory) were employed to examine the process of adjustment to retirement among sample of former professional golfers and football players. Quantitative and qualitative data were collected on such variables as self-esteem, life satisfaction, and morale; and support was found for activity theory.

Webb, W. M., Nasco, S. A., Riley, S., & Headrick, B. (1998). Athlete identity and reactions to retirement from sports. *Journal of Sport Behavior, 21,* 338–362.
 • This study assesses the relationships among the reasons for retirement, athletic identity, psychological process variables (viz., self-esteem and perception of control), and career termination outcome variables (viz., overall life satisfaction, uncertainty regarding postretirement future, and quality of adjustment to retirement) with a sample of 92 high school, collegiate, and professional athletes across 21 sports. Results of correlational analyses revealed that athletic identity was strongly related to the difficulties specific to the retirement event, but that these difficulties were not related to life satisfaction. The reasons for career termination were also found to have a significant effect on the quality of adjustment and uncertainty about the future.

Weinberg, S. K., & Arond, H., (1952). The occupational culture of the boxer. *The American Journal of Sociology, 57,* 460–469.
Weinberg, S. K., & Arond, H., (1969). The occupational culture of the boxer. In J. W. Loy and G. S. Kenyon (Eds.), *Sport, culture, and society.* New York: Macmillan.
 • This study on the postretirement careers of 95 boxers examines the experiences of former champions and leading contenders. Results revealed that retirement brought on emotional problems due to efforts to find and maintain alternate employment and to dramatic decreases in status, prestige, and income. Most of the problems appeared to be associated with injuries, previous dependence on managers, and exorbitant spending habits continuing from active boxing days.

Werthner, P., & Orlick, T. (1982). Transitions from sport: Coping with the end. In T. Orlick, J. Partington, & J. Salmela (Eds.), *Proceedings of the 5th World Congress of Sport Psychology* (pp. 176–183). Ottawa: Coaching Association of Canada.
  • This article suggests that retirement from high-level sport should be seen in terms of a loss of an intense, important relationship. The authors argue that athletes should be taught to cope with this loss so they can prepare for their retirement. In addition, it is suggested that athletes should learn to distinguish themselves as people rather than solely as athletes, whereas the period after their career end should be viewed as an opportunity to develop skills.

Werthner, P. (1985). *Retirement experiences of elite Canadian athletes.* Unpublished master's thesis, University of Ottawa, Canada.

Werthner, P., & Orlick, T. (1986). Retirement experiences of successful Olympic athletes. *International Journal of Sport Psychology, 17,* 337–363.
  • Using the Elite Athlete Retirement Interview Schedule, 28 Canadian Olympic amateur-level athletes who had terminated their sport career were interviewed. Three categories could be identified, including those who had experienced many problems with their career end (31%), those who had experienced some problems (46.6%), and those had experienced almost no problems (21.4%). A total of 25% of athletes assessed that they had reached their goals, 39.3% were not sure, whereas 35.7% assessed they had not reached their goals. Athletes also indicated that their level of satisfaction with their life was at its lowest directly after having decided to end their career, while their level of personal control was the lowest during their international career. The factors that influenced athletes' decision to end their career were as follows: a new focus, the feeling of having achieved what they wanted, coaching, injuries and health problems, problems with the sport organization and/or policy, financial problems, and support from family and friends.

White, C. (1974). After the last cheers, what do superstars become? *Physician and Sportsmedicine, 2,* 75–78.
  • This article outlines the importance of continued exercise upon cessation of a career in elite sport. The relationship between mental and physical well-being is emphasized by drawing upon anecdotal accounts of three former athletes with widely differing postretirement careers.

Williams, J. C. (1991). Socialization experience and identity foreclosure: An exploration of the effects of role disengagement on the personal adjustment of former college athletes (Doctoral dissertation, The University of Connecticut). *Dissertation Abstracts International, 52,* 1094A.

• In this study, results of a discriminate function analysis indicated that social, psychological, educational, and economic variables were related to the degree of personal adjustment experienced by a sample of retired male collegiate athletes. More specifically, educational performance and graduation status were found to be key predictors of adjustment for former athletes in both short- and long-term periods of retirement.

Williams-Rice, B. T. (1990). *After the final snap: Cognitive appraisal and coping among retired intercollegiate football players.* Unpublished master's thesis, University of Idaho, Moscow, USA.

Williams-Rice, B. T. (1996). After the final snap: Cognitive appraisal, coping, and life satisfaction among former collegiate athletes. *Academic Athletic Journal, Spring,* 30–39.

• This study examined the relationship among life satisfaction, coping process, and cognitive appraisal variables with a sample of 52 former collegiate football players. Results suggested that the Lazarus and Folkman's (1984) appraisal process was a stronger predictor of life satisfaction than the use of specific coping strategies, as assessed by Carver, Scheier, and Weintraub's (1989) COPE inventory. Implications for practice are provided, as well as future research directions.

Wolff, R., & Lester, D. (1989). A theoretical basis for counseling the retired professional athlete. *Psychological Reports, 64,* 1043–1046.

• This paper presents a counseling-based intervention designed to assist athletes in coping with retirement from sport. A three-stage model is proposed which consists of cognitive therapy, listening/confronting, and vocational guidance.

Wylleman, P., De Knop, P., Menkehorst, H., Theeboom, M., & Annerel, J. (1993). Career termination and social integration among elite athletes. In S. Serpa, J. Alves, V. Ferreira, & A. Paula-Brito (Eds.), *Proceedings of the VIII World Congress of Sport Psychology* (pp. 902–906). Lisbon: International Society of Sport Psychology.

• The article presents the results of a study on the causes, mediating factors, and consequences of the career end of 117 Flemish Olympic athletes. A total of 45.5% of athletes reported that the lack of preretirement planning and the lack of support from the sport federations and Olympic Committee were most influential upon the way in which they terminated their career.

Yelsa, E. A. (1995). Grief as an emotional reaction of athletes retired from competitive sport (Doctoral dissertation, California School of Professional Psychology). *Dissertation Abstracts International, 57,* 1460B.
• Active athletes, athletes who had retired from sport within one year, and individuals who had experienced the death of a loved one within one year served as participants in this study. Employing the Eysenck Personality Inventory (Eysenck & Eysenck, 1963) and measurements of grief, it was determined that both bereaved individuals and retired athletes experienced higher levels of grief than did competing athletes. Moreover, both bereaved and competing athletes rated higher than retired athletes on measures of neuroticism, and higher levels of neuroticism were found among retired athletes who displayed higher levels of grief.

Zaichkowsky, L., Blann, W., Perna, F., & Danish, S. (1992a, October/November). *From playing career to new career: An in-depth approach.* Paper presented at the annual conference of the Association for the Advancement of Applied Sport Psychology, Colorado Springs, USA.

Zaichkowsky, L., Blann, W., Perna, F., & Danish, S. (1992b, October/November). *Careers and career transition of athletes: Professional, Olympic, and collegiate.* Paper presented at the annual conference of the Association for the Advancement of Applied Sport Psychology, Colorado Springs, USA.

Zaichkowsky, L., Blann, W., Perna, F., & Danish, S. (1992c, October/November). *Career transition needs of professional athletes.* Paper presented at the annual conference of the Association for the Advancement of Applied Sport Psychology, Colorado Springs, USA.
• In this symposium, a number of career transition issues are addressed. First, results from surveys conducted with professional baseball, football, and ice hockey players are reported (see Blann & Zaichkowsky, 1989). Second, the career development efforts sponsored by the United States Olympic Committee are presented. Finally, two studies conducted on the career transition process are outlined.

Zaichkowsky, L., Kane, M. A., Blann, W. & Hawkins, K. (1993). Career transition needs of athletes: A neglected area of research in sport psychology. In S. Serpa, J. Alves, V. Ferreira, & A. Paula-Brito (Eds.), *Proceedings of the VIII World Congress of Sport Psychology* (pp. 785–787). Lisbon: International Society of Sport Psychology.
• Using the Professional Athletes Career Transition Inventory (PACTI) and Professional Athletes Career Transition Inventory for Spouses (PACTI-S),

the authors report on the need of North American athletes for programs during and after their sport career to prepare them for their career termination. Small seminars and individual counseling were found to be most proficient. The authors also provide an overview of the Professional Athletes Career Transition Program (PACTP), consisting of nine modules, which assists athletes in preparing for their career termination.

Zaichkowsky, L., Lipton, G., & Tucci, G. (1997). Factors affecting transition from intercollegiate sport. In R. Lidor & M. Bar-Eli (Eds.), *Proceedings of the IX World Congress of Sport Psychology* (pp. 782–784). Netanya, Israel: International Society of Sport Psychology.

• Two studies were conducted to assess the career transition experience from intercollegiate sport. A total of 274 athletes (148 female; 126 males) initially completed a self-report questionnaire focusing on transition difficulties, and 80 student-athlete alumni participated in a second study that focused on the distress associated with the transition from sport. Results revealed that 20% of the participants experienced transition-related distress. It was also determined that pretransition planning assisted in the overall adjustment. The researchers suggest that intercollegiate institutions need to better assist student-athletes in preparing for their inevitable career transition.

References

Anderson, D. (1996, May). *Lifeskill intervention and elite performance: National Athlete Career and Education Program.* Paper presented at the 13th Annual Conference on Counseling Athletes, Springfield, MA, USA.

Anderson, D. K. (1998). *Lifeskill intervention and elite performances.* Unpublished master's thesis, Victoria University of Technology, Melbourne, Australia.

Asselin, M. C. (1992, November). *Former top athletes in Quebec: Gender differences in withdrawal experience and post-athletic life.* Paper presented at the annual meeting of the North American Society for the Sociology of Sport, Toledo, OH, USA.

Brandmeyer, G. A., & Alexander, L. K. (1989). Gaining access to retired professional ballplayers. *Arena Review, 13,* 28–36.

Brock, S., & Kleiber, D. (1994). Narrative in medicine: The stories of elite college athletes' career-ending injuries. *Qualitative Health Research, 4,* 411–430.

Butlin, P. A. (1980). Is there life after rugby? *Rugby Post, 4 (6),* 15.

Carver, C. D., Scheier, M. F., & Weintraub, J. K. (1989). Assessing coping strategies: A theoretically based approach. *Journal of Personality and Social Psychology, 56,* 267–283.

Charner, I., & Schlossberg, N. K. (1986). Variations by theme: The life transitions of clerical workers. *The Vocational Guidance Quarterly, June,* 212–224.

Danish, S. J., & D'Augelli, A. R. (1980). *Helping skills II: Life development intervention.* New York: Human Sciences.

Danish, S. D., Petitpas, A. J., & Hale, B. D. (1993). Life development intervention for athletes: Life skills through sports. *The Counseling Psychologist, 21,* 352–385.

Deiters, J. A. (1996). *Social psychological correlates of sport commitment and anticipated retirement difficulty among college athletes.* Unpublished master's thesis, University of Northern Colorado, Greeley.

Denison, J. (1994). *Sport retirement: Personal troubles, public faces.* Unpublished doctoral dissertation, University of Illinois, Urbana, USA.

Denison, J. (1996). Sport narratives. *Qualitative Inquiry, 2,* 351–362.

Erikson. E. (1963). *Childhood and society* (2nd ed.). New York: Norton.

Eysenck, H. J., & Eysenck, S. B. G. (1963). *The Eysenck Personality Inventory.* San Diego: Educational and Industrial Testing Service.

Figler, S., & Figler, H. (1984). *Athlete's game plan for college and career.* Princeton: Peterson's Guides.

Fish, M. B., Grove, J. R., & Eklund, R. C. (1997). *Short-term changes in athletic identity as a function of deselection.* Manuscript submitted for publication.

Fortunato, V. (1996). *Role transitions in elite sports.* Unpublished doctoral dissertation, Victoria University of Technology, Melbourne, Australia.

Fortunato, V., & Marchant, D. (in press). Forced retirement from elite football in Australia. *Journal of Personal and Interpersonal Loss.*

Glaser, B. G., & Strauss, A. L. (1965). *Awareness of dying.* Chicago: Aldine.

Gordon, R. L. (1988). Athletic retirement as role loss: A construct validity study of self as process and role behavior. *Dissertation Abstracts International, 49,* 3469B.

Grandisson, A., & Vezina, J. (1997). Psychological consequences of retirement on high level amateur athletes [Abstract]. *Journal of Applied Sport Psychology, 9* (Suppl.), S98.

Harvey, J. H., Weber, A. L., & Orbuch, T. L. (1990). *Interpersonal accounts: A social psychological perspective.* Oxford: Blackwell.

Hathaway, S. R., & McKinley, J. C. (1967). *Minnesota Multiphasic Personality Inventory manual.* New York: Psychological Corporation.

Hinitz, D. R. (1988). *Role theory and the retirement of collegiate gymnasts.* Unpublished doctoral dissertation, University of Nevada, USA.

Hopson, B. (1981). Responses to the papers of Schlossberg, Brammer, and Abrego. *The Counseling Psychologist, 9,* 36–39.

Hurley, E. D., & Mills, B. D. (1993). Do coaches and athletes lose their identity after retirement from sport? *Coaching Volleyball, August, 22–26.*

Kübler-Ross, E. (1969). *On death and dying.* New York: Macmillan.

Lantz, C. D. (1995). *Validation of a conceptual model characterizing college student-athletes' readiness to retire from competitive sport participation.* Unpublished doctoral dissertation, West Virginia University, USA.

Lavallee, D., Sinclair, D. A., & Wylleman, P. (1998). An annotated bibliography on career transitions in sport: I. Counselling-based references. *Australian Journal of Career Development, 7(2),* 34–42.

Lavallee, D., Wylleman, P., & Sinclair, D. A. (1998). An anotated bibliography on career transitions in sport: II. Empirical references. *Australian Journal of Career Development, 7(3),* 32–44.

Lazarus, R. S., & Folkman, S. (1984). *Stress, appraisal, and coping.* New York: Springer.

Lewis, B. A. (1993). The big decision: Retirement looms for all world-class athletes. *American Rowing, 25 (3),* 18–20.

Loppnow, K. (1990). A helping hand to US Athletes: The US Olympic Committee's Career Assistance Program for Athletes. *Olympian, 17,* 34.

Mayocchi, L. (1998). *Transferable skills and the process of skill transfer: The athlete's experience.* Unpublished manuscript, The University of Queensland, Australia.

Mayocchi, L., & Hanrahan, S. J. (1997). *Adaptation to a post-athletic career: The role of transferable skills.* Belconnen, ACT: Australian Sports Commission.

McCann, S. (1995). Ending a sport career. *Olympic Coach, 5 (2),* 8–9.

McNair, I. W., Lorr, M., & Droppleman, L. F. (1971). *Profile of Mood States manual.* San Diego: Educational and Industrial Testing Service.

Missler, S. M. (1996). *Female golfers' transitions from highly competitive sport: A naturalisitc inquiry.* Unpublished doctoral dissertation, The Ohio State University, Columbus, USA.

Murphy, S. M., Abbot, S., Hillard, N., Petitpas, A., Danish, S., & Holloway, S. (1989, October). *New frontiers in sport psychology: Helping athletes with career transition process.* Paper presented at the annual conference of the Association for the Advancement of Applied Sport Psychology, Seattle, USA.

Neyer, M. (1996). Identity development and career maturity patterns of elite resident athletes at the United States Olympic Training Center. *Dissertation Abstracts International, 56, No. 11,* 4328-A.

Owens, S. S. (1994, October). *The relationship between student-athlete identity and career exploration.* Paper presented at the annual conference of the Association for the Advancement of Applied Sport Psychology, Lake Tahoe, NV.

Posthuma, H. (1992). Life after sport: Taking a positive approach to retirement from competition. *Canadian Sports Administrator, 3,* 4.

Reece, S. D., Wilder, K. C., & Mahanes, J. R. (1996). *Program for athlete career transition.* Paper presented at the annual conference of the Association for the Advancement of Applied Sport Psychology, Williamsburg, VA, USA.

Riesterer, U., & Etzel, E. (1992). Retirement from shooting: An inevitable transition. *UIT Journal, 4,* 18–22.

Schlossberg, N. K. (1981). A model for analyzing human adaptation to transition. *The Counseling Psychologist, 9,* 2–18.

Schlossberg, N. K. (1984). *Counseling adults in transition: Linking practice with theory.* New York: Springer.

Sowa, C. J., Yusuf, F. R., & Mass, J. L. (1996, May). *Making the transition: Issues confronting high school student-athletes after graduation.* Paper presented at the 13th Annual Conference on Counseling Athletes, Springfield, MA, USA.

Sparkes, A. C. (1998). Athletic identity: An Achilles' heel to the survival of self. *Qualitative Health Research, 8,* 644–664.

Stambulova, N. (1998, August). Sports career transitions of Russian athletes: Summary of studies (1991–1997). In D. Alfermann (Chair), *Career transitions in sport: Determinants and consequences.* Paper presented at the 24th International Congress of Applied Psychology, San Francisco, CA.

Sussman, M. B. (1972). An analytical model for the sociological study of retirement. In F. M. Carp (Ed.), *Retirement* (pp. 29–74). New York: Human Sciences.

Tate, G. F., & Joshua, M. (1996, May). *Sliding through the system: The development of the US Luge Association's Academic and Career Assistance Program.* Paper presented at the 13th Annual Conference on Counseling Athletes, Springfield, MA, USA.

Tian, M., Li, D., & Zhang, R. (1993). Arrangements for retired elite platers in China and measures to improve it. *Journal of Beijing Institute of Physical Education, 16,* 2–8.

Tuckman, B. W., (1965). Developmental sequence in small groups. *Psychological Bulletin, 63,* 384–399.

Ungerleider, S. (1994, August). *Transition: From the Olympic podium to the workplace.* Paper presented at the International Congress of Applied Research in Sports, Helsinki, Finland.

Urofsky, R. I. (1997, May). *Using athletic identity in working with athletes in transition.* Paper presented at the 13th Annual Conference on Counseling Athletes, Springfield, MA, USA.

Weimer, T. (1987, October/November). *The retirement of former West Virginia University basketball All-Americans: Effects of education and occupational attainment.* Paper presented at the annual conference of the North American Society for the Sociology of Sport, Las Vegas, USA.

Weiss, E. H. (1992). *A qualitative study of the retirement experiences of former professional ice hockey players.* Unpublished doctoral dissertation, University of Connecticut, USA.

Wendel, J. F., & Shefsky, L. E. (1994, May). *Second careers for athletes*. Paper presented at the 20th Annual Sports Lawyers Conference, Scottsdale, AZ, USA.

Wheeler, G., Hutzler, S., Campbell, E., Malone, L., Legg, D., & Steadward, R. D. (1996). *Retirement from disability sport: A cross cultural analysis*. Paper presented at the Paralympic conference, Atlanta, USA.

Wheeler, G. D., Malone, L. A., VanVlack, S., Nelson, E. R., & Steadward, R. D. (1996). Retirement from disability sport: A pilot study. *Adapted Physical Activity Quarterly, 13,* 382–399.

Winston, R., Miller, T., & Prince, J. (1979). *Assessing student development: A preliminary manual for the Student Development Task Inventory and the Student Development Profile and Planning Record.* Athens, GA: Student Development Associates.

Wooten, H. R. (1994). Cutting losses for student-athletes in transition: An integrative transition model. *Journal of Employment Counseling, 31,* 2–9.

Appendix B

European Federation of Sports Psychology (FEPSAC) Position Statement 3: Sports Career Transitions

'Sports career' (SC) is a term for the multiyear sports activities of the individual aimed at high level sport achievements and self-improvement in sport. The effects of SC can be considered from two viewpoints: the narrow view considers only sport achievements (records, places in competitions, sport titles, etc.), whereas the broad view also considers the athletes' personal development.

The SC can be divided into several stages, with each stage characterised by a set of specific demands requiring adjustments by the athletes. The success of the athlete's transition from one SC stage to another depends not only on his/her success at a given stage, but throughout the SC as a whole.

Sports Career Transitions

Research has shown that several transitions can be identified:

- *The beginning of sports specialization* is characterized by adjustments to the demands of the sport, coach, sport group, and new lifestyle. Young athletes must ensure the right choice of sport and show ability to learn sport techniques
- In *the transition to more intensive training* athletes should adjust themselves to the new regime of training loads, improve their techniques and tactical skills, and attempt to achieve stable results in competition.
- *Transition to high-achievement and adult sports* is marked by the athlete attempting to find his/her individual way in sport, to cope with the pressure of selection to important competitions, and gaining respect of a team, opponents, officials, and other sport professionals. It is critical for

the athlete to change his/her lifestyle at this point and make it work in favor of sport achievement.

- *Transition from amateur to professional sport* is marked by adaptation to the specialized requirements and pressures of professional sports, to competition with equally strong opponents, independent training.
- *Transition to the end of the SC* is characterized by the necessity to search for additional self-resources in order to maintain high levels of achievement and preparation for leaving sport.
- *The termination of the SC* is marked by leaving sport and a transition to some other career, as well as adjustments to new status, lifestyle and social networks.

Positive Transitions and Crisis Transitions

Positive transitions take place when an athlete makes a relatively quick and easy adjustment to the demands of a given SC stage. It usually happens in cases where the necessary preconditions (e.g., theoretical and practical knowledge, skills, attitudes, etc.) have been created during the previous stage. Other factors that can ease the course of transition are : athletes' giftedness; high motivation; positive attitude towards training, competitions; active coping with difficulties; trust in coach; and a positive psychological climate.

Crisis transitions take place when the athlete has to make a special effort to successfully adapt to new requirements. Inability to adjust creates symptoms of crisis transition, such as lowered self-esteem, emotional discomfort (e.g., doubt, anxiety, fear), increased sensitivity to failure, disorientation in decision making, and confusion. These are often accompanied by a stagnation or decline in results. Psychological assistance can prevent such negative outcomes, as well as drop out from sport.

Recommendations

Since SC transitions are predictable in the course of the SC, knowledge of peculiarities of each transition is extremely important. The following recommendations should be taken into account not only by sport psychologists, but also coaches, parents and all other people and organisations (e.g., Sport Federations, National Olympic Committees) involved in competitive sport.

1. *Beginning stage.* Inform young athletes about the specifics of training in a given sport; create a comfortable supportive atmosphere in the sport group; use developmentally appropriate methods of training; develop young athletes' interests; encourage them regardless of success or failure, reward effort; give social support in competition, especially in cases of failure.

2. *Transition to intensive training.* Don not force the training process. More forward gradually and smoothly to prevent injuries and overtraining. Teach athletes the basics of psychological preparation for competition; help them find the optimal regime to combine sports, school, and other activities.

3. *Transitions to high-achievement and adult sport.* This is the most difficult one for an athlete since it is linked not only to the sport maturity of an athlete, but also to his/her psychological maturity. The main focus for the sport psychologist here is co-operation with the athlete. Coaches and sport psychologists should advise the athlete, but give him/her the opportunity for independent decision making. The psychological assistance during the transition from amateur to professional sport is similar to that just described.

4. *Transition to the end of the SC.* The athlete becomes more reserves and anxious, and may need social support, expert advice, and counselling, including assistance in searching for a new career.

5. *Termination of the SC.* This should involve helping an athlete into a new career and surroundings. Support of sport organizations for their former athletes plays an important role.

6. The particular methods of psychological assistance to an athlete in the different SC transitions vary, including psychodiagnostic, psychological prevention, mental training, and others. However, their effectiveness is dependent on taking into account the specifics of the sport event, SC stage, athlete's age, gender, and his/her individual traits.

7. Sport psychologists should study the ways in which athletes experience and cope with different SC transitions and then assist in educating the athletes and coaches in providing positive transitions in order to make the athletes' career in sport longer, successful and more enjoyable.

INDEX

Editor Biographies

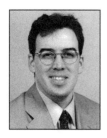 David Lavallee, PhD, is a principal lecturer in the School of Social Sciences at the University of Teesside, England, where he teaches courses in psychology and is the director of the Center for Sport Performance and Applied Research. His educational qualifications include a master's degree in psychology from Harvard University and a doctorate in sport psychology from the University of Western Australia. He is also a chartered psychologist and graduate member of the British Psychological Society. His general area of research and applied interest is in counseling in sport and exercise settings. Currently, David serves on the editorial board of the *Journal of Personal and Interpersonal Loss* (Taylor & Francis), and is a member of the British Psychological Society Sport and Exercise Psychology Section Committee. He is a former All-American soccer player.

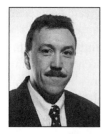 Paul Wylleman, PhD, is an associate professor at the Vrije Universiteit Brussel, Belgium. He teaches psychology of sport, exercise and leisure in the Faculty of Physical Education and Physiotherapy and the Faculty of Psychology and Education at graduate level. He is also the coordinator of the Department of Top-level Sport and Study, where he provides career counseling to elite-level student athletes and where he co-ordinates the Study and Talent Education Program (STEP). After completing his dissertation on talented young athletes' interpersonal relationships at the Vrije Universiteit Brussel he conducted postdoctoral research at the Institute for the Study of Youth Sport at Michigan State University. His research interests are focused on the interpersonal relationships in competitive sport and on the career development of elite athletes. Paul has been heading the Special Interest Group on Career Transitions of the European Federation of Sport Psychology (FEPSAC) since 1993. His publications include *Career Transitions in Competitive Sports*, which he coedited with David Lavallee and Dorothee Alfermann for FEPSAC and different articles in sport psychology journals. He is currently on the editorial board of *The Sport Psychologist* and the *Sportpsychologie Bulletin*. Paul is board member of the Belgian Sport Psychology Federation and serves on the board of FEPSAC as treasurer. Paul is an avid badminton and judo player and downhill skier.

Author Biographies

Dorothee Alfermann, PhD, is a professor of sport psychology at the University of Leipzig, Germany, where she teaches undergraduate and graduate sport psychology. Her research focuses on gender roles in sport, career development of young athletes, and coping processes after injuries and career termination. She is involved in the working group of career transitions of the European Federation of Sports Psychology (FEPSAC), and she is a member of the managing council of the International Society of Sport Psychology (ISSP).

Deidre Anderson has been working with elite athletes for the past 10 years with the Australian and Victorian Institutes of Sport. She has become internationally recognized for her work with elite athletes through the development of a program called the Athlete Career and Education (ACE) Program. The program provides services to some 3,000 athletes throughout Australia. It is also offered to athletes in the United Kingdom through its Sports Institute. Deidre's academic background includes an MA and baccalaureate degrees in both science and arts with postgraduate studies in athlete counseling and social science. Her research has included the impact on the performance of athletes through life-skill development and the balanced approach to coaching excellence. She has been a member of the Australian Advisory Board Drug Education, Victorian Olympic Education Committee, Australian Gymnastics Board and the Sports Industry Training Board. A recipient of many awards for her contribution to elite athletes and coaches, Deidre's expertise is keenly sought after as a keynote speaker and international consultant.

Erika Borkoles is a doctoral student in exercise and sport psychology at Leeds Metropolitan University, England. She previously received a master's degree in exercise and sport psychology from the University of Exeter, England. Erika currently serves as the student representative for the Sport and Exercise Psychology Section of the British Psychological Society.

Britton W. Brewer, PhD, is an associate professor of psychology at Springfield College in Springfield, Massachusetts, where he teaches undergraduate and graduate psychology, conducts research on psychological aspects of sport injury, and coaches the men's cross-country team. He is listed in the United States

Olympic Committee Sport Psychology Registry, 1996–2000, and is a certified consultant, Association for the Advancement of Applied Sport Psychology.

Delight Champagne, PhD, is a professor in the Psychology Department at Springfield College, and serves as director of the Graduate Program in Student Personnel Administration in the Higher Education Program. At Springfield College, she teaches courses in career development, college student development, and counseling with an emphasis on career and life transitions. She has provided consulting services in the LPGA's Transitional Golf Program and the USOC's Career Assistance Program for Athletes and has offered workshops in a variety of educational settings on managing life roles and transitions. Her research and applied work have focused on development and change over the life course.

Ian Cockerill, PhD, is a psychologist with the School of Sport and Exercise Sciences, University of Birmingham, England, where he presently teaches courses in sport psychology and growth, maturation and physical activity. His research focuses principally on the application of psychological theory to the investigation of real-life issues in sport. Ian is a chartered psychologist, an accredited sport and exercise psychologist, and secretary of the British Psychological Society's Sport and Exercise Psychology Section. He also works as a sport psychologist in private practice with athletes across a range of disciplines and up to professional and international standard.

Sean P. Cumming is a doctoral student in sport psychology at Michigan State University. He grew up in the Orkney Islands, off the north coast of Scotland, where he competed in soccer, rugby, and track. Prior to accepting a graduate post at Michigan State, he earned an honors degree in psychology at the University of Edinburgh and a master's degree in exercise and sport psychology at the University of Exeter. Sean currently works for the Institute for the Study of Youth Sports at Michigan State University, where he conducts research in youth sports issues and teaches sport psychology in the coaches' education program for high school coaches, parents, and athletes.

Paul De Knop has a PhD in physical education from the Faculty of Physical Education of the Vrije Universiteit Brussel, Belgium, graduated in leisure studies at the same university and earned a master's degree in sports sociology and sports management from the University of Leicester, England. He is a full-time professor at the Vrije Universiteit Brussel and is the head of the

Youth Advisory Center for Sport, an interdisciplinary research and advisory center. Teaching includes areas of sport, leisure, and physical education from a sociopedagogical perspective. He is the secretary-general of ICSSPE's Sport and Leisure Committee, member of ISCPES, EASM, ICSS and NASS, and president of BLOSO, the Flemish sport administrative body. Research interests include youth and sport, sport and ethnic minorities, sport and tourism, and sport management.

Amanda Edge graduated from the University of Birmingham, England, in 1998 with an honors degree in sport and exercise science. She is an all-around athlete, particularly as a netball player and middle-distance runner. Amanda works as a regional development officer with the Welsh Netball Association.

Martha E. Ewing, PhD, is an associate professor in the Department of Kinesiology at Michigan State University. Her primary research interest is in the area of achievement motivation of youth sport participants. Specifically, she has investigated reasons youth participate in sport and drop out of sport, plus parents' perspectives on pressure that is put on youth to play sports. In addition, she has been involved in the development and delivery of coaches' education to high school and volunteer coaches through the Institute for the Study of Youth Sports. Prior to her taking her doctorate, Marty coached volleyball, basketball, and tennis at the collegiate level.

Dieter Hackfort, PhD, is a professor of sport psychology at the University of the Federal Defence in Munich and head of the Institute for Sport Science and Sports. He earned his doctoral degree from the German Sports University at Cologne. His main areas of research are the development of action theory and empirical methods within the framework of this perspective, emotions in sports, self-presentation, and issues referring to health in sports as well as health by sports. He is a past president of the ASP (the national sport psychological association in Germany), counselor for various national teams/Olympic teams, and editor/coeditor of national and international book series in sport science. Dr. Hackfort has also authored or edited a dozen books, including *Anxiety in Sports: An International Perspective* (with Charles D. Spielberger) and *Research on Emotions in Sport.* He is married and the father of two boys, and his favorite sports are tennis, skiing, and golf.

Stephanie J. Hanrahan, PhD, is a senior lecturer in sport and exercise psychology at The University of Queensland in Australia. She received her doctorate in sport psychology from the University of Western Australia and her MSc in physical education with an emphasis in sport psychology at the University of Illinois. Her BA in psychology (and coaching certification in swimming and volleyball) were obtained at the University of California at Santa Barbara. As a registered psychologist, Stephanie has worked with athletes and coaches from a wide variety of sports—from ballet to football and from bocci to skydiving.

Jamie Kallio is an international-level biathlete and coach who represented Canada at the 1988 Calgary Olympics. He graduated from the University of Ottawa with a master's degree in applied sport psychology. He has presented his biathlon research at North American conferences and is currently a coach and a sport psychology consultant in cross-country skiing and biathlon.

Elizabeth King is currently a doctoral student in counseling psychology at New York University.

Jeffrey J. Martin, PhD, is an associate professor of sport and exercise psychology in the Division of Health, Physical Education and Recreation in the College of Education at Wayne State University in Detroit, Michigan. His research interests include disability sport and the role of physical activity in improving the quality of life for children with disabilities.

Tony Morris, PhD, has a professorial position at Victoria University, Melbourne, Australia. He has been involved in teaching, research and community service work in sport psychology for over 20 years. Tony has supervised more than 60 doctoral and master's degree candidates, several working on career transitions. In addition to his involvement in career transitions and life-skills education since 1990, his longstanding research interests have been imagery, confidence, concentration, stress, and anxiety in sport, and motivation for sport and physical activity. Tony was the first chair of the Australian College of Sport Psychologists. He is currently a member of the Managing Council of the International Society of Sport Psychology and president of the Asian-South Pacific Association of Sport Psychology.

Lisa Mayocchi, PhD, is a consultant in the Training and Development Team at Her Majesty's Treasury, London. She received her doctorate in organizational psychology and her BA (Honors) from The University of Queensland, Australia. In her work at HM Treasury, London, and at Queensland Treasury,

Australia, she has carried out projects on mentoring, change management, and staff training needs. She has also facilitated workshops with a variety of audiences, including the Queensland Academy of Sport's Girls Soccer Team.

John McCarthy, M.Ed., is currently a doctoral student in sport psychology at Boston University. He played professional football after college in camps with NFL teams, the New York Jets in 1985 and the Green Bay Packers in 1987. Afterwards he played in a quasiprofessional league in Italy where he also began to coach. He coached college football for ten years, of which the last eight were at Boston University prior to them dropping their program. John is currently a competitive rower.

Mark Nesti is a senior lecturer in sport psychology at Leeds Metropolitan University, England. He is a member of the British Association of Sport and Exercise Science and a registered psychologist with the British Olympic Association. He conducts research on anxiety in sport and existential-phenomenological psychology.

Wendy Patton, PhD, has worked in career education and career counseling for over 20 years, in the area of curriculum, counseling, and university teaching. She is presently senior lecturer at the Queensland University of Technology, Australia, where she coordinates a master's of education in career guidance and supervises the research of postgraduate students. She has an extensive publishing record and currently edits the *Australian Journal of Career Development*.

Albert J. Petitpas, EdD, is a professor of psychology at Springfield College in Springfield, Massachusetts, where he directs the graduate training program in athletic counseling. He is a fellow and certified consultant of the Association for the Advancement of Applied Sport Psychology. He has provided consulting services to a wide range of sport organizations, including the National Collegiate Athletic Association's Youth Education Through Sport Program, the United States Olympic Committee's Career Assistance Program for Athletes, the Ladies Professional Golf Association's Transitional Golf Program, and the United States Ski Jumping and Nordic Combined teams. His research and applied work focus on assisting athletes in coping with injury and other sport and career transitions.

Susan Ryan is a postgraduate student completing her doctorate in psychology with the Queensland University of Technology in Brisbane, Australia, where she teaches developmental psychology. Her research interests include dancers' identity and career development and psychological aspects of dance medicine. She is a psychological consultant in rehabilitation and career counseling and previously was a teacher of dance for 10 years.

John H. Salmela, Ph.D., is a professor of sport psychology at the University of Ottawa whose research focus is the development of expertise of both coaches and athletes. He is the author of 13 books and over 100 research and professional publications in the field. He has worked as a sport psychologist with a number of Canadian national teams, most particularly in gymnastics. He has also served on the executive boards of the International Society of Sport Psychology and the Association for the Advancement of Applied Sport Psychology.

Dana A. Sinclair, PhD, is a registered psychologist who holds doctorates from the University of Cambridge as well as the University of Ottawa, and is a clinical assistant professor with the Faculty of Medicine at the University of British Columbia. She is currently a psychologist and partner with Human Performance International, Vancouver, Canada. She emphasizes a positive psychology approach in her extensive personal resource consulting practice and focuses on the developmental and clinical aspects of personnel and organizational performance needs/problems in both the corporate and sport arenas. She specializes in the development and maintenance of consistent and effective performance through the application of Mental Management® techniques and works extensively in the areas of performance enhancement, worker motivation, and injury recovery. Dana is a consultant for such corporations as Xerox, Telus, Agra Simons, Raytheon, the NBA's Vancouver Grizzlies, and the NHL's Vancouver Canucks and Philadelphia Flyers, as well as a number of Canadian National and Olympic teams. In addition, she works with a number of provincial teams and individual elite athletes. Dana is a former captain of the Canadian National Women's Field Hockey Team and member of the Cambridge University Women's Ice Hockey Team.

Judy L. Van Raalte, PhD, is an associate professor of psychology at Springfield College in Springfield, Massachusetts, where she teaches undergraduate and graduate psychology, and conducts research on cognitive factors and sport performance. She is listed in the United States Olympic Committee Sport Psychology Registry, 1996–2000, and is a certified consultant, Association for the Advancement of Applied Sport Psychology.

Bradley W. Young completed his master's degree at the University of Ottawa in sport psychology. He is an accomplished middle-distance runner and has competed at the Canadian intercollegiate level. He has made presentations both in Canada and the United States on his research in the development of expertise in middle-distance runners. He is currently teaching high school in Toronto.

Leonard D. Zaichkowsky, PhD, is a professor of education at Boston University. His teaching and research specialty is the psychology of human development and performance. His current research interests include exercise and well-being, career transition of elite performers, development of expertise, and the psychophysiology of peak performance. He has published over 50 articles on sport psychology and has coauthored or edited 6 books on motor development and sport psychology. He is a member of numerous state, national, and international organizations, including the Association for Applied Psychophysiology and Biofeedback, the American Psychological Association, the International Society of Sport Psychology, and the Association for the Advancement of Applied Sport Psychology (past president). He is on the Registry of Sport Psychologists for the U.S. Olympic Committee and is a columnist for *Senior Golfer* magazine and sport psychologist for the Boston Celtics of the National Basketball Association.